Public Health Perspectives on Disability

Donald J. Lollar • Willi Horner-Johnson
Katherine Froehlich-Grobe

Editors

Public Health Perspectives on Disability

Science, Social Justice, Ethics, and Beyond

Second Edition

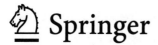 Springer

Editors
Donald J. Lollar
School of Public Health
Oregon Health & Science University
Portland, OR, USA

Katherine Froehlich-Grobe
Baylor Scott and White Institute
for Rehabilitation
Dallas, TX, USA

University of Texas School of Public Health
Dallas Regional Campus, USA

Willi Horner-Johnson
Institute on Development and Disability
Oregon Health & Science University
Portland, OR, USA

OHSU-PSU School of Public Health
Portland, OR, USA

ISBN 978-1-0716-0890-6   ISBN 978-1-0716-0888-3   (eBook)
https://doi.org/10.1007/978-1-0716-0888-3

This Springer imprint is published by the registered company Springer Science+Business Media, LLC,
part of Springer Nature.
The registered company address is: 1 New York Plaza, New York, NY 10004, U.S.A.

Dr. Allan Meyers envisioned a public health world in which disability was an integral part of the public health curriculum in all schools and programs, and that people with disabilities would live more healthy and fulfilled lives as a result. He believed that the foundational areas of public health should include disability applications. His passion, vision, and energy for this topic culminated in a 1998 conference sponsored by the U.S. Centers for Disease Control and Prevention (CDC) led by Dr. Meyers and included a small group of public health academics, practitioners, and CDC Disability and Health staff. The first study on inclusion of disability in public health curricula was completed by him and his students, concluding that "there is a clear need for more systematic and comprehensive coverage of disability in the graduate public health curriculum." He was adamant that all public health students be immersed in disability-focused academic opportunities, including science, policy, and programs. He was tenacious and enthusiastic about this venture and implemented it at Boston University, where he had served for years on the faculty of the School of Public Health. He died prematurely in 2001 before the first edition of this volume was published. We hope that this book moves Allan's vision forward so that public health professionals are better equipped to improve the health and well-being of people with disabilities.

Chris Kochtitzky, MSP, was an urban planner of a unique sort. He did not plan new developments, calculate transit ridership, or host community design charrettes. Rather, he did what urban planners are supposed to do—bring people together to envision and plan for a better future. Instead of a single community, Chris orchestrated urban planning across national, state, and local scales through knowledge dissemination and building multi-sector collaborations that broke down silos and divisions between disciplines of urban planning, public health, aging, disability studies, engineering, architecture, medicine, and more. Chris was a social justice pioneer who helped policy makers and practitioners understand the link between urban planning and public health, especially for people with disabilities and older adults. Working across many departments at the Centers for Disease Control and Prevention, Chris helped to elevate the importance of environmental influences on public health for all people through public health initiatives, standards, funding opportunities, courses in the Rollins School of Public Health at Emory University, and many influential articles and chapters. Chris dedicated 28 years of service at the CDC in pursuit of social justice and healthy equity goals. Chris passed away prematurely before the publication of the new edition of this volume. We hope this book and especially the chapter on environmental public health pass on the meaningful, interdisciplinary ideas and linkages to public health professionals that Chris was passionately committed to, and tirelessly worked towards, throughout his career.

Foreword

Disability has touched or will touch most of us during our lifespan. My teachers about disability are many, beginning with members of my own family, friends, and colleagues. Despite their disabilities and chronic conditions—whether visible to others or not—all of these individuals live each day to their fullest by striving to do all functions of daily living well, maintaining good health, and participating in work and community events to the fullest. In most cases, they would say that they are no different than those without disabilities and do not want to be treated as if they have a medical illness or were different from others. Instead, they acknowledge that they have challenges but can do the things everyone else can do if they have the supports and services in their environments to enable them to function fully in all aspects of living, including work and play. And, with the right supports in their respective family and social environments, they can be very productive and have a good quality of life over their life courses.

As a public health researcher, policy maker, and advocate, however, I continue to experience a large disconnect between the experiences of individuals with disability and the larger public community, including those who formulate policies or conduct research regarding disability. Unfortunately, many still use a medically focused lens on disability and do not address the larger societal context that is needed to support individuals with disability. Although there has been progress made in attitudes and understanding of disability in the past decade since the first edition of this volume was published, there is still much to be done to eliminate discriminatory attitudes about disability and the resulting stigma about individuals with disability in order for all to receive the environmental accommodations needed so all can thrive in all career paths.

Changes in attitude and understanding about disability must happen in disciplines, including medicine, and all sectors of the community that intersect with disability. A public health approach, which this volume uses as a framework for each chapter, is needed to inform how all of us understand disability. A community-based, population-based public health approach will lead to a transformation in the way disability is viewed by the public as well as to improved health and quality of life for all with disabilities. This important volume describes the public health approach to disability from a variety of disciplines, societal sectors, and other perspectives.

Societal Importance of Addressing Disability

The economic and social reasons why individuals with disabilities can no longer be ignored for a productive and successful economy in the United States and globally continue to intensify as the number of individuals with disabilities grows across the lifespan. No longer can we afford to exclude individuals with disabilities and chronic illnesses from productive jobs and well-integrated lives in the community. Globalization trends and aging demographics in the United States imply that every child and youth today be prepared to be a member of a specialized workforce over their lifetime. The chapter on aging and disability by Clark, Twardzik, and Meade as well as those on disability and health programs by Nary and Mullis and federal programs and disability by Hall elaborate on these themes.

During the next few decades, it is expected that there will be much fewer younger workers under 35 years of age for every individual that turns 65, many of whom choose to receive social security benefits. The aging of the "baby boom" generation in the United States continues to increase with an exploding number of elders in the next few decades. This aging population of the future will have an increased incidence of chronic illnesses as well as physical and/or cognitive impairments.

Data from the Behavioral Risk Factor Surveillance System collected in 2016 (Okoro, Hollis, Cyrus, & Griffin-Blake, 2018) revealed that 25% of adults in the United States—61 million—have a disability that impacts major life activities. Mobility, the most common disability, affects 2 in 5 adults age 65 and older. These disabilities can be attributable to chronic illness, intellectual or developmental disabilities, mental illness, injury, or other underlying conditions. Furthermore, the number and percentage of individuals with disabilities and/or chronic conditions vary by the type of condition (e.g., cognitive impairment, physical impairment, sensory impairment), geography (e.g., region, state), and various demographic characteristics (e.g., education, race, gender, age).

Another compelling reason to successfully address the challenges of disability is related to the medical and societal costs associated with disability. It is estimated that 27% of healthcare expenditures were associated with disability in 2006 (Anderson, Armour, Finkelstein, & Wiener, 2010), with Medicaid and Medicare accounting for 69% and 38%, respectively. The major costs of health care related to chronic conditions increasing must address issues associated with disability or supports needed for functioning. The majority of dollars spent on individuals with disabilities in the healthcare and social support systems are spent on expensive treatments and institutionalized settings such as nursing homes and habilitation settings. Much too little is spent on changing the physical and social environments that encourage health promotion and prevention of secondary conditions that are necessary for maximum health and well-being of those with a disability.

The provision of community-based care and services—with an emphasis on environmental supports—must be accelerated with supporting policies at the local, state, and federal levels. Major federal initiatives, such as Medicaid demonstration programs and Title V (of the Social Security Act) funding through the Maternal and Child Health Block Grant, as well as various community-based initiatives, such as Special Olympics and family-led organizations, are needed to propel the funding of community-based options that empower individuals with disabilities to direct and fund the services they need to live productive lives, including full inclusion in work without fear of losing health or other benefits. More resources are needed "upstream" in the "healthcare system" to support more prevention and health promotion services for individuals with disabilities so that major complications and secondary conditions do not develop. In addition, the adoption of laws and regulations that promote inclusion and equity for individuals with disabilities is necessary to make changes for all individuals with disabilities at the population-wide level.

Implementation of the Patient Protection and Affordable Care Act, enacted in law in March 2010, must be protected and expanded to successfully address issues related to disability in the next decade. This healthcare reform legislation continues to offer opportunities for a public health approach to disability in the establishment of health outcomes, conduct of comparative effectiveness research, development of clinical and community prevention initiatives, implementation of health information technology in clinical and public health settings, examination of cost control strategies, and implementation of secondary prevention and health promotion initiatives in the community.

Significance of Sourcebook on Public Health and Disability

This second edition of the sourcebook on public health and disability will enable the study of disability from a public health perspective. Public health, the practice of social justice using science-based strategies to improve population health, has the approaches and congruence of mission that can propel research, practice, and advocacy related to disability in the future. The current inequities in access to prevention and intervention services and policies for individuals with disability are a major social injustice in the United States and globally. The chapter on health equity and intersectionality by Horner-Johnson presents the evidence that people with disabilities are a health disparity population who need focused attention as do other populations suffering with health inequities. Embracing disability as a health disparity can lead to major advances in reducing inequities and maximizing well-being for people with disabilities in the future.

The focus on disability from a public health perspective has slowly grown over the past three decades since the passage of the Americans with Disabilities Act

(ADA) to outlaw discrimination against people living with physical and/or mental disabilities. The national commitment to public health and disability is acknowledged today by the existence of 19 states having a State Disability and Health Program funded by a grant from CDC. These programs, discussed in the chapter by Nary and Mullis, support evidence-based approaches to improve the health and quality of life among people with mobility limitations and/or intellectual disabilities. I am pleased to have started the first office of disability and health in the country in the Massachusetts Department of Public Health in the late 1990s with Deborah Allen and Laura Rauscher, its first director. We were pleased to do one of the first state surveys of all mammography facilities to assure access for women with disabilities and publish the first report on the health status and access for adults with disabilities. Given the strong role public health agencies can play in improving the lives for individuals with disabilities, I do lament the fact that all state public health agencies do not include disability programs after two decades of work. Our vision for individuals with disabilities across the lifespan is being implemented at a much slower pace than we would like, but the struggle for equity for this population across most sectors in society continues.

However, it is encouraging that other sectors, such as the philanthropic community, are explicitly addressing inequities related to individuals with disabilities in their funded initiatives (Besser, 2019). For example, the leaders of the Robert Wood Johnson Foundation and the Ford Foundation are working with 15 foundations on the Presidents' Council on Disability Inclusion in Philanthropy to champion inclusion of disability in own organizations and philanthropic mission.

This second edition will allow for more work in the continual development of principles, programs, and policies needed for building a strong foundation for public health and disability within the United States and globally. The editors of this volume have assembled leading public health experts in the various areas of public health to contribute to this volume, which can be used in courses in schools and programs on public health and related disciplines. There are chapters related to many of the competencies needed to be a public health practitioner and leader: i.e., statistics and epidemiology, social and behavior sciences, environment and health services, law and ethics, maternal and child health, and international health. As discussed in the chapter on disability in the health curriculum by Griffen and Havercamp, this sourcebook can be used in any of the relevant courses in each of the areas of public health or can be used as a text in a course on disability.

A public health systemic approach is needed to guide research, interventions, policies, and advocacy related to disability in order to fully transform health and social systems. Each of the authors explores how disability is related to each of the public health disciplines and sectors. In many cases, it is clear how much needs to be done to embrace disability to move the field of public health and disability forward. This basic sourcebook is an important contribution in the establishment of public health and disability as a key area of study in public health programs and schools.

Major Themes Related to Public Health and Disability

The authors of this book describe disability from their various viewpoints and disciplines, showing major points of overlap in perspectives and approaches as well as revealing areas of tension in how disability is defined and approached. They also reveal what needs to be done to integrate the study of disability in public health over time. These struggles and evolving approaches to the study of disability within public health are not surprising since public health has just begun to embrace disability as a focus area. The evolving transformation and integration of approaches to disability within a public health perspective will take time as the two fields are merged and approached in a unified population-based framework that incorporates social determinants of health and a lifespan perspective.

The following observations or themes about disability and public health, many of which I identified in the Preface to the first volume, need to be addressed and understood more fully in the future. This sourcebook introduces the reader to many of these themes and suggests recommendations for the future in furthering research, interventions, and advocacy related to disability and public health.

- Disability does not equate to a medical illness or condition and must be considered in the total context of function within environmental supports. The shift from a medical focus is critical to understanding disability from a public health perspective. Given the influence and power of the medical system in the United States, this will take steady education and persistence to change how the medical profession and the public perceive disability. Public health professionals need to work closely with their clinical and medical colleagues to change attitudes and approaches to disability from the medical paradigm to a public health one. All of the chapters use this approach in their discussions of the issues.
- A lifespan approach to the study of disability must be embraced. Disability and public health can benefit from a life course perspective since many disabilities begin in childhood and exist into adulthood. In addition, the major transitions in one's life (e.g., entry to school, transition to adulthood, transition to "senior status") present special challenges for individuals with disability. Disability is uniquely impacted by each development stage in an individual's life resulting in differing expectations of one's family and community. The chapters on maternal health by Mitra and Bellil, on child health by Simeonsson, and on aging and disability by Clark, Twardzik, and Meade illustrate disability at various points in the lifespan.
- Environmental, physical, and social supports are key to the definition and approach to disability and the transformation from a medical model. The chapter on environmental health by Eisenberg, Maisel, and Kochtitsky fully explains how the concepts of environment are key to a public health approach. The most recent edition of the World Health Organization's *International Classification of Functioning, Disability and Health (ICF)* fully embraces the environment in its framework for defining disability and functioning. This framework, which is embraced more globally than within the United States, is consistent with the

environmental health field and a social-ecological approach to improving population health. The importance of environment requires advocacy for changing
environments to accommodate and support individuals with disabilities. The ICF
framework supports the notion that it takes a village to support and address
disability.

- Prevention in public health must go beyond primary prevention and reflect secondary prevention and health promotion strategies for individuals with disabilities. The presence of individuals with disabilities in planning prevention
initiatives has refocused the prevention agenda in the states that have disability
and health programs. A focus on prevention and health promotion for individuals
with disabilities is a major factor in preventing additional morbidity and disability and improving quality of life for individuals with disabilities. Public health
uses a science-based and community-centered approach to improve population
health that will not only prevent disabilities but most importantly improve the
lives of all individuals with disabilities in the future if these public health principles and approaches are applied consistently to the study and advocacy related
to disability.

- Disability and public health is a global as well as national movement. Just as
policy toward the inclusion of individuals with disability has been strengthened
in the United States via the Americans with Disabilities Act passed in 1990,
strong support for individuals with disabilities globally has been strengthened by
the United Nations *Convention on the Protection and Promotion of the Rights
and Dignity of Persons with Disabilities* passed in 2007. Within the past decade,
attention on disability has also expanded globally through the leadership efforts
of the World Health Organization. The World Report on Disability by WHO and
the World Bank, released in 2011, was followed up by a WHO Global Disability
Action Plan for 2014–2021. The WHO efforts recognize disability as a global
public health and human rights issue, as well as a development priority. In addition, the International Classification of Functioning (ICF) was used as the basis
of a World Health Survey on disability, which is estimated to be about 15% of the
world's population. This first international human rights treaty in the twenty-first
century, the ICF framework, the World Report on Disability, and international
programs related to disability are described in depth in the chapter on global
public health and disability by Lollar and Chamie.

- Disability should be considered as a major demographic descriptor and not a
health outcome. Disability should be included as a descriptor in public health
surveillance, management information systems, and program outcomes in the
future in order that disparities in health outcomes and social participation
between those with and without disabilities can be documented and monitored.
Just as public health currently focuses on health disparities among racial and
ethnic groups and between those in poverty or not, there should also be a focus
on inequities by the existence of a disability or not. The documentation of disparities in health and other outcomes can be used to improve programs and policies for individuals with disabilities. This approach to disability as an important
demographic description, which is currently acknowledged in Healthy People

2020 and 2030, is fully discussed in the chapter on epidemiology and biostatistics by Andresen and Bouldin.

- Public health departments at the federal, state, and local level need to embrace disability in all its programs and policies. A major initiative funded by the Centers of Disease and Control has successfully funded programs for disability and health in state health departments since the early 1990s. These programs, described in the chapter by Nary and Mullis, have established offices and coordinators for disability and health, developed and implemented health promotion programs for individuals with disabilities, and established disability descriptors in public health surveillance systems. Public health departments should develop policies and programs using the three core functions and ten essential services in public health. These core activities are described in many of the chapters, including the one on emergency preparedness and response by Kailes and Lollar.

- Statistical and epidemiological methods need to be developed to be used in research and evaluation related to individuals with disabilities. For example, consistent and "standardized" approaches to the definitions of disability across the lifespan need to be developed and used consistently in public health research and surveillance systems. Unfortunately, the definitions used in research across the various phases of the lifespan are not consistent, which makes it difficult to develop policy and track progress across the lifespan. More consistent use of the ICF in public health policies, programs, and research could help to standardize a public health approach to disability.

- Schools and programs in public health should include the study of disability in required courses for the Master of Public Health (MPH) as well as other courses in the public health curriculum. This sourcebook includes a chapter on disability in the health curricula by Griffen and Havercamp as well as chapters for each of the core areas of public health as well as those for key specialized areas of public health (e.g., maternal and child health and international health). In addition, schools of public health should consider including a track on disability and public health.

- Education and awareness are a critical component of a public health strategy to transform how each of us views "disability." A major campaign is needed to eliminate the stigma surrounding disability so that an individual with a disability is seen as the person first. Any campaign launched would need to include persons with disabilities who are thriving and leading productive lives in many areas. Public resources need to be allocated to this major campaign against discrimination and stigma related to all forms of disability, including those related to mental health challenges. This stigma can also be reduced by inclusion of more individuals in the workplace and community activities.

- Individuals with disabilities and families of children with disabilities need to be involved in all things affecting them from their individual health care to the policies and community supports that are developed at the organizational and system levels. Adopting the principles and concepts of community-based participation is critical to all programs and research related to individuals with disabilities. These principles of participation by individuals with disability should also be required in all programs, whether funded by public or private resources. Inclusion of individuals with disabilities and families of children with disabilities will lead to changes in attitudes and reduction in stigma as well as the implementation of policies, programs, and research that will lead to the most productive and healthy outcomes for children and adults with disabilities. As individuals with disabilities state "NOTHING ABOUT US WITHOUT US."

In summary, this second sourcebook is a valuable resource about the growing field of public health and disability. The adoption and use of this volume will enable the study of disability policy, programs, and research from a public health perspective. Inclusion of disability in public health courses will lead to more awareness and less stigma about disability as well as better health outcomes and functioning for individuals with disabilities. One hope for this edition focused on public health and disability is that it will play a modest role in creating the twenty-first century as the "Age of Disability"—the century in which the medical illness approach to disability is redefined and a public health approach which addresses inequities in all facets of the lives of people with disability is implemented to improve their health and well-being across the lifespan.

Deborah Klein Walker
Adjunct Professor
Boston University School of Public Health and
Tufts University School of Medicine
Cambridge, MA, USA
December 2019

References

Anderson, W. L., Armour, B. S., Finkelstein, E. A., & Wiener, J. M. (2010). Estimates of state-level health-care expenditures associated with disability. *Public Health Reports, 125*(1), 44–51.

Besser, R. (2019, December 2). *Disability inclusion: Shedding light on an urgent health equity issue*. Robert Wood Johnson Foundation Culture of Health Blog. Retrieved from https://rwjf. ws/201CDvE

Krahn, G. L., Walker, D. K., & Correa-de-Araujo, R. (2015). Persons with disabilities: An unrecognized health disparity population. *American Journal of Public Health, 105*(S2), S198–S206.

Okoro, C. A., Hollis, N. D., Cyrus, A. C., & Griffin-Blake, S. (2018). Prevalence of disabilities and health care access by disability status and type among adults—United States, 2016. *Morbidity and Mortality Weekly Report, 67*(32), 882–887.

Contents

About the Editors

Donald J. Lollar, EdD is Professor Emeritus of Public Health, School of Public Health, Oregon Health & Science University (OHSU). Dr. Lollar was the Associate Director for Research and Academic Affairs in the OHSU Institute on Development and Disability and directed the OHSU University Center for Excellence in Developmental Disabilities. Prior to his OHSU tenure, he was a Senior Health Scientist in the National Center for Environmental Health (NCEH) and the National Center on Birth Defects and Developmental Disabilities (NCBDDD) at the US Centers for Disease Control and Prevention (CDC) in Atlanta, Georgia. During his 15-year association with CDC, Dr. Lollar directed the Office on Disability and Health at NCEH and NCBDDD Office of Extramural Research. He has written extensively in the area of public health and disability, emphasizing the need for disability to be an integral part of public health education and training, culminating in the inclusion of people with disabilities in public health science, policy, and programs. He has published in *Public Health Reports,* the *Annual Review of Public Health,* the *Journal of Developmental and Behavioral Pediatrics,* and *Rehabilitation Psychology.* He was a practicing psychologist for 25 years before coming to CDC. Dr. Lollar received his MS and EdD degrees in Rehabilitation Counseling from Indiana University.

Willi Horner-Johnson, PhD is an Associate Professor in the collaborative Oregon Health & Science University and Portland State University School of Public Health and in OHSU's Institute on Development and Disability. Dr. Horner-Johnson received her graduate training in community psychology at the University of Illinois at Chicago, where she studied attitudes toward community inclusion of individuals with intellectual disabilities and coauthored a curriculum on recognizing and addressing abuse and maltreatment of people with disabilities. Since joining OHSU in 2001, her research has focused on disparities in health and access to health care as they impact youth and adults with disabilities. She has particular interests in reproductive health of women with disabilities, intersectionality of disability with other marginalized identities, and measurement of health-related quality of life in the context of disability. She directs the Oregon Office on Disability and Health, a

CDC-funded project to monitor and promote the health of individuals with disabilities in Oregon. She is active in disability-related professional organizations nationally and internationally and is a Past-Chair of the Disability Section of the American Public Health Association.

Katherine Froehlich-Grobe, PhD is Acting Director of Research at Baylor Scott and White Institute for Rehabilitation where she has been since 2016, having spent 16 years in academia at the University of Kansas Medical Center, the University of Kansas, and the University of Texas School of Public Health where she maintains an adjunct faculty appointment and continues teaching a course on Disability and Public Health. Dr. Froehlich-Grobe received her graduate training in behavioral psychology and has spent her professional career conducting research to enhance access to and engagement in health behaviors for community-dwelling individuals who live with disabilities. Her research program has focused on developing and testing evidence- and theory-based strategies to promote behavior change around dietary intake and physical activity for individuals with physical disabilities with support from the NIH, CDC, NIDILRR, and private foundations. Dr. Froehlich-Grobe's research has explored social determinants of health, specifically perceived and environmental barriers to exercise that people with disabilities face. She has conducted several intervention studies that target reducing exercise barriers that wheelchair users encounter including lack of available and affordable transportation and accessible equipment combined with teaching behavioral self-management strategies to initiate an exercise program.

Contributors

Elena M. Andresen, PhD Oregon Health & Science University, Portland, OR, USA

Andrea Betts, MPH Health Promotion and Behavioral Sciences, The University of Texas School of Public Health, Dallas, TX, USA

Erin D. Bouldin, PhD Public Health Program, Department of Health and Exercise Science, Appalachian State University, Boone, NC, USA

Mary Chamie, PhD United Nations Statistics Division (former), Demographic and Social Statistics, New York, NY, USA

International Disability Statistics Consultant, Portland, OR, USA

Philippa Clarke, PhD School of Public Health and Institute for Social Research, University of Michigan, Ann Arbor, MI, USA

Megan Douglas, PhD Baylor Scott and White Institute for Rehabilitation, Dallas, TX, USA

Clive D'Souza, PhD Department of Industrial and Operations Engineering, University of Michigan, Ann Arbor, MI, USA

Yochai Eisenberg, PhD Department of Disability and Human Development, University of Illinois at Chicago, Chicago, IL, USA

Katherine Froehlich-Grobe, PhD Baylor Scott and White Institute for Rehabilitation, Dallas, TX, USA

University of Texas School of Public Health, Dallas Regional Campus, USA

Bill Gaventa, M.Div. Collaborative on Faith and Disability, Waco, TX, USA

Adriane Griffen, DrPH, MPH, MCHES®, CNED Association of University Centers on Disabilities, Silver Spring, MD, USA

Jean P. Hall, PhD Department of Applied Behavioral Science, Institute for Health & Disability Policy Studies and Research & Training Center on Independent Living, University of Kansas, Lawrence, KS, USA

Susan Havercamp, PhD, FAAIDD, NADD-CC Nisonger Center, The Ohio State University, Columbus, OH, USA

Willi Horner-Johnson, PhD Institute on Development and Disability, Oregon Health & Science University, Portland, OR, USA

OHSU-PSU School of Public Health, Portland, OR, USA

June Isaacson Kailes, MSW Disability Policy Consultant, Playa del Rey, CA, USA

Vivian Lasley-Bibbs, MPH Office of Health Equity, Kentucky Department of Public Health, Frankfort, KY, USA

Linda Long-Bellil, PhD, JD University of Massachusetts Medical School/ Commonwealth Medicine, Shrewsbury, MA, USA

Donald J. Lollar, EdD School of Public Health, Oregon Health & Science University, Portland, OR, USA

Jordana Maisel, PhD Center for Inclusive Design and Environmental Access, School of Architecture and Planning, University at Buffalo, Buffalo, NY, USA

Katherine McDonald, PhD Department of Public Health, Syracuse University, Syracuse, NY, USA

Michelle Meade, PhD Department of Physical Medicine and Rehabilitation, University of Michigan, Ann Arbor, MI, USA

Monika Mitra, PhD Lurie Institute for Disability Policy, Brandeis University, Waltham, MA, USA

Lindsey Catherine Mullis, MS Kinesiology and Health Promotion, Human Development Institute, Kentucky Disability and Health Program, University of Kentucky, Lexington, KY, USA

Dot Nary, PhD Developmental and Child Psychology, Research and Training Center on Independent Living, Institute for Health and Disability Policy Studies, Kansas Disability and Health Program, Life Span Institute, University of Kansas, Lawrence, KS, USA

Christa Ochoa, MPH Baylor Scott and White Institute for Rehabilitation, Dallas, TX, USA

Kathleen Sheppard-Jones, PhD Human Development Institute, University of Kentucky, Lexington, KY, USA

Kristina L. Simeonsson, MD, MSPH Department of Pediatrics, Brody School of Medicine, East Carolina University, Greenville, NC, USA

Rune J. Simeonsson, PhD, MSPH School of Education, University of North Carolina at Chapel Hill, Chapel Hill, NC, USA

Devan Stahl, PhD Department of Religion, Baylor University, Waco, TX, USA

Erica Twardzik, MS School of Public Health and School of Kinesiology, University of Michigan, Ann Arbor, MI, USA

Anne Valentine, MA, MPH Lurie Institute for Disability Policy, Brandeis University, Waltham, MA, USA

Silvia Yee, JD Disability Rights Education and Defense Fund, Berkeley, CA, USA

Part I
Core Public Health Topics

Chapter 1
Introduction

Donald J. Lollar, Willi Horner-Johnson, and Katherine Froehlich-Grobe

Disability has been and continues to be communicated to most public health practitioners as one of the three negative health outcomes, alongside morbidity and mortality, that should be reduced or prevented. There was a natural progression that leads to this public health prevention emphasis, beginning with public health's initial mission related to reducing mortality through population-based interventions. Mortality was then joined by morbidity as a major thrust of public health science and programs. Disability was later added as a public health theme, focusing on the prevention and reduction of disability. Disability, however, has an added dimension—the large numbers of individuals who develop or experience a disabling condition and continue to live. If magnitude and severity of conditions drive public health attention, then the health of this population is the naturally occurring next emphasis in the evolution of public health.

A goal of this volume is to assist schools of public health to educate students more fully about this crosscutting area. If an emerging area of academic study is to find its place in an established professional discipline, it must first and foremost be grounded in that discipline. As part of that foundation, the basic conceptual and practice-based relationships should be established between the emerging and established areas of study. The emerging area must then show its capacity to highlight perspectives, approaches, and methodologies that expand and strengthen the established discipline. Simultaneously, then, the established discipline is stretched to encompass the fledgling focus, on the one hand, while its core is being broadened, deepened, and renewed. Such is the case with disability emerging as a crosscutting field within the established discipline of public health.

D. J. Lollar (✉)
School of Public Health, Oregon Health & Science University, Portland, OR, USA
e-mail: lollar@ohsu.edu

W. Horner-Johnson
Institute on Development and Disability, Oregon Health & Science University, Portland, OR, USA

OHSU-PSU School of Public Health, Portland, OR, USA

K. Froehlich-Grobe
Baylor Scott and White Institute for Rehabilitation, Dallas, TX, USA

University of Texas School of Public Health, Dallas Regional Campus, Dallas, USA

© Springer Science+Business Media, LLC, part of Springer Nature 2021
D. J. Lollar et al. (eds.), *Public Health Perspectives on Disability*,
https://doi.org/10.1007/978-1-0716-0888-3_1

This volume will present the case for disability as an area of concentration in the field of public health. Basic public health concepts will be stretched and strengthened by disability. *Healthy People 2010* addressed three principles in Chap. 6, *Disability and Secondary Conditions*:

1. Disability does not equate to illness
2. The environment is a crucial factor (either a facilitator or a barrier) in the health and well-being of people with disabilities
3. People with disabilities, like any targeted population, should be intimately involved with any activities affecting them – or, in the parlance of the disability community, "Nothing about us without us." (DHHS, 2001)

Each chapter will challenge the reader to expand their public health concepts and be creative in developing opportunities for public health science, policies, and interventions.

Since the initial edition of *Public Health Perspectives on Disability* was published a decade ago, there have been numerous other advances in the acknowledgment of disability as a public health construct and people with disabilities as a public health target. During the past decade a case definition of "disability" as a demographic variable has finally been established, using six functional items in health and other surveys used in the USA. Many public health professionals and students, however, may not know that both Healthy People 2010 and 2020 (DHHS, 2001, 2011) include a chapter entitled *Disability and Secondary Conditions*. These chapters set the goals for inclusion of people with disabilities in the national health agenda. The Disability Section of the American Public Health Association has doubled in size over the past 10 years. *Disability and Health Journal* is a thriving peer-reviewed health journal focused on advancing knowledge in disability and health, including global health, quality of life, and specific conditions as they relate to disability. The World Health Organization's World Report on Disability was published in 2012 providing a global perspective for the inclusion of people with disabilities in the core public health functions of assessment, policy development, and assurance (WHO, 2011). The Affordable Care Act amended the Public Health Service Act to require the development of data-collection standards that include five demographic categories: race, ethnicity, sex, primary language, and *disability status*. Finally, the Public Health Accreditation Board (PHAB) plans to include disability in Version 2.0 of its standards for accreditation, projected to be released in 2021 (Public Health Accreditation Board, 2018. See Chapter 16 on Building Workforce Capacity). In spite of all of these pronouncements, activities, and directions, still there is a paucity of on-the-ground disability-inclusive public health. Public health professionals often have little exposure to this growing demographic group during graduate training, even though prevalence figures indicate approximately 26% of Americans live with the limitations of a disabling condition (CDC, 2020).

The mission of this second edition is to educate public health professionals about the current substantive issues for public health science, policy, and programs to improve the health of people living with disabling conditions. This group of Americans number around 61 million and yet remain a silent minority in public health agencies and activities. Americans living with disabilities are not receiving the attention or the services commensurate with their public health needs, even though disability has been described as a universal phenomenon that affects most every family (Zola, 1994).

1.1 Foundations of Public Health Education

The second Institute of Medicine report on public health was published in 2003. *The Future of the Public's Health in the 21st Century* provides basic constructs which support the inclusion of disability in public health, the most basic of which is the notion that "health problems must be examined in the context of defined populations" (IOM, 2003a, 2003b; p. 362). The chapters of this volume focus on the assumption that public health students and workers need to be aware of the characteristics of the large defined population of those living with disabilities. The IOM committee's recommendation that academic institutions increase learning opportunities for students through integrated interdisciplinary activities is particularly relevant for health professionals in medicine; nursing; rehabilitation; psychology; allied therapies such as occupational, speech, and physical; and social work. Public health, in conjunction with health professions, balances the individual clinical experiences with the population-based prevention approaches of public health (DeFries, Andresen, & Classen, 2008; Lollar, 2008).

In addition, the public health emphasis on environmental influences on health is integral to the field of disability. As the IOM report indicates, health does not occur in a vacuum. The environment interacts with the individual at various levels to influence health and functioning. And health status then affects the individual's participation in life's activities, such as work or school or, for children, play. The disability framework, as will be noted later, expands the definition of environment so that societal attitudes, systems, and policies are given attention equal to physical and human-made environments as barriers or facilitators of health and functioning. While the IOM report primarily described the socio-ecological model as addressing health disparities in racial and ethnic minority groups, rural and urban communities, or communities that differ by poverty, the concepts are equally applicable to understanding health disparities impacting people with disabilities.

A third theme from the IOM report is the critical relationship between the health-care delivery system in this country and public health. People with disabilities are one bridge between the two. Data show that people with disabilities use a disproportionate percentage of health care relative to their percent of the population—15% of the population accounting for 46% of medical expenditures (Hough, 2000). Public health programs encouraging health promotion and preventing secondary conditions among this population may substantially reduce health care costs, *if* those programs are accessible to people with disability. Public health research and programs are needed to address this and related issues, but training in disability is required for public health workers to accurately frame science, policy, and programs and to understand disability experience and culture.

Finally, the IOM report addresses the growing issue of health disparities among racially and ethnically diverse populations in our society. Examples of how disparities are characterized include (a) lack of representation of the minority group among healthcare professionals, (b) lack of skill among healthcare workers to provide culturally competent care, and (c) the inherent context of pervasive inequities that lead to "stereotypes, biases, and uncertainties that result in unequal treatment" (IOM, 2003a, p. 37). While these characteristics are applied to racial groups, they are just as easily applied to public health activities in disability and health. Inclusion of people with disabilities in implementation of the ten essential public health services is required, and graduates from public health programs should have understanding of how this can be implemented.

As indicated, if an emerging area is to find its place in an established discipline, it must show both connection to and expansion of the field. We will go into more detail to highlight numerous basic issues and activities that indicate the need for a new perspective on disability in the public health curriculum—a redefinition. These include public health's historical perspective on disability, the status of disability-related public health data, and federal and state public health activities addressing individuals living with disability. These will be framed by the functions of public health outlined in *The Future of Public Health*, the seminal Institute of Medicine report (IOM, 1988), namely, assessment, policy development, and assurance. Understanding public health functions in the context of public health education allows the integration of disability at both conceptual and practical levels.

Disability also provides a connection to the future of public health and brings the discipline into alignment with international definitions used in health care, research, and public health. Case definitions for public health mortality and morbidity are routinely attached to the classification of diseases from the World Health Organization (WHO)—the *International Classification of Diseases (ICD)* (WHO, 2019). WHO approved a second classification in 2001, providing a conceptual framework, classification, and coding system addressing functioning and disability—the *International Classification of Functioning, Disability and Health: ICF* (WHO, 2001). The term "disability" in ICF is used as an umbrella term that includes body impairments, activity limitations, or participation restrictions. To these function-centered domains was added a unique and crucial new classification—environment. With this addition, functional status can be placed in the context of environmental factors—coded as either barriers or facilitators of a person's functioning. Public health functions are also stretched and enhanced by attention to functional descriptors, beyond diagnosis, and the impact of environments on functioning.

With the growing need to consider not just acute but chronic conditions, with the aging of the population (see Chap. 11), and with improved medical interventions, it is difficult to overstate the importance of incorporating functioning, operationalized by the *ICF* into the public health armamentarium. Disability, a crosscutting public health field most dramatically defined by the *ICF*, provides a practical and theoretical foundation for future public health students to understand the integrated nature of environment and human health and functioning. ICF conceptual dimensions distinguish among body functions and structures, person-level limitations of activities, and participation in society. Environment is included in the *ICF* as a factor affecting all the other dimensions. In this regard, the ICF disability and IOM public health models begin to converge (Andresen, 2004; IOM, 2003a, 2003b). The future of public health data for disability is closely tied with the use of the *ICF* system. As public health expands in response to a changing world, disability has the capacity to provide relevant concepts and data for that expansion.

1.2 Barriers to Inclusion

There are barriers, however, to the inclusion of disability in public health activities. It is possible that public health professionals can often have similar attitudes to that of the general public. As with other minority groups, challenging these negative attitudes is crucial to the inclusion of a group into the mainstream. Jones and Bard (2019) have delineated several of those attitudes. People with disabilities are often seen as second-class citizens, inferior to the rest of the population. These perceptions go beyond, and may be layered on top of, discrimination related to gender, race, ethnicity, or sexual orientation. People with disabilities are at times pitied and therefore patronized by the able-bodied population. Others treat people with disabling conditions, particularly those who are working and participating in the community, as heroes, brave, and special. People with disabilities wish no elevated status, only the opportunity to live their lives. Stereotyping also occurs, for example, when it is assumed that someone who is blind will have musical skills or that individuals with developmental disabilities are always gentle and kind. Individual differences are not recognized. Finally, many able-bodied individuals live in fear of interacting with people with disabilities, fearful that they will say or do the wrong thing. An antidote for many of these misconceptions is increased interactions with people with disabilities, recognizing that they want the same opportunities for participation, social relationships, work, school, and community living as everyone else.

These dynamics have contributed to a tension between the notion that disability is a universal phenomenon and the reality that people with disabilities are a minority group (Hahn, 1997). With this ambiguity it is easy to understand the lack of attention paid to this population in public health. Practically, however, a knowledge gap is created between the potential public health science, policy, and programs and the public health professionals responsible for implementing these activities. The challenge to public health education is to train new professionals and already-employed public health practitioners to understand the issues affecting the health and well-being of people with disabilities.

1.3　Changes During the Decade: Assessment

Improvements in medical treatment and prevention efforts created substantial gains in life span during the twentieth century from 49 to 72 years (CDC, 1999). With this increase in life expectancy has come a concomitant increase in the number of people living with disabilities. The first objective in the *Disability and Secondary Conditions* chapter in HP 2010 called for a standardized set of questions to identify people with disabilities to be included in any survey of health and well-being. A question set has now been selected and incorporated into several existing surveys. This set may not be the final answer for case definition but is a strong beginning.

The set of six questions identifies some 61 million Americans experiencing functional difficulties associated with disability (CDC, 2020). As a result of the sheer number of individuals and families affected by disability and associated conditions—chronic illness, traumatic injuries, birth defects, aging, or developmental disabilities—traditional public health perspectives have gradually given way to an acknowledgment of the need for greater attention to disability. This new definition allows cleaner data to be used for both prevalence and disparities. Intersectionality and international data are also stronger. Several chapters in this volume will include implications of the six-question set, including epidemiology/biostatistics, health equity, and international public health.

In recent years, disability advocates have placed increasing emphasis on improving the health of people with disabilities. Further, they are challenging the deeply rooted notion that people with disabilities are by definition ill or unhealthy. This basic and often unstated fallacy still pervades much of public health's disability-related efforts and remains at the core of resistance to the inclusion of people with disabilities in public health activities. In fact, recent data from the Centers for Disease Control and Prevention (CDC) Behavioral Risk Factor Surveillance System (BRFSS) indicate that 61% of people self-identified with disabilities report excellent, very good, or good health (MMWR, 2008). This would dispute the assumption that people with disabilities are ill or unhealthy. On the other hand, there is a clear disparity between 61% of people with disabilities and 91% of the general population reporting the same levels of positive health. This presents a challenge for public health scientists and policy makers. How do we improve the health of this section of the population? Assessment, of course, is only the first step in public health activities.

1.4　Changes During the Decade: Policy

Inclusion represents a crucial policy direction integrating public health and disability. In the IOM report *"Who will keep the nation healthy?"* (IOM, 2003b), emphasis on community-based participation in developing research, programs, and policies is clear. It would be unthinkable to develop public health data or materials on Hispanics, African-Americans, the LGBTQ community, or other minorities without the participation of these groups. Why should it be different for people with disabilities? Reality suggests that it is! Yet the field of public health has broadened, deepened, and expanded because of this principle. It has become more diverse. Public health professionals who themselves live with disabilities already enrich the field. Purposeful recruitment of students with disabilities can further build upon that enrichment.

The nation's health agenda for the decade beginning in 2020 will again include a chapter entitled *Disability and Health*. The *Healthy People* agenda in both HP 2020 and HP 2030 (DHHS, 2011, 2019) also highlights the need to eliminate health disparities among subpopulations. While race/ethnicity has rightly attracted attention related to disparities, people with disabilities are an oft-overlooked minority for whom substantial disparities exist. Remember that 61 million Americans live with disabilities. Key adverse health indicators like obesity, reduced physical activity, and smoking are more prevalent among people with disabilities than in the general population. The Disability, Intersectionlity, and Inequity chapter (Chap. 4) in this volume focuses on the extent of these and other disparities. This highlights the notion that when there is poignant public health data, there must be public health professionals who understand the needs, culture, and nuances of the population in order to address the inequity with well-developed programs. This is, on the whole, not currently the case among either experienced or newer public health professionals.

Disparities include those in clinical preventive services, which often fall through the gap between primary and specialty medical staff. Since people with disabilities often require specialty services, they may see their specialist more frequently than a primary care provider. The specialist assumes preventive services will be provided by the primary care physician, while the primary care professional sees the person infrequently and so does not focus on preventive care. Care coordination policies are needed to address this gap.

1.5 Changes During the Decade: Assurance

There has been a considerable reduction in the number and focus of Healthy People objectives from 2010 to 2030. However, of the six 2030 Disability and Health objectives, five were retained from the HP 2010 chapter for disabilities (DHHS, 2019). The current objectives include the following:

DH-2030-1 Increase the proportion of nationally-representative, population-based surveys that include in their core a standardized set of questions that identify people with disabilities.

DH-2030-2 Reduce the proportion of adults with disabilities aged 18 and older who experience delays in receiving primary and periodic preventive care due to cost

DH-2030-3 Increase the proportion of children and youth with disabilities who spend at least 80 percent of their time in regular education programs

DH-2030-4 Reduce the proportion of people with disabilities who receive long-term care services that live in congregate care residences with seven or more people

DH-2030-5 Increase the proportion of all occupied homes and residential buildings that have visitable features

DH-2030-6 Reduce the proportion of adults with disabilities aged 18 years and older who experience serious psychological distress

A crucial but often overlooked element in the public health and disability objectives is the need for intersectoral communication, cooperation, and coordination. Objective 2 addresses clinical preventive services, requiring medical sector communication. Objective 3 focuses on education as a crucial element of health among children and youth. Reducing congregate care (Objective 4) for individuals living with developmental disabilities or chronic health conditions requires interaction and coordination with various alternative living circumstances. New Objective 5 addresses issues of universal design, which requires working with city planners and architects. Finally, Objective 6 focuses on mental health issues. Community mental health centers are conceptually, if not practically, an extension of public health departments. Close coordination is needed to meet this objective. Frankly, most of these sectors can be as isolated from one another as can be public health departments. The challenge, however, is to be sufficiently acquainted with the population so that this intersector interaction can be positive and productive.

Just as the six-question identifier of people with disabilities provides major progress in the assessment function of public health, so universal design provides substantial growth in the public health function of assurance. Universal design principles have been significantly developed and implemented throughout the country and globally to improve the physical and learning environments for all individuals but are especially useful when implemented to improve the lives of people with disabilities. Several chapters in this volume, including the Environmental chapter (Chap. 5) and the Work chapter (Chap. 15) will highlight the ways in which public health can use universal design on behalf of individuals living with disabling conditions.

Specifically, public health professionals can pay attention to environmental accommodations and public infrastructure that contribute substantially to healthy living for people with disabilities. This includes ensuring the accessibility of technology, health information, and systems that are to be accessed by people with physical, sensory, and cognitive disabilities. This includes electronic health records and personal health records as well as wearable technologies and home monitoring systems. Working in concert with city planners and architects, public health professionals can assist in designing homes and communities that are fully accessible to individuals with disabilities.

1.6 Conclusion

For the editors of this volume, it would be a wonderful outcome if those reading this chapter already have begun the task of learning about disability as a construct and working with people with disabilities in their public health activities. For younger or older professionals, an "aha" experience, realizing the needs and opportunities of this population, would be a "win." This book contains a rich and diverse set of information providing the foundation for working alongside people with disabilities to improve their health and well-being. We hope you will find ideas and directions that will stretch and strengthen your public health science, policy, and programs. Most of all we sincerely hope you will consider your attitudes and behavior toward people living with disabilities.

References

Andresen, E. M. (2004). Public health education, research, and disability studies: A view from epidemiology (invited commentary). *Disability Studies Quarterly, 24*. Retrieved from http://www.dsq-sds-archives.org/_articles_html/2004/fall/dsq_fall04_andresen.asp

Centers for Disease Control and Prevention. (1999). Ten great public health achievements—United States, 1900-1999. *Morbidity and Mortality Weekly Report, 28*(12), 1.

Centers for Disease Control and Prevention (2020). *Disability statistics overview*. Retrieved from https://www.cdc.gov/ncbddd/disabilityandhealthdisability.html

Department of Health and Human Services. (2001). *Healthy People 2010*. Washington, DC: DHHS.

Department of Health and Human Services. (2011). *Healthy People 2020*. Washington, DC: DHHS.

Department of Health and Human Services. (2019). *Healthy People 2030*. Washington, DC: DHHS.

DeFries, E. L., Andresen, E. M., & Classen, S. (2008). The intersection of public health data and rehabilitation practice. *Topics in Geriatric Rehabilitation, 24*, 185–191.

Hahn, H. (1997). Advertising the acceptably employable image: Disability and capitalism. In L. J. Davis (Ed.), *The disability studies reader* (pp. 172–186). London: Routledge Kegan Paul.

Hough, J. F. (2000, June 25). *Estimating the health care utilization costs associated with persons with disabilities: Data from the 1996 Medical Expenditure Panel Survey (MEPS)*. Presentation at the Annual Meeting, Association for Health Services Research, Los Angeles, California.

Institute of Medicine. (1988). *The future of public health*. Washington, DC: National Academy.

Institute of Medicine. (2003a). *The future of the public's health in the 21st century*. Washington, DC: National Academy.

Institute of Medicine. (2003b). *Who will keep the public healthy? Educating public health professionals*. Washington, DC: National Academy.

Lollar, D. J. (2008). Rehabilitation psychology and public health: Commonalities, barriers, and bridges. *Rehabilitation Psychology, 53*(2), 122–127.

Jones, J., & Bard, C. E. (2019, September 12). *Getting comfortable with disability*. Presentation, Human Development Institute, University of Kentucky, Lexington, KY.

Morbidity and Mortality Weekly Report. (2008). Racial/ethnic disparities in self-rated health status among adults with and without disabilities—United States, 2004–2006. *Centers for Disease Control and Prevention, 57*, 1069–1073.

Public Health Accreditation Board (2018). *Inclusive health expert panel meeting*. Retrieved from https://phaboard.org/wp-conent/upleads/2.0.

World Health Organization. (2019). *Manual of the International Classification of Diseases, Injuries, and Causes of Death*. Geneva: WHO.

World Health Organization. (2001). *International Classification of Functioning, Disability, and Health: ICF*. Geneva: WHO.
World Health Organization. (2011). *World report on disability*. Geneva: WHO.
Zola, I. (1994). Toward inclusion: The role of people with disabilities in policy and research in the United States: A historical and political analysis. In M. Rioux & M. Bach (Eds.), *Disability is not measles: New research paradigms in disability* (pp. 49–66). Toronto, ON: Institut Roeher.

Chapter 2
Epidemiology and Biostatistics

Elena M. Andresen and Erin D. Bouldin

2.1 Introduction

Epidemiology and biostatistics are two of the foundations of public health science and practice (Institute of Medicine, 1988). Graduate and undergraduate degrees in schools of public health all include some level of training in these basic disciplines. As epidemiologists, we consider the training to be vital to provide future researchers and practitioners of public health with the analytic reasoning and interpretation skills to (1) understand and interpret research publications, (2) plan and execute research and evaluation studies, (3) provide scientific information about causal evidence, (4) use information about risk factors and cause to shape programs and policies, and (5) identify which interventions are most effective and for what groups. When teaching the complexity of analytic reasoning in epidemiology, we often search for relevant, real-world examples that permit us to impart both methods and broader public health content. Disability epidemiology provides a rich opportunity on both counts. It offers intellectually stimulating examples on issues that span the disciplines of both epidemiology and biostatistics. These issues, some of which are discussed in this chapter, relate to everything from pragmatic problems in field research to theoretical frameworks about the impact of risk factors across multiple levels of personal and environmental influences. Special populations, including people with disability (PWD), also offer an opportunity to examine and grapple with the public health challenge of disparities and, through that challenge, to help the disciplines of epidemiology and biostatistics evolve. Unfortunately, there is an

E. M. Andresen (✉)
Oregon Health & Science University, Portland, OR, USA
e-mail: andresee@ohsu.edu

E. D. Bouldin
Public Health Program, Department of Health and Exercise Science, Appalachian State University, Boone, NC, USA
e-mail: bouldinel@appstate.edu

© Springer Science+Business Media, LLC, part of Springer Nature 2021
D. J. Lollar et al. (eds.), *Public Health Perspectives on Disability*,
https://doi.org/10.1007/978-1-0716-0888-3_2

13

uneasy and sometimes even disrespectful relationship between the disability world and the world of public health, including epidemiology, when such an interface exists at all.

This chapter provides examples of the opportunities and limitations of the discipline of epidemiology as a tool for research and teaching about disability. Biostatistical techniques are discussed as they facilitate or impede disability research, but this chapter does not purport to offer an expansive overview of statistical methods. The chapter is intended for public health students or practitioners with some basic epidemiology training, and therefore it does not attempt to explain basic epidemiology and biostatistics, except where relevant to specific examples related to etiology and outcomes research. There are excellent epidemiology methods textbooks that cover traditional methods and analysis issues in substantially more depth (e.g., Gordis, 2014; Koepsell & Weiss, 2014; Rothman, 2012; Rothman, Greenland, & Lash, 2008; Szklo & Nieto, 2012).

For epidemiologists, we hope to evoke interest in a new sub-discipline. Epidemiology, like other disciplines, has its "lumpers" and "splitters." Is someone trained in epidemiology just an epidemiologist? Or should they always apply an adjective to explain their particular area of interest, expertise, and research? Most meetings of epidemiologists include proceedings grouped by specialty topics such as cancer, genetics, and maternal and child health (see, e.g., agendas for meetings of the *Society for Epidemiologic Research* at https://epiresearch.org/annual-meeting/). Disability epidemiology also has a small group of professionals who cluster within the definition. Like any area of science, disability epidemiology requires—and is still developing—spirited debate about its contents, breadth, rigor, and nature. As discussed later in this chapter, the concepts and content of disability epidemiology derive naturally from a number of other epidemiology disciplines (e.g., injury, maternal and child health, aging, and outcomes research). Despite some differences in methods and focus, neither biostatical nor epidemiology principles alter remarkably as one moves from one content area to another. In this spirit, we offer examples that can be shared in introductory and methodology courses in epidemiology. Rather than limit consideration of disability to special courses, it would strengthen the training of epidemiologists to have public health and research examples on disability topics in general coursework. In addition to methodological examples in this chapter, there are a number of potential practice problems that we hope instructors will use as part of training examples, homework, or exams and quizzes.

2.2 Defining and Some Parameters of Disability Epidemiology

Epidemiology has expanded its scope beyond the narrow focus on disease or illness to look at health events, health states, and health differences (Porta, 2008). Although disability epidemiology has not been defined explicitly, the scope of general epidemiology would suggest that the definition should certainly include study of basic elements of descriptive epidemiology (who, what, where), etiological determinants of physical impairments and functional limitations, and the frequency and predictors of different outcomes experienced by people with disabilities. And while epidemiology is concerned with identifying distributions and determinants of health outcomes, it also uses this information to intervene to improve the health of populations. Some have argued that the field of epidemiology generally has become too focused on precisely measuring the frequency and modeling the causes of disease at the expense of rigorously identifying solutions that work to improve communities' health while eliminating health inequities (Galea, 2013; Galea & Keyes, 2018). Therefore, disability epidemiology might also include studies of policies or interventions with the potential to improve participation, function, and quality of life among people with disability. All of these questions incorporate the common epidemiology study designs and methods. Questions that ask students to consider study designs using disability topics are included in the Appendix. Additional descriptive disability epidemiology examples also are included in the section on surveillance and secondary data sources.

Importantly, disability must be defined as a state that is largely independent of health and health status. As described by the World Health Organization model of disability below (the ICF), disability is a state that is inexorably connected to the environment in which people live. That is, with a properly accommodated social, built, and policy environment, a person with functional limitation would also participate fully and would enjoy improved health outcomes. The conceptual separation of health and disability is clearly described in the *Healthy People 2010* and *Healthy People 2020* chapters on disability (Centers for Disease Control and Prevention, 2001). Prominent in these documents are the following basic assumptions about disability:

> "Disability is a demographic descriptor rather than a health outcome. It should be used to monitor disparities in health outcomes and social participation." (Healthy People, 2010: Centers for Disease Control and Prevention, 2001)

> "A diagnosis of impairment or disabling condition does not define individuals, their talents and abilities, or health behaviors and health status. Consistent with the World Health Organization's (WHO) model of social determinants of health, Healthy People 2020 recognizes that what defines individuals with disabilities, their abilities, and their health outcomes more often depends on their community, including social and environmental circumstances." (Healthy People, 2020: Centers for Disease Control and Prevention, n.d.)

Defining disease, health outcomes, health states, or health events for purposes of disability epidemiology are further challenges. The temporal nature of these events or states is important. A disease or health outcome may be an *event* that occurs at a specific point in time. For example, an automotive crash that results in injury, a suicide attempt, or a birth injury would be classified as events. A disease also may be a *state* that characterizes an individual during some time period. That is, it has duration. For these conditions or diseases, the particular time of onset (or diagnosis) is often of interest. Examples include depression, Parkinson's disease, disability, or a particular level of health-related quality of life (HRQoL). A disease or health state also has a course that helps to define how it is dealt with in epidemiologic studies.

Some diseases occur only once and the individual does not (given current medical understanding) recover, e.g., Alzheimer's disease and Parkinson's disease. However, the *impact* of the state, disease, or characteristic is not necessarily static and may change over time. For disability epidemiology, this dynamic state fits well into the concepts of the International Classification of Functioning, Disability and Health (ICF: World Health Organization [WHO], 2001a). For a person with a spinal cord injury (SCI), there may be no change in the biological description of their injury level and neurologically defined impairment as time passes. But there might be substantial variation over the course of their lifetime in the impact of SCI, especially as impairments are affected by environmental variables. Other conditions can affect an individual multiple times, e.g., upper respiratory tract infections, depression, or myocardial infarction (MI or heart attack). A disease or health condition can be secondary to some primary condition, for example, if a person has a spinal cord injury, our interest may be in the occurrence of secondary conditions and health events, such as pressure sores, urinary tract infections, etc.

In epidemiology, the course of a disease or condition is important because the measures of excess risk from an exposure or experience require some understanding of a person's or population's risk status. An individual is either "at risk" or "not at risk" for a given disease or event at a given time. "At risk" does not necessarily imply "at high risk" relative to others: it means that there is a nonzero chance of developing a disease. "Not at risk" means an individual is considered to have a zero chance of developing the disease. So, for example, a person with a spinal cord injury (SCI) may be at risk for a urinary tract infection (UTI), and this risk is higher, on average, than that of a person who is fully ambulatory; but the latter is also "at risk," even if the risk is much smaller. Different risks based on individual, relationship, or community characteristics are what we measure in epidemiology to identify risky exposures and define groups with need of specific intervention(s). An individual's "at-risk" status may change over time. In the example above (urinary tract infection), it is particularly important to discover if there are *intervenable* risk factors that place some people with spinal cord injury at special risk for an adverse outcome. In other words, we need to discover what risk factors there are in addition to the primary impairment of SCI. Added to this mix of factors that describe a person's possibly elevated "at-risk" status for disability is the need to measure and understand the environment. For example, having a personal care assistant may have a large impact on the occurrence of pressure sores for a person with SCI, and good transportation and accessible food stores contribute to the nutritional status of a person who is blind. Some variables that shape the association between SCI and UTI may not turn out to be ones on which we can intervene, but may give us insight into groups with extra risk and corresponding need for careful monitoring. Examples of risk factors that cannot be changed may include age, gender, and race or ethnicity.

In addition to methodological and measurement considerations, people working within the field of disability also should be attuned to disability frameworks. Public health has long explained itself as a discipline aimed at finding causes of disease and identifying interventions to prevent disease, impairment, and disability. The heavy emphasis on primary prevention as the goal of these efforts has often translated, explicitly or implicitly, into a goal of "preventing" people with diseases, impairments, or disabilities. Epidemiologists need to expand their definition of etiology to include PWD as another population in which we have an interest in improving outcomes across the full range of health risks (Andresen, 2004). Specifically, epidemiologists need to embrace research about the outcomes of impairment and disability. Spinal cord injuries occur, and people with these injuries lead productive lives. The determinants of successful outcomes—people fully integrated into their chosen lifestyles—are also a proper arena for epidemiologic research and biostatistical methods. However, we cannot expect nor do we want a retraction of the research efforts into understanding and preventing events like spina bifida from nutritional deficits, or of spinal cord injuries that result from traffic crashes, or examinations into the causes of strokes or hearing loss. The point is to state clearly that prevention does not have to mean prevention of *people*; but the process of making personal or societal changes that can change the incidence or severity of impairments.

Involving people with disability in research is one aspect of assuring that research is designed and conducted in a way that does not confuse the prevention of poor health states with the prevention of people or experiences. Although there was a time when participants were uninformed about the nature of scientific investigations to limit bias, today informed consent is a requirement for ethical research. Many researchers, including epidemiologists and biostatisticians, embrace the practice of participatory research. Indeed, disability research was at the vanguard of this transition with the disability community's expectation that participants will be involved in the design, conduct, and interpretation of research: "Nothing about us without us" (Charlton, 1998). There are different approaches to including community members in the research process, and describing these is beyond the scope of this chapter, but there are ample examples from disability and other fields to guide researchers in the process (e.g., Hagey, 1997; Nicolaidis et al., 2019; Wallerstein, Duran, Oetzel, & Minkler, 2017).

An increasingly important segment of clinical epidemiology seeks to define and incorporate patient-centered or patient-generated outcomes into research questions by including patients with experience in planning and conducting studies (e.g., Frank, Basch, Selby, & Patient-Centered Outcomes Research Institute, 2014; Gilliam et al., 1997). Indeed, the 2010 Affordable Care Act (ACA) mandated the creation and funding of a research office focused on patient-reported outcomes, known as the Patient-Centered Outcomes Research Institute (PCORI). We revisit the issues of research participation and ethics and involving the community in epidemiologic research at the end of this chapter. See also Chap. 11 that discusses disability and ethics in detail.

In summary, disability epidemiology includes the usual aspects of epidemiologic investigations. These include descriptive and analytic epidemiology and the full spectrum of events and health states that arise in all epidemiologic work. Many definitions of disability exist and have been used for different purposes. It is critical for epidemiologists and biostatisticians who are new to the field of disability to consider the history of disability research and the needs of people with disabilities when designing and conducting research.

2.3   Contributing Epidemiology Disciplines and Interdisciplinary Collaboration

Disability epidemiology derives much of its content and methodology from traditional epidemiology and other well-established disciplines. Content areas tend to be defined either by a medical model for classifying diseases or by methodological discipline. For example, injury epidemiologists and epidemiologists working in content areas like gerontology and neurological diseases contribute to the issues often dealt with in disability epidemiology, such as challenges in collecting information from respondents with cognitive or communications impairments.

As noted earlier, disability epidemiology is a loosely defined discipline. There are no societies of similar scientists nor are there scientific epidemiology journals where one would examine the ongoing work of the discipline (in contrast to other branches of epidemiology that produce such journals as *Neuroepidemiology*; *Epidemiology and Infection*; *Paediatric and Perinatal Epidemiology*; *Cancer Epidemiology, Biomarkers & Prevention*; and *Social Psychiatry and Psychiatric Epidemiology*). However, there is a journal for the broader aspects of public health with substantial numbers of epidemiology articles, *Disability and Health Journal* (https://www.journals.elsevier.com/disability-and-health-journal/). Interdisciplinary and interprofessional research often results in better research products, both in terms of the design of studies and in their influence on public health and clinical practice. There are several avenues for forging and nurturing these interdisciplinary and interprofessional connections and they can begin in the classroom. Interprofessional education (IPE) within clinical disciplines was endorsed by the Institute of Medicine as a way to improve the safety and quality of health care (Institute of Medicine (IOM), 2003a, 2003b). It has support from multiple organizations including the World Health Organization (1988) and the American Public Health Association (2008). The Interprofessional Education Collaborative has published core competencies for interprofessional collaborative practice to guide these efforts (Interprofessional Education Collaborative, 2016). For those already in practice, professional organizations offer opportunities for interdisciplinary work. Relevant examples for this chapter include the American Public Health Association's Disability Section, which has members from diverse backgrounds and perspectives who all work toward improving the health and quality of life of people with disabilities, and the American Association on Health and Disability, which works to improve health and wellness policies and programs for people with disabilities across the lifespan and to reduce health disparities.

2.4 Disability Surveillance Data and Secondary Analysis

2.4.1 Introduction

Many public health questions and program plans regarding disability are based on ongoing surveillance systems. This section provides an overview of some of the sources for data regarding disability and their use and problems. A variety of surveillance sources are used to answer questions about disability prevalence, and these are the focus for this section. In addition, the general topic of sources for secondary data analysis is covered here and in the Appendix. Federal and state surveillance systems offer data that can be used for preliminary analytic work on a broad array of disability and health topics. Entire careers can be built around analysis of these data. For many epidemiologists, the complex sampling designs that produced these data sets and the resulting sampling weight and statistical variance complexity may require additional statistical training or working with a survey statistician. The quality of data and uses and limitations of such systems also are described on the web sites for each surveillance source. As the examples below demonstrate, most of these data resources have yet to be fully analyzed in relation to disability epidemiology and health outcomes associated with disability.

2.4.2 Measures and Classification of Disability

2.4.2.1 Surveillance Measures

As a nation, we need to know various characteristics of our population in order to monitor our progress and allocate resources. We may have a relatively simple question, "How many people are there in the United States with disabilities?", but the answer depends on (1) our definition of disability and (2) the mechanism we choose for collecting the information. As described by Adler (1996) and Altman (2014), there are many ways to measure disability. Interestingly, surveillance classification questions carry implications that can clash with disability advocacy and politics. A broadly defined question will add to the population size that is claimed for the advocacy community, giving the issues of concern to this community greater social weight. Yet many of those counted by a broadly applicable question will not view themselves as having a disability, nor will they be viewed by others as such. Their inclusion in a count could have the effect of diluting the force with which disability concerns are expressed. In addition, broad measures may limit the user's ability to identify groups with particular types of disability. Questions that are worded narrowly, however, may exclude people who are seen and see themselves as part of the disability numerator. Decisions about the choice of questions that provide the data for public health need to reflect the exact purpose of the surveillance. In general,

Table 2.1 Percentage of persons who indicated they were limited in any way in any activity in a study of PWD (Nanda & Andresen, 1998)

Group	Total interviewed	% who answered "yes" to screening question on limitation
Traumatic brain injury	16	50.0
Spinal cord injury	195	91.3
Parkinson's disease	26	80.8
Multiple sclerosis	16	75.0
Nursing home residents	44	66.0
Assisted living settings	212	50.0

surveillance measurements opt for a very broad and inclusive classification system. A few examples help demonstrate these issues.

Table 2.1 shows how one measure of disability works (Nanda & Andresen, 1998). The question "Are you limited in any way in any activities because of physical, mental, or emotional problems?" was used by the CDC's Behavioral Risk Factor Surveillance System for a number of years (e.g., Andresen, Prince-Caldwell, Akinci, Brownson, Jackson-Thompson, & Crocker, 1999). If we wished to "count" people who had a traumatic brain injury (TBI), the fact that only 50% of them said "yes" to having a limitation would be a problem. On the other hand, the fact that only 50% of people with TBI reported limitations is a good sign: they distinguish between their disability and the limitation that might result from TBI. However, for policy and program planning, an accurate and clear "count" is needed. The Appendix includes questions that exemplify the effect of using broad or narrow definitions of disability/mobility impairment on the sensitivity and specificity of Behavioral Risk Factor Surveillance System (BRFSS) data.

Epidemiologists are generally comfortable that definitions and classifications may be different depending on a specific question or need. However, the simple goal of counting people with disabilities makes it problematic to have many definitions. The report generated as part of *Healthy People 2010* (Centers for Disease Control and Prevention, 2001) specifically recommends consistent definitions, universal collection of disability status, and methodological studies to help provide more accurate and useful data, and the *Healthy People 2020 Disability and Health* objectives (Centers for Disease Control and Prevention, n.d.) begin with a goal to increase the use of a common set of questions to identify disability.

In 2011 the US Department of Health and Human Services (DHHS) issued guidance regarding minimum data standards for several demographic characteristics, including disability (U.S. Department of Health and Human Services, 2011). This effort was required as part of the ACA in order to consistently measure health disparities. Specifically, the DHHS recommended a set of disability measures developed for use on the US Census Bureau's American Community Survey (ACS) that evaluate the presence of a vision, hearing, cognitive, mobility, self-care, or independent living disability. The questions have a dichotomous yes/no response set.

Box 2.1 Measuring Disability Using Washington Group on Disability Statistics Short Set on Functioning (The International Disability Data Collection Standard for Censuses and Surveys) and the American Community Survey Disability Questions (The US Department of Health and Human Services Disability Data Collection Standard)
Washington Group Short Set on Functioning (WG SS-F).

1. Do you have difficulty seeing, even if wearing glasses?
2. Do you have difficulty hearing, even if using a hearing aid?
3. Do you have difficulty walking or climbing stairs?
4. Do you have difficulty remembering or concentrating?
5. Do you have difficulty (with self-care such as) washing all over or dressing?
6. Using your usual (customary) language, do you have difficulty communicating, for example, understanding or being understood by others?

Response options are no, no difficulty; yes, some difficulty; yes, a lot of difficulty; and cannot do at all. The recommended cutoff for calculating disability is any "a lot of difficulty" or "cannot do at all/unable" response across the six functioning domains.

Source: Washington Group on Disability Statistics (2017), http://www.washingtongroup-disability.com/

American Community Survey Disability Questions (ACS)

1. Are you deaf or do you have serious difficulty hearing?
2. Are you blind or do you have serious difficulty seeing, even when wearing glasses?
3. Because of a physical, mental, or emotional condition, do you have serious difficulty concentrating, remembering, or making decisions? *Asked of people age 5 years or older.*
4. Do you have serious difficulty walking or climbing stairs? *Asked of people age 5 years or older.*
5. Do you have difficulty dressing or bathing? *Asked of people age 5 years or older.*
6. Because of a physical, mental, or emotional condition, do you have difficulty doing errands alone such as visiting a doctor's office or shopping? *Asked of people age 15 years or older.*

Response options are yes or no for each question. The recommended cutoff for calculating disability is any "yes" response across the six functioning domains.

Source: U.S. Department of Health and Human Services (2011)

Respondents who indicate any "yes" to one of the six questions are considered to have disability (Box 2.1). These questions are now used in many surveillance systems and data collection efforts; the CDC's Disability and Health website lists the surveys that include the items on its website (https://www.cdc.gov/ncbddd/disabilityandhealth/datasets.html).

In addition to the US effort, the United Nations formed the Washington Group on Disability Statistics (WG) in 2001, a city group which addresses the need for cross-culturally comparable disability measures and supports national statistical offices and organizations in the standard collection and use of disability statistics. (http://unstats.un.org/unsd/methods/citygroup/washington.htm). The group has developed several question sets designed to measure disability, including a six-item version that is similar to the ACS (see Box 2.1; Madans, Loeb, & Altman, 2011). Both question sets ask about hearing, vision, mobility, cognition, and self-care but in slightly different ways. The content of the sixth question diverges on the two measures: the ACS set assesses independent living, while the Washington Group set measures communication. Acknowledging that disability is not a dichotomous state, the Washington Group set assesses degree of difficulty using a four-category response set and has produced recommended cut points for defining the population with disability.

2.4.2.2 Detailed Classification Systems: The ICF

The current theoretical model of disability is multidimensional, incorporating individual and environmental factors (World Health Organization [WHO], 2001a). The World Health Organization's *International Classification of Functioning, Disability and Health* (ICF) provides a framework and a coding scheme that captures information on domains of body functions (e.g., hearing functions; code b210), body structures (e.g., structure of inner ear, cochlea; code s2600), activities and participation (e.g., conversation; code d350), and environment (e.g., sound; code e250: individual attitudes of strangers; code 2445). In its full application, the measurement is complex and not readily applied to large-scale surveillance surveys, especially if the purpose of the surveillance system is to provide information to a broad spectrum of public health practitioners. The ICF provides a set of codes for minimal health systems or surveys (World Health Organization, 2001a, page 253) that, though brief relative to the full ICF, are still somewhat daunting for surveillance purposes. However, the ICF was recommended, at least in principle, as the classification system for coding functional status in medical encounters data by the *National Committee on Vital and Health Statistics* (Department of Health and Human Services, 2001). In addition, the ICF is proposed as the unifying framework for disability measurement in public health (Lollar, 2002; Lollar & Crews, 2003).

Questionnaires that are substantially longer than usual surveillance tools have been developed for classifying people according to the ICF. The WHO developed and tested a comprehensive tool for measuring disability and the environment: the WHO Disability Assessment Schedule (WHODAS II; World Health Organization,

2001b). Given some practical limitations of this measure (e.g., length and adminis-tration burden), the WHO updated the measure to WHODAS 2.0 in 2010 (World Health Organization, 2018). This instrument provides a profile of functioning across six activity domains, as well as a general disability score. There are 36-item and 12-item versions of the WHODAS 2.0, and both ask respondents to rate how much difficulty they have engaging in specific activities on a scale from 0 (no difficulty) to 4 (extreme difficulty). In general, given the complexity and training issues for even clinical applications, the research applications of the full ICF are likely to remain in clinical rehabilitation and outcomes arenas and not surveillance systems (e.g., see Grimby & Smedby, 2001, and Reed et al., 2008). The DHHS minimum data standards encompass four of the six domains represented in the WHODAS 2.0.

2.4.3   Selected Data Sources

In this section, we describe a few of the data sources available in the United States that include measures of disability. There are many other possibilities beyond those listed here, including in surveys conducted by the Departments of Education, Justice, and Labor, to name a few. The ones we note below have been used with some frequency to produce disability estimates and/or to study disability and there-fore we include them here to illustrate possibilities.

2.4.3.1   The Behavioral Risk Factor Surveillance System (BRFSS)

The Behavioral Risk Factor Surveillance System (BRFSS) is an annual survey con-ducted in all US states and territories (Centers for Disease Control and Prevention, 2013; Mokdad, 2009). Currently, it is the primary source for data regarding disability for states, but also contributes to national estimates and analysis of disability. The BRFSS is supported and supervised by the Centers for Disease Control and Prevention (CDC) although states may use their own funds to add optional sections to the survey or increase sample size among particular population groups. The BRFSS is a random-digit-dialed telephone survey that covers health behaviors, med-ical diagnoses, demographic variables, and health-related quality of life (HRQoL).

Beginning in 2001, the core BRFSS data for all states, DC, and territories included two questions on disability mentioned in the examples above. With these additions, which permitted identification of people with disabilities and ascertain-ment of information about their specific sociodemographic characteristics, health status, and health risks, the BRFSS became a valuable source of national- and state-level information about disability. In 2013, the BRFSS adopted the DHHS questions to identify disability. For 3 years, both the old and new questions were asked of all respondents. Beginning in 2016, the old disability questions moved to an optional module on the BRFSS, and the core demographics section now includes the new set of six items.

In addition to asking respondents about disability, the BRFSS includes questions related to caregiving for people with disabilities. Core questions for the 2000 BRFSS included items measuring caregiving provided to older adults with disability; 15.6% of respondents reported they provided caregiving to someone aged 60 or older (McKune, Andresen, Zhang, & Neugaard, 2006). In addition, 28 states added a supplemental module on caregiving to the BRFSS in 2000 and/or 2001 (Fig. 2.1). This provided new information on the BRFSS respondents who said they needed either personal care assistance or assistance with routine needs and how adequate the caregiving assistance was (Jamoom, Andresen, Neugaard, &

This optional module was asked of respondents who said "yes" to either of the following questions on the core survey:

1. Are you limited in any way in any activities because of physical, mental, or emotional problems?

2. Do you now have any health problem that requires you to use special equipment, such as a cane, a wheelchair, a special bed, or a special telephone?

---

3. Because of any impairment or health problem, do you need the help of other persons with your PERSONAL CARE needs, such as eating, bathing, dressing, or getting around the house?

Earlier you reported that due to your impairment you need some assistance from another person with your PERSONAL CARE needs...

---

10. Who usually helps you with your personal care needs, such as eating, bathing, dressing, or getting around the house?

---

11. Is the assistance you receive to meet your personal care needs: (usually, sometimes, or rarely adequate)?

---

4. Because of any impairment or health problem, do you need the help of other persons in handling your ROUTINE NEED, such as everyday household chores, doing necessary business, shopping, or getting around for other purposes?

Earlier you reported that due to impairment you need some assistance from another person with ROUTINE needs...

---

12. Who usually helps you with handling your routine needs, such as everyday household chores shopping, or getting around for other purposes?

---

13. Is the assistance you receive to meet your routine needs: (usually, sometimes, rarely adequate)?

Fig. 2.1 Selected items from the Quality of Life and Care Giving optional module for the Behavioral Risk Factor Surveillance System (2000, 2001). Source: Behavioral Risk Factor Surveillance System Questionnaire, 2001 from National Center for Chronic Disease Prevention and Health Promotion, Division of Population Health. (2019). https://www.cdc.gov/brfss/questionnaires/index.htm

McKune, 2008). In more recent years, caregiving has been promoted as a public health issue (Talley & Crews, 2007), and some states now report on the prevalence and correlates of caregiving (Bouldin, Akhtar, Brumback, & Andresen, 2009; Horner-Johnson, Dobbertin, Kulkarni-Rajasekhara, Beilstein-Wedel, & Andresen, 2015; McGuire, Bouldin, Andresen, & Anderson, 2010; Neugaard, Andresen, DeFries, Talley, & Crews, 2007). In 2009, a caregiving question was again included on the core BRFSS and asked in all US states and territories. This time, the question asked about care for people of any age. The prevalence of caregiving using this measure was 24.7% (Anderson et al., 2013). Between 2015 and 2018, 44 states, the District of Columbia, and Puerto Rico included the optional caregiving module on their BRFSS.

The BRFSS offers remarkable opportunities for epidemiologic questions and analytic practice for graduate students. These might include questions used in the context of a specific health behavior (e.g., physical activity, smoking), specific diagnoses (e.g., arthritis, diabetes), or disparities in healthcare access. Appendix provides a number of epidemiology methodology practice questions using BRFSS data and questions.

2.4.3.2 The National Health Interview Survey (NHIS)

The National Center for Health Statistics (NCHS) conducts the annual National Health Interview Survey (NHIS). Since 2009, NHIS has included the ACS and/or WG SS-F disability measures (see https://www.cdc.gov/nchs/nhis/data-question-naires-documentation.htm for a list of questionnaires by year). Between October 2008 and December 2009, the disability questions were asked of both the respondent and about family members, but that practice was discontinued. Currently, respondents only report disability for themselves. NHIS includes questions on a variety of topics, including healthcare utilization, prescription medication use, immunization, physical and mental health conditions, and social functioning. During some years, data on additional topics like sleep, the physical environment, and behaviors like smoking, alcohol use, and sun protection also are collected on the survey.

During 1994 and 1995, the NHIS also included a supplement on disability (NHIS-D). NHIS-D data entail face-to-face interviews with 202,000 adults and children (using parent proxies for child subjects). Follow-up interviews collected data on 33,000 persons with disability. NHIS-D findings provided an exceptional opportunity to examine healthcare utilization and access among people with disability, especially in comparison to the general population. Other disability-related topics addressed in the supplement were chronic conditions, impairments, functional limitations, activities of daily living (ADLs, which are basic self-care activities), instrumental activities of daily living (IADLs, which are more complex self-care activities), the use of assistive technology, transportation, personal assistance services, labor force participation, workplace accommodations, and disability benefits. Although these data are now quite old, they provided a wealth of information for detailed reports describing disability among children and youth (Druss et al., 2000; Druss & Rosenheck, 2000; Hogan, Msall, Rogers, & Avery, 1997; Newacheck et al., 1998) and on specialty topics among adults, for example, injury (Guerrero, Sniezek, & Sehgal, 1999), sensory impairment (Hoffman, Ishii, & Macturk, 1998), and personal assistant services (LaPlante, Harrington, & Kang, 2002).

NHIS-D data also have been used to examine disparities in health care. For example, women with functional limitations were found to have lower screening rates for Papanicolaou tests and mammograms (Centers for Disease Control and Prevention, 1998; Iezzoni, McCarthy, Davis, Harris-David, & O'Day, 2001). Disparities in health insurance coverage for children with chronic conditions were reported from these data (Silver & Stein, 2001). Russell and colleagues reported on increasing use of assistive technology over the period ending with the 1994 NHIS (Russell, Hendershot, LeClere, Howie, & Adler, 1997). While it would be useful for a new supplement to be fielded like the NHIS-D, NHIS surveys always include some data that can address disability and disability experiences (http://www.cdc. gov/nchs/nhis.htm).

2.4.3.3   The Medical Expenditure Panel Study (MEPS)

MEPS data collection is supported by the Agency for Healthcare Research and Quality (AHRQ). MEPS data provide a broad set of measurements of health status and diagnoses, healthcare use and expenditure, and issues about access to care (Cohen, 2002; Cohen et al., 1996-1997). MEPS data consist of four components. The Household Component (HC) collects data on a sample of families and individuals who comprise households drawn from a nationally representative subsample of households that participated in the prior year's NHIS. The Medical Provider Component (MPC), which covers hospitals, physicians, and home healthcare providers, supplements information from HC respondents. The Insurance Component (IC) consists of two subcomponents. The first consists of data from the household sample on the health insurance held by and offered to HC respondents. The second component comprises data collected from a sample of business establishments and governments throughout the United States. MEPS also periodically includes a Nursing Home Component (NHC). MEPS now includes the standard DHHS disability questions.

Disability analyses based on MEPS have examined ethnic disparities in function (Vásquez et al., 2018), child disability and expenditures (Chan, Zhan, & Homer, 2002; Newacheck, Inkelas, & Kim, 2004), healthcare issues in mental health disability (Druss & Rosenheck, 2000; Egede, Zheng, & Simpson, 2002; Nguyen, Chan, & Keeler, 2015; Olfson et al., 2002), preventive service use (Horner-Johnson, Dobbertin, Lee, & Andresen, 2014; Reichard, Stolzle, & Fox, 2011), delaying necessary health care (Reichard, Stransky, Phillips, McClain, & Drum, 2017), complimentary medicine therapies used by PWD (Druss & Rosenheck, 2000), and home health care (Mullner, Jewell, & Mease, 1999; Pérez Jolles & Thomas, 2018). Several groups have demonstrated the value of these data as a basis for understanding access to care and healthcare costs (e.g., Kennedy, Wood, & Frieden, 2017; Mitra, Findley, & Sambamoorthi, 2009; Yelin, Herrndorf, Trupin, & Sonneborn, 2001). Future studies using MEPS data could explore issues related to disability that crosscut diagnostic categories and represent definitions of disability in line with the ICF. MEPS data provide a unique opportunity to assess economic and other impacts associated with disability, especially because of the population perspective of the data that allow comparisons between PWD and others (see http://www.ahrq.gov/data/mepsix.htm).

2.4.3.4   The Census Bureau Resources

The United States Bureau of the Census provides data on disability drawn from four primary sources: the decennial census of population, the American Community Survey, the Survey of Income and Program Participation, and the Current Population Survey. Two of these data resources are briefly described here (see also http://www.census.gov/).

The US Census, conducted at 10-year intervals, is not primarily a health surveillance tool, and yet it provides denominator data for use in population research, policy and political analysis, and resource allocations. In 1990 and 2000, the long form of the census included questions on functional status and disability, permitting better estimation of disability prevalence. The Census 2000 questions addressed instrumental and basic activities of daily living (ADL/IADLs, i.e., self-care, mobility), activity limitations, working, and sensory impairments (Andresen, Fitch, McLendon, & Meyers, 2000). The American Community Survey (ACS) began in 2005 as a way to collect representative data in between census years. The US Department of Health and Human Services disability measures described above were first tested as part of the 2006 ACS and became standard in 2008 (United States Census Bureau, 2017). Census data, even from the sample-based long form, are representative and applicable to very small areas—as small as neighborhoods. In fact, small local area comparisons may need to rely on the census or ACS because of the difficulty of using state (BRFSS) and national (NHIS) data for estimates at smaller geographic regions (Andresen, Diehr, & Luke, 2004).

The Survey of Income and Program Participation (SIPP) is a multistage-stratified sample of the US civilian noninstitutionalized population. The SIPP is a continuous series of national panels, with sample size ranging from approximately 14,000 to 36,700 households. The duration of each panel ranges from 3 to 5 years. Interviews are conducted in-person and by telephone. All household members 15 years old and over are interviewed with proxy responses permitted when household members are not available. SIPP data include detailed information on cash and noncash income and data on taxes, assets, liabilities, and participation in government programs along with information about the social characteristics of individuals and families. The SIPP survey was substantially redesigned in 2014; part of the change included adding the six DHSS disability questions. In addition, the survey asks three questions about work-related disability, and it also queries the respondent about disability among children in the household (United States Census Bureau, 2018).

These brief examples of Census Bureau data and publications hint at their utility in disability epidemiology. In particular, the data might be subjected to complex analyses beyond surveillance statistical reports of prevalence and descriptive epidemiology.

2.5   Selected Methodological Issues in Disability Research

2.5.1   Introduction

Disability research raises unique methodological issues. Four that are discussed in the section that follows are sample size, measurement, multi-level studies, and the process of field research. As often happens in relation to methodology decisions, there are trade-offs among solutions. For example, methods to include representative PWD in research efforts often involve increased costs. Efforts to increase sample sizes may require a less costly (and less precise) measurement strategy. Epidemiology is usually concerned with precise measurements (e.g., exposures and case definitions) to estimate valid exposure-outcomes relationships of interest. However, in order to increase sample sizes for statistical precision, it may be necessary to combine people with different impairments. These issues, and potential conflicts between solutions, are discussed in more detail below.

2.5.2   Sample Size

In epidemiology, if a condition is not relatively common, it is hard to conduct statistically useful research on it. The following examples based on hearing impairment/loss in children show why this is true. Hearing impairment among infants and young children is challenging to detect and surveillance statistics equally hard to estimate. The CDC's programs of research on this topic include an active surveillance registry for the Metropolitan Atlanta area (MADDSP). Severe hearing impairment among children aged 3 to 10 was estimated as 1.1 per 1000 children (Van Naarden, Decoufle, & Caldwell, 1999), and the estimate was higher for African American male children (1.4/1000). If we wished to study this problem in more detail and understand the contributors to higher risk of hearing impairment, it would require over 445,000 children to be sure that we were confident that there is a statistically significant difference between 1.4/1000 and 1.1/1000. That is, hearing impairment is not common, and it would take a very large sample of children to determine if it is truly more frequent among African Americans. But let's say we wanted to look at a new suspected cause of hearing loss in children (some new pregnancy exposure,

Table 2.2 Does "exposure X" cause hearing impairment in children? A cohort study example. How many subjects (children/mothers) would it take to make sure we know this statistically?[a]

Exposure effect size Relative risk (RR)	Total study sample size[b]
1.1	3,030,000
1.5	150,000
2.0	46,300
5.0	6200
10.0	2300

[a]$p = 0.05$, power $= 0.80$, equal number of exposed and unexposed; frequency of hearing impairment in the unexposed $= 1.1/1000$ children/mothers
[b]Sample size estimates in this calculation have been rounded since the numbers were so large

Table 2.3 Does "exposure X" cause hearing impairment? A case-control study example. How many subjects (children/mothers) would it take to make sure we know this statistically?[a]

Exposure effect size odds ratio (OR)	Total sample size (*cases only*)	Total sample size with 3:1 controls per case (*cases only*)
1.1[b]	37,400 *(18,700)*	49,500 *(12,380)*
1.5	1914 *(957)*	2472 *(618)*
2.0	614 *(307)*	776 *(194)*
5.0	78 *(39)*	116 *(29)*
10.0	44 (22)	52 (13)

[a]$p = 0.05$, power $= 0.80$; base frequency of exposure in control children/mothers is set in this example at 10%. This example is based on an unmatched study design
[b]Sample size estimates in this row were rounded since the numbers were so large

e.g., a new popular dietary supplement among pregnant women that about 10% of pregnant women use). Table 2.2 shows how many children with and without the exposure would be needed to detect a significant difference based on exposure status (i.e., conclude that the exposure *caused* hearing impairment in statistical terms). The measure of effect in this hypothetical cohort is the relative risk (RR). You can reproduce this sort of exercise using *EpiInfo*, a statistical program available from the CDC (https://www.cdc.gov/epiinfo/index.html). Clearly, this could be a cost-prohibitive study if the effect size were modest. For example, to answer the question on causation based on a RR of 1.5, the study would have to enroll over 150,000 children/mothers to follow up and ascertain outcomes when children are between 3 and 10 years of age.

In some instances, rare events can be studied more efficiently by case-control methods. Table 2.3 shows the sample size required for case-control studies with the same effect sizes (here the odds ratio approximation to the relative risk, or OR). In this example, we also could take advantage of including a higher control-to-case ratio since we know that hearing impairment is rare and enrolling cases (children/mothers) will be difficult. If we use a single control per case, we can accomplish the same study with a medium effect size of 1.5 as our cohort above with 1914 subjects (and 957 cases). Increasing the control ratio to 3 per case, we would need a slightly larger *total* sample size, but only 618 cases of children with hearing impairment. The problems of case-finding, enrolling and interviewing subjects, ascertaining exposure with accuracy, and the potential for problems of recall bias might still make this a difficult study. And it is important to note that hearing impairment, while rare, is still a common event compared to other specific impairments. For example, about 54 people per one million Americans sustain (and survive) a spinal cord injury each year, making this a rare event that is difficult to study on the population level (National Spinal Cord Injury Statistical Center, 2019). These examples underscore the problem of conducting disability research, especially with the aim of ascertaining etiology of specific impairments.

2.5.3   Measurement Issues (Classification and Bias)

As noted above, combining groups is one strategy to overcome the problem of small samples. For example, we might combine specific diagnoses into functional categories such as mobility, communication, or learning/cognition impairments. This is part of the rationale for the ICF classification system of the WHO. The trade-off here is that heterogeneity of exposures and outcomes may bias relationships toward the null (no effect). For a study on etiology, combining people with different impairments will obscure causes. Such varied diagnoses as Parkinson's disease, multiple sclerosis, HIV/AIDs, and spinal cord injury can all lead to mobility impairments but entail very different etiology. Thus, grouping people with mobility impairments in a study of etiology would obscure the very different causal pathways that can produce this outcome. For a study on secondary conditions, or outcomes research, this grouping of impairments may be fine as long as proper consideration is paid to differences of other characteristics and risk factors, such as severity.

In epidemiology, we generally prefer homogenous measures of both exposures and outcomes precisely because blending across disparate groups can mask effects. A real difference (measured, e.g., by a relative risk) may be missed because of fuzzy classification. A real excess risk may be underestimated. For example, an important current question about risk of secondary conditions is whether people with mobility conditions, and specifically people who use wheelchairs, are at higher risk of particular secondary conditions like pressure sores. If we include people who use wheelchairs for diverse reasons, we may mask the differential effects of wheelchair use among subgroups. Table 2.4 shows how this can work. If we include all 126 people in our sample of 239 who are "exposed" to wheelchair use, we do, indeed, see that they have an increased risk of having skin problems (pressure sores, skin ulcers, etc.). The gender and age-adjusted risk is 4.3; this is a pretty strong effect (and the 95% confidence intervals exclude 1.0 so it is statistically significant). But people can use a wheelchair for many reasons. People with spinal cord injury (SCI) use wheelchairs because of paralysis, which could entail a much higher risk. If we define the exposed group as the 83 people with SCI, we see that the risk increases to

Table 2.4 Risk of skin problems associated with wheelchairs in a heterogeneous group of people with disability

Exposure group	Group sample number	Skin problems		Adjusted odds ratio[a]	95% confidence interval
		Number	%		
No wheelchair (reference)	113	9	8.0	–	–
All wheelchair users	126	39	31.0	4.3	(1.7–10.9)
People with spinal cord injury who use a wheelchair	83	30	36.1	10.0	(1.7–59.8)

[a]Odds ratios are adjusted for age and gender

more than 10 times baseline. In fact, the heterogeneous group masked the very high effect of wheelchair use among people with SCI. Some studies may need to use more homogeneous groups rather than broad heterogeneous classifications to elucidate such exposure-outcome casual questions. In this example, we fortunately would conclude that there is risk for even the heterogeneous group; but clearly the causal inference one would draw is stronger for people with SCI.

Another concern about misclassification stems from the issue of who is reporting. In some studies, it may be convenient or even necessary to ask a proxy to report on the health status, impairment level, or quality of life of a person with a disability rather than asking the person directly. For example, a researcher may want to collect information from someone with a cognitive or communication disability but lack the tools or resources to do so and therefore instead ask someone who knows the person well to answer on their behalf. Previous research shows that this is likely to create misclassification of function, pain, and quality of life (e.g., Andresen, Vahle, & Lollar, 2001; Magaziner, Zimmerman, Gruber-Baldini, Hebel, & Fox, 1997; Yasuda et al., 2004). In general, proxies tend to over-report impairments and disability and under-report quality of life and pain compared to the respondents themselves. Proxies tend to report most accurately on physical domains like mobility and least accurately on psychological domains like depressive symptoms. Evidence suggests that when the proxy is also the caregiver, the level of burden or stress that caregiver is experiencing can impact how different their ratings are compared to the person themselves (e.g., Neumann, Araki, & Gutterman, 2000). While there are examples of situations in which agreement tends to be better—for example, among people immediately following a stroke (e.g., Jette et al., 2012) or people with cognitive impairment (e.g., Bravo, Sene, & Arcand, 2017)—the body of evidence suggests researchers should carefully weigh the benefits and drawbacks of using information collected from a caregiver, spouse, friend, or healthcare provider to classify someone as experiencing impairments, limitations, pain, and disability. Misclassification from proxy responses may result in bias, and the direction of that bias can be difficult to predict depending on the domain measured and the relationship of the proxy to the person with disability.

2.5.4 Multi-level Studies

Epidemiologists, historically, tended to eschew research where associations are made between variables based on grouped data, that is, those that are "ecological" in design. In a purely ecological study, we compare people at an ecological level in terms of exposure and outcome. The problem of inferences about cause-and-effect relationships from grouped data is called *ecological fallacy*.

However, when exposures really do operate at an ecological level as do many that have a potential impact on PWD (e.g., especially environmental ones, such as disability awareness media campaigns, laws, severity of winter weather, wheelchair accessible public transportation), there is a strong argument for applying a combined ecological- and individual-level study design (e.g., Adams, Eisenman, & Glik, 2019; Von Korf, Koepsell, Curry, & Diehr, 1992). In fact, the IOM recommends combined—personal and environment—models of public health training and thinking as a high priority (Institute of Medicine, 2003a, 2003b), although this typically refers to understanding the social influences on health for racial and ethnic minority groups. Aside from a need for more complex statistical analysis (i.e., mixed variance estimates), there are relatively few barriers to multi-level studies in disability epidemiology. The ICF includes codes for specific aspects of environment as experienced by individuals. Measures and models that are truly multi-level can provide a very rich area of research for understanding variations in levels of participation of PWD. At present, this kind of work is in its early years, with some examples published (e.g., Devereux, Bullock, Gibb, & Himler, 2015; Vaughan et al., 2017). Still, few disability-relevant ecological-level measures have been defined.

2.5.5   Field Methods in Disability Epidemiology

Allan Meyers used the phrase "Enabling our Research" to describe what is needed to support the health assessment of people with disability (Meyers & Andresen, 2000). He also advocated what he termed "universal design" in research methods and measures borrowing the phrase from architecture and interior design. These ideas reflect the observation that is often a challenge to include PWD in research and that they are often, therefore, excluded from research. A study conducted by Barnett and Franks (1999) underscored just one aspect of this problem. They demonstrated that deaf people were substantially less likely to own a telephone and were therefore excluded from participation in surveys conducted by telephone. At the time, deaf people who did have telephones used TTYs, which sounded to the caller like a fax machine and also led to exclusion. In the present day, cellphone technology could reduce this exclusion, but it would require a different strategy (e.g., text-based and web-linked survey or use of video relay services).

In general, field research, meaning finding subjects and collecting data from them, entails specific disability-related challenges. These include, but are not limited to, (1) communication (e.g., telephone survey methods) and (2) validity of questions from general surveys when applied to disability groups. Below is a descriptive list of how these issues affect research (Meyers & Andresen, 2000).

- Standard sampling methods do not reach the same proportions of PWD as people without disabilities.
- If they are included in a sample, some PWD may be excluded by standard modes of questionnaire administration and interviews; others may be able to participate only to a limited extent.

- Even when PWD are included in a sample and are able to complete instruments, many questionnaires include questions and measures that are offensive or simply irrelevant to PWD.

Ideally, there should be full participation of people with disabilities in epidemiologic research, whether they are the primary focus of a particular study or just one statistically identified subgroup in broader population research. Consider the problem of a tradition of excluding women and older adults from randomized trials of heart disease prevention and treatment therapies. The result has been a need to play "catch up" in order to provide meaningful information for women (e.g., see Bennett, 1993; Buring & Hennekens, 1994; and Gurwitz, Col, & Avory, 1992). The Women's Health Initiative (WHI) was an effort by the National Institutes of Health to address the lack of data for women. Over a 15-year period from 1991 to 2005, a series of studies focused on understanding and preventing the major causes of death and disability among post-menopausal women (heart disease, breast and colorectal cancer, and osteoporosis) and led to major changes in clinical practice and, subsequently, health outcomes (Office on Women's Health, 2014). Long-term follow-up continues today. This same point applies to people with disabilities. The full population perspective on the health of Americans has to include PWD to be complete, especially with the changing age structure that includes larger proportions of older adults. Further, the health of PWD of all ages is a public health priority, and inclusion of PWD in surveillance and research must be a component of the successful conduct of public health functions aimed at health objectives for PWD. Enablement of disability research is an ethical, legal, and methodological imperative.

2.6 Protection of Human Subjects in Disability Public Health Research

In general, research that is inclusive of people with disability is not different in terms of human subjects' issues than other research. However, Human Subjects Institutional Review Boards (IRBs) often incorporate a category of special concern for research participants with disability without guidance for people with particular types of needs or support. This kind of broad categorization of protection reminds us of the decades of research that excluded women of child-bearing age so as to protect them and their possible fetuses. The unstated assumption seemed to be that women did not know how to protect themselves and could not participate in informed consent and decide themselves if they wished to participate. While this is not likely to be the explicit reason for having PWD in a category of IRB concern, considering special circumstances remains important for public health researchers.

It is possible that persons of legal age may include individuals with cognitive or intellectual impairment or limited English language fluency. Public health researchers should embrace self-determination as a core ethic for human subjects research and acknowledge that legal assent/consent may require additional safeguards. Stineman and Musick proposed guidelines and recommendations in their 2001 review, which serves as an excellent resource for educators and researchers (Stineman & Musick, 2001). Informed consent procedures may include brief cognitive screening to determine subjects' capacity to understand and freely give consent (e.g., using the MMSE (Fields & Calvert, 2015)), use of literacy screening tests (Aldoory, Ryan, & Rouhani, 2014), and/or oral and electronic formats of consent procedures (Naghibi Sistani, Montazeri, Yazdani, & Murtomaa, 2013). They may also include brief questionnaires to assure respondents understand the information provided during the consent process.

In some cases, proxy consent or supported decision-making may be needed (Horner-Johnson & Bailey, 2013; Kohn, Blumenthal, & Campbell, 2013; and see, e.g., http://supporteddecisionmaking.org). However, researchers should not assume that a diagnosis of intellectual disability, brain injury, or other condition associated with cognitive impairment means the person cannot make an informed decision. Horner-Johnson and Bailey (2013) demonstrated that nearly all people with intellectual disabilities they screened for a health promotion research study could understand and describe five fundamental aspects of the study: purpose, activities, confidentiality, the voluntary nature of participation, and their right to withdraw (Horner-Johnson & Bailey, 2013). Only about half of participants could accurately identify the risks in the low-risk study in question (Horner-Johnson & Bailey, 2013), suggesting that higher-risk studies may require additional strategies for ethically including people with intellectual disabilities. Such strategies could include involvement of a trusted support person to help the potential research participant weigh the risks and benefits of participation (Horner-Johnson & Bailey, 2013).

To approve research under the federal regulations, an IRB should determine that subject selection is equitable and be particularly cognizant of the special problems of research involving vulnerable populations including persons with cognitive impairment or other mental health disability. There is no standard definition of who is vulnerable as a person with cognitive impairment, and there are no additional safeguards codified in regulation. However, states may have statutes that specify who can consent for incapacitated or decisionally impaired adults. Researchers should consider their IRBs as a partner in the protection of human subjects' process, consult with them about their plans, and consider IRB feedback to determine if additional safeguards should be included in the study to protect the rights and welfare of research participants with disability. Pragmatically, experienced disability researchers know that some cross-education on research and PWD may be needed to facilitate the sense of partnership with IRB staff and committees (White, Klatt, Gard, Suchowierska, & Wyatt, 2005).

2.7   Future Directions and the Role of Epidemiology

This chapter has described classic epidemiology methods and their relevance and benefit to research involving disability populations, issues, and outcomes. A number of methodological difficulties are present: for example, epidemiologists may express concern over the heterogeneous nature of disability classification as an "event" or "state." Another area of concern for epidemiologists is the evolving theoretical nature of the disabling process, which overlaps with the subject of classification. Currently, the WHO's ICF is the most widely used framework for disability epidemiology. While it offers a view of disability consistent with public health's conception of health relating to multiple levels of the social-ecological framework, it has limitations. For example, Mitra and Shakespeare (2019) point out that the ICF does not consider the full environmental context in which people live and work—the social determinants of health—and also that it offers a somewhat limited representation of well-being (i.e., that it does not include quality of life). While epidemiologists often lack training in theory directly, they can be helpful in this effort to evaluate and amend disability models or framework through the design and conduct of quantitative studies and by developing high-quality measures that align with theoretical models.

In order to build the field of disability epidemiology, training on the topic and collaboration with other professions will be necessary. The Council on Education for Public Health (CEPH), the accrediting body for schools and programs of public health, includes working effectively on interprofessional teams (MPH) and proposing interprofessional approaches to improving public health (DrPH) as foundational competencies for students (Council on Education for Public Health, 2016). Assignments, projects, or discussions on topics related to disability lend themselves well to achieving these objectives since there are clear connections to rehabilitation medicine, city planning, construction, and law, among other disciplines. Disability and function are also good examples of measures, which could contribute to the CEPH learning objective that students be able to list major causes and trends of morbidity and mortality (Council on Education for Public Health, 2016). Finally, people with disabilities experience many health disparities relative to people without disabilities (see Chap. 3 for more details). Examples suggested in this chapter could be used to contribute to the CEPH competency that students "discuss the means by which structural bias, social inequities and racism undermine health and create challenges to achieving health equity at organizational, community and societal levels" (Council on Education for Public Health, 2016).

Finally, a general area of research that has grown substantially in the past decade but may still make some epidemiologists uneasy is the notion of involving the research population in the research process.

Some prominent epidemiologists have called for the field to move toward focusing more on the consequences of our policies and programs so that we may improve the health of the public. This effort may require scientists to translate their findings so that policy makers and the public can understand the potential for action that the research suggests. Related to this is the recognition that excluding people with disabilities from randomized trials and other efforts has resulted in a lack of data that can be used to develop evidence-based programs and policies for people with disabilities. The need for inclusion ranges from the questions in our public health surveillance systems (Fox, Bonardi, & Krahn, 2015) to the design of trials aimed at improving public health (Hinton, Kraus, Richards, Fox, & Campbell, 2017). Incorporating universal design concepts into the design of research studies could substantially improve the inclusion of people with disabilities in research (Rios, Magasi, Novak, & Harniss, 2016; Williams & Moore, 2011). Examples include recruiting using multiple modes (e.g., fliers, audible announcements on radio or TV, and targeted recruitment through disability organizations) and allowing for different modes of response (e.g., telephone, written, video relay, Internet). Expanding inclusive practices in research will not only improve our knowledge about disability but also result in more representative studies in general. Lastly, discipline-specific guides regarding the ethics of including communities and subjects' perspectives in research now can be incorporated into the new imperative for community-based participatory research for scientific and ethical reasons (Institute of Medicine, 2003a, 2003b). The challenges of disability research that confront epidemiology also provide substantial impetus for expanding methodological innovation, extending traditional epidemiological thinking, and learning from our knowledgeable subjects and communities.

2.8   Epilogue

During our years of training epidemiologists and researchers and discussing how epidemiology views (or does not view) disability, we have encountered mostly right-minded and caring professionals and students who find the barriers that people with disabilities face inexcusable. The belief in social justice reigns strong in public health communities. It is therefore surprising, and even shocking to many, that the basic concept of "prevention" might be taken as a problem in public health thinking (Andresen, 2004). Two kinds of examples help us make this issue concrete.

The first example comes from public health history of defining prevention: until the past decade, health departments included "disability prevention" as part of their names. The Division of Human Development and Disability of the Centers for Disease Control and Prevention instead uses current mainstream terminology in naming their branches "Disability and Health Promotion" and "Child Development and Disability." A visit to their website will provide an education to students and practitioners alike as to the full public health and research agendas in disability (see http://www.cdc.gov/ncbddd/dh/default.htm). It also offers access to an array of disability-related data from the BRFSS through its Disability and Health Data System (https://www.cdc.gov/ncbddd/disabilityandhealth/dhds/index.html)

The second example speaks to the common response of good people that "of course" they do not mean they seek to prevent people. We use an example from a new article in *The New York Times* to make the point that PWD may not be paranoid about the use of the term "prevention" (McBryde Johnson, 2003). A woman with a developmental disability, Harriet McBryde Johnson, shared her story about her experience in a debate with Princeton Professor Peter Singer. Professor Singer has advocated for the possibility of euthanizing babies who whose lives he deems to be cognitively impaired enough to not be "persons." The cover magazine read "Should I have been killed at birth? The case for my life." In public health we can all answer her question easily and with spirit ("No, Harriet! Your life has meaning and value."). We simply have to think more deeply about what would provide for equity, inclusion, and participation of people with disability in public health and epidemiologic research.

Acknowledgments This work is supported, in part, by funding from the Centers for Disease Control and Prevention (CDC; grant # U48/CCU710806) for the Methods Core of the Saint Louis University Prevention Research Center. The authors gratefully acknowledge the primary methodological coursework that provides the foundation for this chapter from Drs. Noel Weiss and Thomas Koepsell at the University of Washington School of Public Health (Koepsell & Weiss, 2014). However, Drs. Weiss and Koepsell bear no responsibility for errors or interpretations that deviate from their teachings. The authors also appreciate the assistance of the following individuals in the preparation of this work: Tori Vahle, M.P.H.; Janet Tang, M.P.H.; Tricia McLendon, M.P.H.; and Tegan Boehmer, Ph.D. We are grateful to Julie D. Weeks, Ph.D., for her advice and assistance related to the ACS and Washington Group disability measures discussed in the chapter. The students of Dr. Andresen's graduate course in disability epidemiology at the Saint Louis University School of Public Health also furnished valuable comments, questions, and editing; their time and patience have made this a better product.

2.9. Appendix: Incorporating Disability Examples into Epidemiology Coursework: Questions and Examples

1. Prevalence, Odds Ratios, Stratified Analysis (Confounding or Effect Modification), Study Design, and Causal Inference

    As a project for a disability epidemiology course, M.P.H. students Tori Vahle and Mary Gould analyzed data from special surveys in Missouri adapted from the Behavioral Risk Factor Surveillance System (BRFSS). These were random-digit-dialed telephone surveys conducted in six Missouri counties between 1995 and 1997. The sample consisted of a total of 3343 adults: 1380 from rural and 1963 from nonrural areas. Disability was defined as "limited in any way in any activities because of any impairment or health problem."

    (a) The Table 2.5 shows the crude results of the study. Is there an increased prevalence of disability in rural areas compared to urban areas?

    Answer: The odds ratio for this table is 1.14 (95% confidence interval [CI] = 0.96, 1.34).

Table 2.5 Risk of disability
by urban/rural residence

Residence	Limited/disability?	
	Yes	No
Rural	344	1036
Urban	444	1519

Table 2.6 Risk of disability by residence and age

Age group	Limited (disability)		Not limited	
	Rural	Urban	Rural	Urban
18–64	132	314	840	1244
65–99	210	128	190	254

(b) The data were also stratified by age. Table 2.6 shows these data (note: age is missing for 31 subjects). Accounting for age, how does the odds ratio change compared to your answer based on Table 2.5 and answer a. above? Why?

Answer: The rural population is older than the urban population; we can see that 20% of the urban group is over age 65 and 29% of the rural population is over age 65. Since disability increases with age (due to increasing chronic conditions), the crude odds ratio is biased high just because of the older age of rural adults. The age-adjusted OR is 0.98 (95% CI = 0.83, 1.17). However, if one examines the stratum-specific results, it appears that the results are reversed for the two age groups. For younger adults, the effect of living in a rural area is protective (OR = 0.62, 95% CI 0.50, 0.78), but for older adults, it is associated with an increased risk (OR = 2.19, 95% CI 1.63, 2.96). This kind of effect modification finding (age modifies the effect of rural residence) would need to be checked for statistical significance (we can tell it would be, since the 95% CI of the two stratum-specific estimates do not overlap) and also to be sure the difference makes sense (preferably, it would have been hypothesized in advance). If we had not hypothesized this finding in advance, we'd be cautious about interpreting it as effect modification. Perhaps we'd recommend this for further follow-up in future studies. See Tables 2.7 and 2.8 for the stratum-specific results.

(c) The results of the cross-sectional study above seem to suggest that rural residence is associated with an increased risk of disability in older adults and protective in younger adults. What kind of study would make the causal inference stronger for this hypothesis? Since we cannot assign people randomly to their geographic residence, this will have to be an observational design.

Answer: These cross-sectional data raise concerns about causal inference because we don't know if residence preceded disability. There may be reasons that that people may have moved to a different kind of setting. It is plausible that a person might move to a city for its healthcare, social, or transportation services if they had a disability. If so, the prevalence odds ratio we calculated above underestimates the association of rural living and disability. Or, perhaps,

Table 2.7 Younger adults (aged 18–64): risk of disability by urban/rural residence

	Limited/disability?	
Residence	Yes	No
Rural	132	840
Urban	314	1244

OR = 0.62 (95% CI 0.50, 0.78)

Table 2.8 Older adults (aged 65+): risk of disability by urban/rural residence

	Limited/disability?	
Residence	Yes	No
Rural	210	190
Urban	128	254

OR = 2.19 (95% CI 1.63, 2.96)

people with disability might stay in the rural area and be less likely to move because they had strong social support in the rural area. In this case, the lower prevalence of disability in urban areas might be falsely high and the rural excess inflated because of the exodus of people without disability. Whether or not either is true, they both pose potential problems to thinking that rural residence causes disability in older adults because of inconsistent temporality of the exposure (residence) and outcome. A stronger study design would be to examine cohorts of people, initially free of disability, to see which group was more likely to incur a disability. This is likely to be a question also that could benefit from a less heterogeneous outcome: for example, maybe sensory impairments are more likely to occur in one setting or another, but mobility impairments may be similar. Cohorts are, unfortunately, very expensive study designs; a very specific hypothesis about residence (the components of rural living that increase the risk of disability, e.g.) would probably take place over a long time period and require a large sample size and many different types of rural and urban settings.

2. Relative Risk, Classification, and Confounding.

Andresen, Fouts, Romeis, and Brownson (1999) analyzed the risk of disability among different ethnic groups of women in the United States. The data were based on a national stratified random-digit-dialed sample of women aged 40 and older; most questions were derived from the modules of the Behavioral Risk Factor Surveillance System, including disability definitions. One measure of disability was defined from a woman's report that she was "limited" and also that she needed personal care assistance with activities such as eating, bathing, dressing, or getting around the house (classified as having activities of daily living dependence, or ADL). In another analysis, women were asked to describe their overall health status as excellent, very good, good, fair, or poor. Tables 2.9 and 2.10 show the responses of women who were Native American or Alaskan natives compared to white women. Participants included 774 white and 739

Table 2.9 Risk of ADL dependency for ethnic minority women

	ADL dependent?	
	Yes	No
Native women	25	431
White women	13	761
Total	38	1192

Table 2.10 Risk of lower health status for ethnic minority women

	Fair/poor health status?	
	Yes	No
Native women	157	300
White women	156	617
Total	313	917

Native American women; because of some missing responses, not all analyses included all women who were interviewed. Are Native American women more likely to be disabled according to ADLs? Are they more likely to be in fair/poor health (for this problem, answers are grouped as fair/poor versus good-excellent)? Can you think of reasons that these results might differ? Consider that the average age of white women was 57.3 and that of Native American women was 54.4 (*t*-test for difference $p < 0.01$). What additional analysis would you recommend to make sure these results were not biased by age? Why?

Answers: In the first table (Table 2.9), the relative risk (RR) for ADL dependency for Native American women is 3.26 (95% confidence intervals [CI] of 1.69, 6.32; statistical significance, $\chi^2_{MH} < 0.01$) compared to white women. In the second table (Table 2.10), Native American women are more likely to be in fair/poor health, but the estimate is not as large (RR = 1.70 and 95%CI 1.41, 2.06; statistical significance, $\chi^2_{MH} < 0.01$). Since these are prevalence data, some might argue for analysis using the odds ratio (OR); however, race/ethnic group is clearly temporally prior to the health status/disability determination, so we are less concerned about the problem of cross-sectional data here.

It is hard to compare directly the two RR estimates; while ADL dependency is one appropriate classification for disability, it is not synonymous with health status. Therefore we might expect that disability and health status have a relationship, but that they would not be overlapping definitions. A woman might require ADL assistance for mobility impairment, but consider her health status to be excellent or very good.

The problem of confounding by age is very likely here. Since various chronic conditions and mobility impairments increase with age (a prime example is arthritis), and Native American women are, on average, younger than white women in this sample, our calculated estimates of the risk of poor outcomes may be confounded by age. If we conducted a stratified analysis with age, we would expect that the RRs we calculated may be biased low and that the age-adjusted RRs should be somewhat larger.

3. Classification and Proxy Response.

Table 2.11 Agreement of people and their family member proxies on dependence in bathing (needs any help)

PWD response	Proxy response	
	Yes	No
Yes	21	5
No	7	44

In a reliability study of adults with disability and proxy respondents, we found that people with disability (PWD) and family members—who also answered for them—disagreed about the level of functional impairment of the PWD themselves (Andresen et al., 2001). The tables below show how their answers compare for one measure of dependence (needing help bathing) and the report of pain as a secondary condition. Calculate the percent agreement, κ, and difference in the response (proportion) of the proxy from the person with disability (Table 2.11).

Answers: The summary answer is listed below (and calculation of κ also described). Proxies do agree with PWD about needing assistance with bathing, although the κ is not in the "excellent" (above 0.75). Overall, their responses *overestimated* the need for assistance compared to the person with a disability. These results are common to tests of proxy response: the reliability is better for objective compared to subjective variables. The direction of differences also is common: proxies consider the PWD to be more "disabled" than they are.

Variable	% Agreement	κ	% yes responses		Proxy difference
			PWD	Proxy	
Need assistance bathing?	84.3	0.66	33.8	36.4	+ 2.6%

Calculating formulas for percent agreement and κ (*for a completed treatment of these methods, see Fleiss, Levin, and Paik,* 2004):

(a) Calculating overall percent agreement.

PWD response	Proxy response		Total
	Yes	No	
Yes	P_{11}	P_{12}	$P_{1.}$
No	P_{21}	P_{22}	$P_{2.}$
Total	$P_{.1}$	$P_{.2}$	Total = 1.0

Percent agreement, or percent observed, is $P_0 = P_{11} + P_{22}$

But this is misleading because some agreement is due to chance alone. We therefore calculate the expected agreement (by multiplying the column and row totals for

Table 2.12 Agreement of people and their family member proxies on dependence in bathing (needs any help)

	Proxy response		
PWD response	Yes	No	Total
Yes	0.272		
No		0.571	
Total			1.0

Table 2.13 Agreement of people and their family member proxies on dependence in bathing (needs any help)

	Proxy response		
PWD response	Yes	No	Total
Yes	0.123		0.338
No		0.421	0.662
Total	0.364	0.636	1.0

each cell, as in calculating chi-square statistics) and then summarize the agreement that is *beyond chance*, as a proportion of all that is possible. That defines the κ statistic (below). The examples are calculated below (Table 2.12).

Observed agreement is $P_0 = 0.272 + 0.571 = 0.843$

Or about 84% of the proxy-PWD sets agree on whether or not the PWD needs assistance in bathing.

(b) Calculating expected agreement (Table 2.13).

	Proxy response		
PWD response	Yes	No	Total
Yes	$P_{1.} P_{.1}$	$P_{1.} P_{.2}$	$P_{1.}$
No	$P_{2.} P_{.1}$	$P_{2.} P_{.2}$	$P_{2.}$
Total	$P_{.1}$	$P_{.2}$	1.00

Percent expected is $P_e = P_{1.} P_{.1} + P_{2.} P_{.2}$

Percent expected agreement is $0.123 + 0.421 = 0.544 = P_e$

Or over 50% of the agreement is expected by chance alone!

(c) Calculating κ. κ is the measure of "beyond chance" agreement. That is, accounting for chance, how much more agreement do we observe (as a proportion of 100 better than chance)?

$$\kappa = \left(P_o - P_e\right) / \left(1.0 - P_e\right)$$

Agreement about dependence in bathing, this would be:

$(0.843 – 0.544) / (1.0 – 0.544) = 0.66$. The κ is 0.66, or agreement of PWD and their proxies is 65% better than chance. This would be considered "good" agreement.

4. Study Designs

For each of the following research questions, consider the issues of (1) frequency of the outcomes; (2) feasibility and practicality, in measuring the outcome and/or exposures; (3) the issues of resulting causal inference; (4) the stage at which the question is directed (descriptive, hypothesis generating, hypothesis testing); and (5) the potential for sources of existing data. Suggest the best study design and explain the reasons for your choice.

(a) Cleft lip (with or without cleft palate) occurs in about 1 to 2 births/1000 in Northern European countries and in people of these backgrounds in the United States. How would you investigate the hypothesis that a woman's exposure to certain medications during early pregnancy may increase the risk of these birth outcomes?

(b) Among adults with high-level spinal cord injury (SCI—affecting motor control of upper limbs), there is a large amount of variability in the incidence of upper respiratory infections (URI). While there is evidence that URI is increased compared to the general population, it is not clear if certain kinds of URIs are more common or if URI is just more serious when it does occur (bringing it to medical attention). Because you are part of a large, pre-paid healthcare plan, you have access to a large clinical group of people with the appropriate SCI classification and (1) can assume each person will attend a general medical clinic at least once a year and (2) their other clinical, emergency, and hospital visits are available in the same medical care system; what kind of study would you perform to determine more exactly the nature and risk factors for URI in people with SCI compared to the other plan enrollees?

Answers

(a) This fairly uncommon outcome may best be studied early on by a case-control study. Medications taken during pregnancy may be recalled with some accuracy by mothers in this design. Considerable care would need to be taken to assure that case mothers were not better at recalling their histories (or telescoping in exposures at other times); a validity study, perhaps using medical records and prescription records, would assist in finding out the overall accuracy of reports and if it were "differential" by case status. Because pregnancy is of short duration, it also may be possible to do a cohort study; this would be especially true for exposures of interest that are uncommon (e.g., a specific medication used to treat infections). Any of these designs would be somewhat difficult if asking about over-the-counter medications; however, diligent work on obtaining exposure information and/or getting women to record such information (specifically based on interviews at their first prenatal visit, e.g.) might overcome these difficulties.

(b) This might be a good opportunity to use the records and billing data of healthcare plan in a cohort study; potentially much of this work could be accomplished by database analysis, with no further data collection from individuals. If substantial data cleaning or database construction is required (e.g., combining pharmacy records, office visit records, hospital billing, etc.), you might want to use data on all enrollees with SCI and a sample of others. An alternate or auxiliary effort could be a survey of enrollees classified by exposure, as (1) all enrollees with SCI, compared with (2) a sample of other enrollees, matched possibly for age and gender. They would be surveyed, perhaps on several occasions, about their incidence of URI, symptoms severity, and office and/or hospital visits. In either design, the potential for differential misclassification and identification of URIs exists. One would want to ascertain data accuracy (e.g., respiratory infections noted and coded accurately and the same for SCI and others?), and a validity sub-study may be needed. The direction probably is in the direction of better ascertainment for enrollees with SCI, but you would want to confirm this.

5. Utilizing Publicly Available Data Sources.

   Most of the surveillance data sources that include disability mentioned in this chapter are publicly available. The BRFSS disability data are easily accessible through the Disability and Health Data System (https://www.cdc.gov/ncbddd/disabilityandhealth/dhds/index.html). The data portal provides tools for users to run basic analyses without downloading the data itself, and results can be output as figures or tables. Use the Disability and Health Data System to answer the questions below. Include table(s) or figure(s) to summarize your findings.

   (a) Identify the overall prevalence of disability and disability by type (i.e., vision, hearing, cognitive, mobility, self-care, or independent living disability) in your state.

   (b) Explore demographic subgroups within the population to assess whether there are differences in disability prevalence. For example, you might look at specific age groups, people with different race or ethnicity classification, or people with different levels of socioeconomic status.

   (c) Examine at least one health outcome and evaluate whether there are differences by disability status or type in the state.

      Answers

      Answers will, of course, depend on the state in which students live, the year(s) of data available through the Disability and Health Data System at the time the assignment is completed, and the demographic characteristics the student chooses. As the instructor, you may choose to limit these parameters to assure you can easily confirm their work.

References

Adams, R. M., Eisenman, D. P., & Glik, D. (2019). Community advantage and individual self-efficacy promote disaster preparedness: A multilevel model among persons with disabilities. *International Journal of Environmental Research and Public Health, 16*(15), E2779. https://doi.org/10.3390/ijerph16152779

Adler, M. (1996). *People with disabilities: Who are they? Beyond the Water's Edge: Charting the course of managed care for people with disabilities.* Washington DC: Office on Disability, Aging and Long-Term Care Policy/ASPE/Department of Health and Human Services.

Aldoory, L., Ryan, K., & Rouhani, A. (2014). *Best practices and new models of health literacy for informed consent: Review of the impact of informed consent regulations on health literate communications* (p. 81). Institute of Medicine. Retrieved from http://nationalacademies. org/hmd/~/media/Files/Activity%20Files/PublicHealth/HealthLiteracy/Commissioned%20 Papers%20-Updated%202017/Aldoory%20et%20al%202014%20Best%20Practices%20 and%20new%20models%20of%20health%20literacy%20for%20informed%20consent.pdf

Altman, B. (2014). Definitions, concepts, and measures of disability. *Annals of Epidemiology, 24*, 2–7.

American Public Health Association. (2008). *Promoting interprofessional education (policy number 20088).* Retrieved from https://www.apha.org/policies-and-advocacy/public-health-policy-statements/policy-database/2014/07/23/09/20/ promoting-interprofessional-education

Anderson, L. A., Edwards, V. J., Pearson, W. S., Talley, R. C., McGuire, L. C., & Andresen, E. M. (2013). Adult caregivers in the United States: Characteristics and differences in well-being, by caregiver age and caregiving status. *Preventing Chronic Disease, 10*, E135.

Andresen, E. M., Fouts, B. S., Romeis, J. C., & Brownson, C. A. (1999). Performance of health-related quality-of-life instruments in a spinal cord injured population. *Archives of Physical Medicine and Rehabilitation, 80*, 877–884.

Andresen, E. M., Prince-Caldwell, A., Akinci, F., Brownson, C. A., Hagglund, K., Jackson-Thompson, J., & Crocker, R. (1999). The Missouri Disability Epidemiology and Health Project. *American Journal of Preventive Medicine, 16*(3 Suppl), 63–71. https://doi.org/10.1016/ s0749-3797(98)00151-2

Andresen, E. M., Fitch, C. A., McLendon, P., & Meyers, A. (2000). Reliability and validity of disability questions for U.S. Census 2000. *American Journal of Public Health, 90*, 1297–1299.

Andresen, E. M., Vahle, V. J., & Lollar, D. (2001). Proxy reliability: Health-related quality of life (HRQoL) measures for people with disability. *Quality of Life Research, 10*, 609–619.

Andresen, E. M. (2004). Public health education, research, and disability studies: A view from epidemiology (invited commentary). *Disability Studies Quarterly, 24*. Retrieved from http:// www.dsq-sds-archives.org/_articles_html/2004/fall/dsq_fall04_andresen.asp

Andresen, E. M., Diehr, P., & Luke, D. A. (2004). Public health surveillance of low-frequency populations. *Annual Review of Public Health, 25*–52.

Barnett, S., & Franks, P. (1999). Telephone ownership and deaf people: Implications for telephone surveys. *American Journal of Public Health, 89*, 1754–1756.

Bennett, J. C. (1993). Inclusion of women in clinical trials—Policies for population subgroups. *New England Journal of Medicine, 329*, 288–292.

Bouldin, E. D., Akhtar, W., Brumback, B., & Andresen, E. (2009). *Characteristics of caregivers and non-caregivers—Florida, 2008.* Gainesville, revised April 8, 2009. Retrieved from http:// fodh.phhp.ufl.edu/publications/

Buring, J. E., & Hennekens, C. H. (1994). Randomized trials of primary prevention of cardiovascular disease in women. An investigators view. *Annals of Epidemiology, 4*, 111–114.

Bravo, G., Sene, M., & Arcand, M. (2017). Reliability of health-related quality-of-life assessments made by older adults and significant others for health states of increasing cognitive impairment. *Health and Quality of Life Outcomes, 15*, 4. https://doi.org/10.1186/s12955-016-0579-3

Centers for Disease Control and Prevention. (1998). Use of cervical and breast cancer screening among women with and without functional limitations—United States, 1994-1995. *Morbidity and Mortality Weekly Report, 47*, 853–856.

Centers for Disease Control and Prevention. (2001). *Healthy People 2010, objectives report (Chapter 6: Disability and secondary conditions).* Atlanta, GA: Centers for Disease Control and Prevention.

Centers for Disease Control and Prevention (n.d.). *Healthy People 2020 topics and objectives: Disability and health*. Retrieved September 1, 2019 from https://www.healthypeople.gov/2020/topics-objectives/topic/disability-and-health/objectives

Centers for Disease Control and Prevention. (2013, August 15). *The BRFSS Data user guide*. Retrieved from https://www.cdc.gov/brfss/data_documentation/pdf/UserguideJune2013.pdf

Chan, E., Zhan, C., & Homer, C. J. (2002). Health care use and costs for children with attention-deficit/ hyperactivity disorder: National estimates from the medical expenditure panel survey. *Archives of Pediatric and Adolescent Medicine, 156*, 504–511.

Charlton, J. I. (1998). *Nothing about us without us: Disability oppression and empowerment*. Berkeley: University of California Press.

Cohen, S. B. (2002). The Medical Expenditure Panel Survey: An overview. *Effective Clinical Practice, 5*(3 Suppl), E1.

Cohen, J. W., Monheit, A. C., Beauregard, K. M., Cohen, S. B., Lefkowitz, D. C., Potter, D. E., … Arnett, R. H. (1996-1997). The Medical Expenditure Panel Survey: A national health information resource. *Inquiry, 33*, 373–389.

Council on Education for Public Health. (2016). *Accreditation Criteria—Schools of Public Health & Public Health Programs*. Silver Spring, MD: Council on Education for Public Health.

Department of Health and Human Services. (2001). *National Committee on Vital and Health Statistics. Classifying and reporting functional status*. Hyattsville, MD. Retrieved from www.ncvhs.hhs.gov

Devereux, P. G., Bullock, C. C., Gibb, Z. G., & Himler, H. (2015). Social-ecological influences on interpersonal support in people with physical disability. *Disability and Health Journal, 8*(4), 564–572.

Druss, B. G., Marcus, S. C., Rosenheck, R. A., Olfson, M., Tanelian, T., & Pincus, H. A. (2000). Understanding disability in mental and general medical conditions. *American Journal of Psychiatry, 167*, 1485–1491.

Druss, B. G., & Rosenheck, R. A. (2000). Use of practitioner-based complementary therapies by persons reporting mental conditions in the United States. *Archives of General Psychiatry, 57*, 708–714.

Egede, L. E., Zheng, D., & Simpson, K. (2002). Comorbid depression is associated with increased health care use and expenditures in individuals with diabetes. *Diabetes Care, 5*, 464–470.

Fields, L. M., & Calvert, J. D. (2015). Informed consent procedures with cognitively impaired patients: A review of ethics and best practices. *Psychiatry and Clinical Neurosciences, 69*(8), 462–471. https://doi.org/10.1111/pcn.12289

Fleiss, J. L., Levin, B., & Paik, M. C. (2004). Statistical Methods for Rates and Proportions, Third Edition. New York, NY: John Wiley & Sons, Ltd. https://doi.org/10.1002/0471445428

Fox, M. H., Bonardi, A., & Krahn, G. L. (2015). Expanding public health surveillance for people with intellectual and developmental disabilities. *International Review of Research in Developmental Disabilities, 48*, 73–114.

Frank, L., Basch, E., Selby, J. V., & Patient-Centered Outcomes Research Institute. (2014). The PCORI perspective on patient-centered outcomes research. *JAMA, 312*(15), 1513–1514.

Galea, S. (2013). An argument for a consequentialist epidemiology. *American Journal of Epidemiology, 178*, 1185–1191.

Galea, S., & Keyes, K. M. (2018). What matters, when, for whom? Three questions to guide population health scholarship. *Injury Prevention, 24*(Supplement 1), i3–i6.

Gilliam, F., Kuzniecky, R., Faught, E., Black, L., Carpenter, G., & Schrodt, R. (1997). Patient-validated content of epilepsy-specific quality-of-life measurement. *Epilepsia, 38*, 233–236.

Gordis, L. (2014). *Epidemiology (5th edition) with student consult online access*. Philadelphia: Elsevier W.B. Saunders.

Grimby, G., & Smedby, B. (2001). ICF approved as the successor of ICIDH. *Journal of Rehabilitation Medicine, 33*, 33–34.

Guerrero, J. L., Sniezek, J. E., & Sehgal, M. (1999). The prevalence of disability from chronic conditions due to injuries among adults ages 18-69 years: United States, 1994. *Disability and Rehabilitation, 21,* 187–192.

Gurwitz, J. H., Col, N. F., & Avory, J. (1992). The exclusion of the elderly and women from clinical trials in acute myocardial infarction. *Journal of the American Medical Association, 268,* 1417–1422.

Hagey, R. S. (1997). The use and abuse of participatory action research. *Chronic Diseases in Canada, 18,* 1–4.

Hinton, C. F., Kraus, L. E., Richards, T. A., Fox, M. H., & Campbell, V. A. (2017). The guide to community preventive services and disability inclusion. *American Journal of Preventive Medicine, 53,* 898–903.

Hoffman, H. J., Ishii, E. K., & Macturk, R. H. (1998). Age-related changes in the prevalence of smell/taste problems among the United States adult population. Results of the 1994 Disability Supplement to the National Health Interview Survey (NHIS). *Annals of the New York Academy of Sciences, 855,* 716–722.

Hogan, D. P., Msall, M. E., Rogers, M. L., & Avery, R. C. (1997). Improved disability population estimates of functional limitation among American children aged 5-17. *Maternal and Child Health Journal, 4,* 203–216.

Horner-Johnson, W., & Bailey, D. (2013). Assessing understanding and obtaining consent from adults with intellectual disabilities for a health promotion study. *Journal of Policy and Practice in Intellectual Disabilities, 10*(3).

Horner-Johnson, W., Dobbertin, K., Lee, J. C., & Andresen, E. M. (2014). Disparities in health care access and receipt of preventive services by disability type: Analysis of the medical expenditure panel survey. *Health Services Research, 49*(6), 1980–1999.

Horner-Johnson, W., Dobbertin, K., Kulkarni-Rajasekhara, S., Beilstein-Wedel, E., & Andresen, E. M. (2015). Food insecurity, hunger, and obesity among informal caregivers. *Preventing Chronic Disease, 12,* E170. https://doi.org/10.5888/pcd12.150129

Iezzoni, L. I., McCarthy, E. P., Davis, R. B., Harris-David, L., & O'Day, B. (2001). Use of screening and preventive services among women with disabilities. *American Journal of Medical Quality, 16,* 135–144.

Institute of Medicine (IOM). (1988). *The future of public health.* Washington, DC: National Academy Press.

Institute of Medicine (IOM). (2003a). Who will keep the public healthy? In K. Gebbe, K. Rosenstock, & L. M. Hernandez (Eds.), *Educating public health professionals for the 21st century.* Washington, DC: National Academy Press.

Institute of Medicine (IOM). (2003b). *Health professions education: A bridge to quality* (A. C. Greiner & E. Knebel, Eds.). Washington, DC: National Academy Press.

Interprofessional Education Collaborative. (2016). *Core competencies for interprofessional collaborative practice: 2016 update.* Washington, DC: Interprofessional Education Collaborative.

Jette, Alan M, Ni, P., Rasch, E. K., Appelman, J., Sandel, M., Terdiman, J., & Chan, L. (2012). Evaluation of Patient and Proxy Responses on the Activity Measure for Postacute Care—PubMed. *Stroke, 43*(3), 824–829. https://doi.org/10.1161/STROKEAHA.111.619643

Jamoom, E. W., Andresen, E. M., Neugaard, B., & McKune, S. L. (2008). The effect of caregiving on preventive care for people with disabilities. *Disability and Health Journal, 1,* 51–57.

Kennedy, J., Wood, E. G., & Frieden, L. (2017). Disparities in insurance coverage, health services use, and access following implementation of the Affordable Care Act: A comparison of disabled and nondisabled working-age adults. *Inquiry, 54,* 0046958017734031. Retrieved from https://www.ncbi.nlm.nih.gov/pmc/articles/PMC5798675/

Koepsell, T. D., & Weiss, N. S. (2014). *Epidemiologic methods. Studying the occurrence of illness* (2nd ed.). New York: Oxford University Press.

Kohn, N. A., Blumenthal, J. A., & Campbell, A. T. (2013). *Supported decision-making: A viable alternative to guardianship?* (SSRN Scholarly Paper ID 2161115). Social Science Research Network. Retrieved from https://papers.ssrn.com/abstract=2161115

LaPlante, M. P., Harrington, C., & Kang, T. (2002). Estimating paid and unpaid hours of personal assistance services in activities of daily living provided to adults living at home. *Health Services Research, 37*, 397–415.

Lollar, D. J. (2002). Public health and disability: Emerging opportunities. *Public Health Reports, 117*, 131–136.

Lollar, D. J., & Crews, J. E. (2003). Redefining the role of public health in disability. *Annual Reviews of Public Health, 24*, 195–208.

Madans, J. H., Loeb, M. E., & Altman, B. M. (2011). Measuring disability and monitoring the UN convention on the rights of persons with disabilities: The work of the Washington group on disability statistics. *BMC Public Health, 11*, S4. https://doi.org/10.1186/1471-2458-11-S4-S4

Magaziner, J., Zimmerman, S. I., Gruber-Baldini, A. L., Hebel, J. R., & Fox, K. M. (1997). Proxy reporting in five areas of functional status: Comparison with self-reports and observations of performance. *American Journal of Epidemiology, 146*, 418–428.

McBryde Johnson, H. (2003). Unspeakable conversations or how I spent one day as a token cripple at Princeton University. *New York Times*. Section 6:50–55, 74, 78–79.

McKune, S., Andresen, E. M., Zhang, J., & Neugaard, B. (2006). *Caregiving: A national profile & assessment of caregiver services & needs*. Americus, GA: Rosalyn Carter Institute for Caregiving. Retrieved from http://www.rosalynncarter.org/publications

McGuire, L. C., Bouldin, E. L., Andresen, E. M., & Anderson, L. A. (2010). Examining modifiable health behaviors, body weight, & use of preventive services among caregivers & non-caregivers aged 65 years & older, Hawaii, Kansas, & Washington using BRFSS, 2007. *Journal of Nutrition Health and Aging*. Retrieved from http://www.springerlink.com/content/f5614366818084j6/

Meyers, A. R., & Andresen, E. M. (2000). Enabling our instruments: Accommodation, universal design, and assured access to participation in research. *Archives of Physical Medicine and Rehabilitation, 81*(12 supplement 2), S5–S9.

Mitra, S., & Shakespeare, T. (2019). Remodeling the ICF. *Disability and Health Journal, 12*(3), 337–339. https://doi.org/10.1016/j.dhjo.2019.01.008

Mitra, S., Findley, P. A., & Sambamoorthi, U. (2009). Health care expenditures of living with a disability: Total expenditures, out-of-pocket expenses, and burden, 1996 to 2004. *Archives of Physical Medicine and Rehabilitation, 90*(9), 1532–1540. https://doi.org/10.1016/j.apmr.2009.02.020

Mokdad, A. H. (2009). The behavioral risk factors surveillance system: Past, present, and future. *Annual Review of Public Health, 30*, 43–54.

Mullner, R. M., Jewell, M. A., & Mease, M. A. (1999). Monitoring changes in home health care: A comparison of two national surveys. *Journal of Medical Systems, 23*, 21–26.

Nanda, U., & Andresen, E. M. (1998). Performance of measures of health-related quality of life and function among disabled adults. *Quality of Life Research, 7*, 644.

National Spinal Cord Injury Statistical Center. (2019). *Spinal cord injury. Facts and figures at a glance*. Birmingham, AL: National Spinal Cord Injury Statistical Center. Retrieved from https://www.nscisc.uab.edu/Public/Facts%20and%20Figures%202019%20-%20Final.pdf

Neugaard, B., Andresen, E. M., DeFries, E. L., Talley, R. C., & Crews, J. E. (2007). The characteristics of caregivers and care recipients: North Carolina, 2005. *Morbidity and Mortality Weekly Report, 56*, 529–532.

Neumann, P. J., Araki, S. S., & Gutterman, E. M. (2000). The use of proxy respondents in studies of older adults: Lessons, challenges, and opportunities. *Journal of the American Geriatrics Society, 48*, 1646–1654.

Newacheck, P. W., Strickland, B., Shonkoff, J. P., Perrin, J. M., McPherson, M., McManus, M., … Arango, P. (1998). An epidemiologic profile of children with special health care needs. *Pediatrics, 2*, 117–123.

Newacheck, P. W., Inkelas, M., & Kim, S. E. (2004). Health services use and health care expenditures for children with disabilities. *Pediatrics, 114*(1), 79–85. https://doi.org/10.1542/peds.114.1.79

Nguyen, M. T., Chan, W. Y., & Keeler, C. (2015). The association between self-rated mental health status and total health care expenditure: A cross-sectional analysis of a nationally representative sample. *Medicine, 94*(35), e1410.

Nicolaidis, C., Raymaker, D., Kapp, S. K., Baggs, A., Ashkenazy, E., McDonald, K., … Joyce, A. (2019). The AASPIRE practice-based guidelines for the inclusion of autistic adults in research as co-researchers and study participants. *Autism, 23*(8), 2007–2019.

Naghibi Sistani, M. N., Montazeri, A., Yazdani, R., & Murtomaa, H. (2013). New oral health literacy instrument for public health: Development and pilot testing. *Journal of Investigative and Clinical Dentistry, 5*(4), 313–321.

Office on Women's Health, U.S. Department of Health and Human Services. (2014). *30 achievements in women's health in 30 years (1984–2014)*. Washington D.C.: U.S. Department of Health and Human Services. Retrieved from https://www.womenshealth.gov/30-achievements/25

Olfson, M., Marcus, S. C., Druss, B., Elinson, L., Tanielian, T., & Pincus, H. A. (2002). National trends in the outpatient treatment of depression. *Journal of the American Medical Association, 287*, 203–209.

Pérez Jolles, M., & Thomas, K. C. (2018). Disparities in self-reported access to patient-centered medical home care for children with special health care needs. *Medical Care, 56*(10), 840–846.

Porta, M. (2008). *A dictionary of epidemiology* (5th ed., p. 81). New York: Oxford.

Reed, G. M., Dilfer, K., Bufka, L. F., Scherer, M. J., Kotzé, P., Tshivhase, M., & Stark, S. L. (2008). Three model curricula for teaching clinicians to use the ICF. *Disability and Rehabilitation, 30*, 927–941.

Reichard, A., Stolzle, H., & Fox, M. H. (2011). Health disparities among adults with physical disabilities or cognitive limitations compared to individuals with no disabilities in the United States. *Disability and Health Journal, 4*(2), 59–67. https://doi.org/10.1016/j.dhjo.2010.05.003

Reichard, A., Stransky, M., Phillips, K., McClain, M., & Drum, C. (2017). Prevalence and reasons for delaying and foregoing necessary care by the presence and type of disability among working-age adults. *Disability and Health Journal, 10*(1), 39–47.

Rios, D., Magasi, S., Novak, C., & Harniss, M. (2016). Conducting accessible research: Including people with disabilities in public health, epidemiological, and outcomes studies. *American Journal of Public Health, 106*(12), 2137–2144.

Rothman, K. J., Greenland, S., & Lash, T. L. (2008). *Modern epidemiology* (3rd ed.). Philadelphia, PA: Lippincott, Williams & Wilkens.

Rothman, K. J. (2012). *Epidemiology: An introduction* (2nd ed.). New York: Oxford University Press.

Russell, J. N., Hendershot, G. E., LeClere, F., Howie, L. J., & Adler, M. (1997). Trends and differential use of assistive technology devices: US, 1994. *Advance Data, 292*, 1–9.

Silver, E. J., & Stein, R. E. (2001). Access to care, unmet health needs, and poverty status among children with and without chronic conditions. *Ambulatory Pediatrics, 1*, 314–320.

Stineman, M. D., & Musick, D. W. (2001). Protection of human subjects with disability: Guidelines for research. *Archives of Physical Medicine and Rehabilitation, 82*, S9–S14.

Szklo, M., & Nieto, E. J. (2012). *Epidemiology. Beyond the basics* (3rd ed.). Gaithersburg, MD: Aspen Publishers.

Talley, R. C., & Crews, J. E. (2007). Framing the public health of caregiving. *American Journal of Public Health, 97*, 224–228.

United States Census Bureau. (2017). *How disability data are collected from the American Community Survey*. Retrieved September 30, 2019, from https://www.census.gov/topics/health/disability/guidance/data-collection-acs.html

United States Census Bureau. (2018). *How disability data are collected from The Survey of Income and Program Participation*. Retrieved December 30, 2019, from https://www.census.gov/topics/health/disability/guidance/data-collection-sipp.html

U.S. Department of Health and Human Services. (2011). Implementation guidance on data collection standards for race, ethnicity, sex, primary language, and disability status. Retrieved from https://aspe.hhs.gov/basic-report/hhs-implementation-guidance-data-collection-standards-race-ethnicity-sex-primary-language-and-disability-status

Van Naarden, K., Decoufle, P., & Caldwell, K. (1999). Prevalence and characteristics of children with serious hearing impairment in metropolitan Atlanta, 1991-1993. *Pediatrics, 103*, 570–575.

Vásquez, E., Germain, C. M., Tang, F., Lohman, M. C., Fortuna, K. L., & Batsis, J. A. (2018). The role of ethnic and racial disparities in mobility and physical function in older adults. *Journal of Applied Gerontology, 39*(5), 502–508.

Vaughan, M. W., Felson, D. T., LaValley, M. P., Orsmond, G. I., Niu, J., Lewis, C. E., … Keysor, J. J. (2017). Perceived community environmental factors and risk of five-year participation restriction among older adults with or at risk of knee osteoarthritis. *Arthritis Care & Research, 69*(7), 952–958.

Von Korf, M., Koepsell, T., Curry, S., & Diehr, P. (1992). Multi-level analysis in epidemiologic research on health behaviors and outcomes. *American Journal of Epidemiology, 135*, 1077–1082.

Wallerstein, N., Duran, B., Oetzel, J., & Minkler, M. (Eds.). (2017). *Community-based participatory research for health: Advancing social and health equity* (3rd ed.). San Francisco, CA: Jossey-Bass.

Washington Group on Disability Statistics. (2017). *The Washington Group Short Set on functioning (WG-SS)*. Retrieved from http://www.washingtongroup-disability.com/wp-content/uploads/2016/12/WG-Document-2-The-Washington-Group-Short-Set-on-Functioning.pdf

White, G. W., Klatt, K., Gard, M., Suchowierska, M., & Wyatt, D. (2005). *Empowerment through research: A primer to guide understanding and use of research to make a difference*. Lawrence, KS: University of Kansas; NIDRR Research and Training Center on Independent Living.

Williams, A. S., & Moore, S. M. (2011). Universal design of research: Inclusion of persons with disabilities in mainstream biomedical studies. *Science Translational Medicine, 3*(82), 82cm12.

World Health Organization. (1988). *Learning together to work together for health: Report of a WHO Study Group on Multiprofessional Education of Health Personnel: The team approach*. World Health Organization Technical Report Series. Geneva: WHO . Home page and full document https://apps.who.int/iris/handle/10665/37411

World Health Organization. (2001a). *International Classification of Functioning, Health and Disability*. Geneva: WHO. Home page and full document http://www.who.int/icidh/

World Health Organization. (2001b). *Disability Assessment Schedule (WHODAS II)*. Geneva: WHO. Home page and full document http://www.who.int/icidh/whodas

World Health Organization. (2018). WHO | WHO Disability Assessment Schedule 2.0 (WHODAS 2.0). World Health Organization. http://www.who.int/classifications/icf/whodasii/en/

Yasuda, N., Zimmerman, S., Hawkes, W. G., Gruber-Baldini, A. L., Hebel, J. R., & Magaziner, J. (2004). Concordance of proxy-perceived change and measured change in multiple domains of function in older persons. *Journal of the American Geriatrics Society, 52*, 1157–1162.

Yelin, E., Herrndorf, A., Trupin, L., & Sonneborn, D. (2001). A national study of medical care expenditures for musculoskeletal conditions: The impact of health insurance and managed care. *Arthritis and Rheumatology, 44*, 1160–1169.

Chapter 3
Social Determinants of Health and Disability

Katherine Froehlich-Grobe, Megan Douglas, Christa Ochoa, and Andrea Betts

3.1 Identifying Social Determinants of Health

Tremendous attention at national and international levels has focused on social determinants of health, as public health professionals have grappled with understanding and reducing health disparities. According to the World Health Organization, "social determinants of health are the conditions in which people are born, grow, live, work, and age. These circumstances are shaped by the distribution of money, power, and resources at global, national, and local levels. The social determinants of health are mostly responsible for health inequalities—the unfair and avoidable differences in health status seen within and between countries." Social determinants include factors such as social class or socioeconomic position; social support, social networks, and social cohesion; access to health care; job stress or exposure to crime or adverse childhood experiences; insufficient affordable housing; and numerous other social factors that have powerful influences on health (Adler et al., 1994;

Ms. Betts was supported by a predoctoral fellowship, University of Texas Health Science Center at Houston (UTHealth), School of Public Health Cancer Education and Career Development Program (National Cancer Institute/NIH Grant T32 CA057712). *Disclaimer*: The content is solely the responsibility of the authors and does not necessarily represent the official views of the NCI or NIH.

K. Froehlich-Grobe (✉)
Baylor Scott and White Institute for Rehabilitation, Dallas, TX, USA

University of Texas School of Public Health, Dallas, TX, USA

M. Douglas · C. Ochoa
Baylor Scott and White Institute for Rehabilitation, Dallas, TX, USA
e-mail: Megan.Douglas1@bswhealth.org; Christa.Ochoa@bswhealth.org

A. Betts
Health Promotion and Behavioral Sciences, The University of Texas School of Public Health, Dallas, TX, USA

© Springer Science+Business Media, LLC, part of Springer Nature 2021
D. J. Lollar et al. (eds.), *Public Health Perspectives on Disability*,
https://doi.org/10.1007/978-1-0716-0888-3_3

Institute of Medicine, 2001). British epidemiologist Marmot et al. (Marmot, Rose, Shipley, & Hamilton, 1978; Marmot, Shipley, & Rose, 1984; Marmot et al., 1991) observed steep gradients between income and health status among British civil servants in the Whitehall studies. They identified health outcomes as being associated with an array of factors beyond income which included social, cultural, and occupational status as well as environments. Similar associations have been observed across the globe, including the USA (Dwyer-Lindgren et al., 2017; Gregorio, Walsh, & Paturzo, 1997; Lantz et al., 1998; Wing et al., 1987), Canada (Berthelot, Wilkins, & Ng, 2002; Billete & Hill, 1978; Ross et al., 2012; Wilkins, Tjepkema, Mustard, & Choinière, 2008), and European countries (Mackenbach et al., 2017). In recent decades, research into social determinants has exploded in attempt to disentangle the complex mechanisms responsible for these social gradients affecting health status. While ongoing research has examined factors responsible for these disparities in various contexts at state and country levels, the World Health Organization has established a guiding framework for researchers, policymakers, and governments across the globe to address social determinants of health.

   This chapter is divided into three sections: Sect. 3.2 presents a brief historical context of the rapidly evolving research into social determinants of health. Section 3.3 discusses conceptualizations of disability which evolved in parallel. Section 3.4 introduces evidence demonstrating how social determinants shape the health status of populations broadly and for populations of people who experience disability specifically. Finally, the chapter concludes with recommendations for future research directions to strengthen the evidence base of social determinants of health for people with disabilities.

3.2   Evolving Understanding of Social Determinants of Health

Bronfenbrenner's theory of the ecology of human development (Bronfenbrenner, 1977, 1979) provides the foundational concepts for social determinants of health, delineating the reciprocal relationship between behavior and the environment. Bronfenbrenner offered an expansive view of the environment that reflected the interconnected systems which emanate outward from the individual to society. These systems encompass physical environments such as the home, church, school, and neighborhood, as well as relationships between people and institutions within those systems. These relationships influence and are in turn influenced by the social and cultural environments within the community and larger society. Additional environmental components recognized by Bronfenbrenner include mass and social media, educational systems, economic systems, political systems, government, laws, and social services (Fig. 3.1).

   Although Bronfenbrenner originally developed his ecological systems theory as a framework to understand factors that impact child development, his work, and that

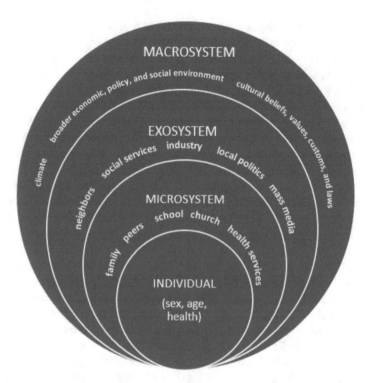

Fig. 3.1 Depiction of Bronfenbrenner's interconnected ecological systems that emanate outward from the individual

of others in this domain has since been adapted into what is now known as the *social ecological model*. This model emphasizes the importance of the complex interaction between multiple levels of influence (individual, community, society, etc.) and has given researchers a framework to study and begin to understand the complex mechanisms underlying social determinants of health. Today the social ecological model is commonly applied across numerous public health issues, from violence prevention (National Center on Injury Prevention and Control, n.d.) to dietary choice (U.S. Department of Health and Human Services and U.S. Department of Agriculture, 2015).

Subsequently, Link and Phelan (1995) discussed the need to understand associations between social connections and wellness and articulated that access to resources underlies the *fundamental causes* of diseases. The authors contended that these fundamental causes influence multiple risk factors and multiple disease outcomes because access to resources such as money or social connectedness influence whether individuals can avoid risk for morbidity and mortality. This notion of a "fundamental cause"—that upstream factors cause health outcomes—is central to the social determinants of health view. According to Link and Phelan, the structure of medical and public health systems, which predominantly focus on treating health problems and encouraging personal action to avoid health risks, leads only to change in those with access to resources needed to avoid health risks. Thus, by addressing the fundamental cause and eliminating the source of the problem where it occurs, governments and policymakers can improve the health of everyone. Braveman, Egerter, and Williams (2011) clearly illustrated this concept by describing a scenario in which people get sick due to drinking from a polluted water source. Those with resources can purchase water filters or buy bottled water, but those unable to afford those strategies continue to be exposed and fall ill. On the other hand, eliminating the source of the contamination, which is the factory located upriver that is dumping toxic chemicals, would prevent the chemicals from entering the water and protect all citizens downstream from exposure to the contaminants.

In accordance with this simplified example, the accumulated body of evidence to date (Braveman, Cubbin, Egerter, Williams, & Pamuk, 2010; Commission on Social Determinants of Health, 2008; Yen & Syme, 1999) clearly demonstrates that "the contexts in which people live, learn, work, and play influence both the choices available to them and their ability to choose paths leading to good health. In many instances, the barriers to good health exceed an individual's abilities, even with the greatest motivation to overcome these obstacles..." (p. S5) (Braveman, Egerter, & Mockenhaupt, 2011). Emerging evidence has demonstrated that conditions in socioeconomically disadvantaged neighborhoods, such as inadequate housing (i.e., occupied housing that has moderate or severe physical problems), crime, noise, pollution, lack of services, and limited green spaces, are related to poorer health (Pickett & Pearl, 2001; Steptoe & Feldman, 2001). Other social factors that are linked to poorer health include discrimination (Williams, 1999; Williams, Mohammed, Leavell, & Collins, 2010) and stress (McEwen, 1998; Seeman, Epel, Gruenewald, Karlamangla, & McEwen, 2010; Seeman, McEwen, Rowe, & Singer, 2001). Further, children may have fewer opportunities for physical activity when they live in urban neighborhoods with high crime, no sidewalks, poorly maintained parks, few after-school programs, and parents or guardians who work hourly wage jobs, as compared to children who live in suburban neighborhoods with low crime, well-maintained parks, numerous after-school programs, and parents or guardians working in salaried positions with flexible hours.

Since finding evidence of a socioeconomic gradient for health outcomes, where greater disease burden is observed among individuals at the lower end of the income ladder, researchers have begun to investigate the mechanisms by which this inequity occurs. Adler and Newman (2002) offered an analysis of the component parts of *socioeconomic status* (SES) to examine the multiple pathways through which SES influences health. The authors identify education, income, and occupation as the three SES components, each of which provides different resources and relationships to various health outcomes. They contend that education may be the most basic component, as it shapes future job opportunities and earning potential, while also providing people with knowledge and life skills. Higher income allows people to obtain better nutrition, housing, school, recreational opportunities, and health care. They note that occupation can have a more complex association with resources due to differing levels of prestige, qualifications, rewards, and job characteristics, yet they note that autonomy and control at work is a factor strongly linked to health status. These three component factors operate individually and collectively in ways that are related to environmental exposures, social networks and social cohesion, architectural and aesthetic features of communities, access to and quality of health care, lifestyle behaviors, and chronic stress to support or negatively impact health. Thus, it has become more evident over time that contextual factors play a key role in people's ability to engage in healthy behaviors based on opportunities and resources in the environment.

3.3   Extending the Investigation of Social Determinants of Health to Populations with Disability

Although there is ample evidence about how social determinants impact health broadly, there remains a disconnect between public health researchers recognizing the myriad of factors that affect the health of various minority populations (e.g., African Americans, Native Americans, the LGBTQ community) and an appreciation of how these same factors impact the health of people with disabilities. Health professionals outside the fields of disability and rehabilitation tend to accept that health disparities observed among people with disabilities reflect a truism that people with disabilities have poorer health, higher rates of depression, and are more sedentary (Grosse, Lollar, Campbell, & Chamie, 2009; Rock, 2000). Whereas professionals within the fields of disability and rehabilitation recognize that a myriad of modifiable factors impact people's access to the locations, activities, equipment, services, and behaviors critical to their achieving the highest level of health possible. The perception that people with disabilities de facto have poorer health conforms with the medical model of disability, which views disability as residing within the person and is logically consistent with the notion that they will therefore have poor health. Inherent to the medical model perspective is a view of people with disabilities who continue on with their life and earn a college degree, work, get married, raise children, and follow their passions as inspirational stories of people who overcame great adversity. This "supercrip" narrative, as it is commonly known in the disability community, engenders seeing successful people with disability as "defying their disability" (Charlton, 2000; Hardin & Hardin, 2004; Silva & Howe, 2012). The reality is that most people who are born with or acquire disability due to injury or disease eventually adjust to their new life (Martz, Livneh, Priebe, Wuermser, & Ottomanelli, 2005). People living with disabilities recognize that barriers they encounter do not reflect their limitations, but rather that they live in environments that do not support strategies they have adopted to function, such as using a wheelchair for locomotion or sign language for communication.

3.3.1 Evolving Conceptualizations of Disability

Conceptualizations of disability have been evolving since 1965 following Saad Nagi's (1965) publication that recognized four distinct, yet interrelated concepts in which he defined "disability" as referring to *limitations a person experiences in performing socially defined roles and responsibilities* expected during that developmental stage, in contrast to disability being a function of physical limitations. Nagi (1964, 1965, 1969) noted that these socially defined roles and responsibilities are further defined by the sociocultural and physical environments and are generally organized around life activities such as family and interpersonal relationships, education, work, employment, or other economic pursuits, in addition to other domains such as recreation and self-care. This was conceptually and functionally different from the current colloquial use of the word "disability," in which people allude to concepts of pathology (infection, trauma, degenerative disease, or other etiology), impairment (abnormal function of anatomical, physiological, mental, or emotional systems), and functional limitation (changes that result in limitations in performing tasks such as reaching, walking, seeing).

This evolution of thinking about disability as a construct separate from pathology and impairment has proceeded in parallel with the development and application of the social ecological model to health. Numerous conceptual models of disability have been offered over the years, each of which furthered the field's thinking about how the environment impacts the function and health of individuals living with disability. One useful heuristic that built upon earlier models was put forward by Brandt and Pope in Chap. 3 of the 1977 Institute of Medicine (IOM) report *Enabling America* (1997). This model offers two useful constructs of the person-environment fit, where people generally "fit" within their physical and social environment (see Panel 1 Fig. 3.2 (top), which is recreated from their model to illustrate these concepts). Panel 2 depicts that in the disabling process, a person's needs exceed what is available in their environment, and that the enabling process (i.e., rehabilitation) provides two pathways to allow the person to fit back within their environment, depicted in Panel 3. One is functional restoration, where medical treatment restores a person's function; the other is environmental modification, where the environment is enlarged to address the person's needs through actions like providing a wheelchair, widening doorways, or building ramps. The second useful construct of the model is viewing the physical and social environment as a mat, where disability occurs at the intersection of the person and their environment; see Fig. 3.2 (bottom). Resilient environments support the person's needs though providing assistive technology, having accessible physical environments, and supportive relationships, while environments with fewer of these resources pose barriers for the person to participate in their environment and achieve optimal health.

A more recent and widely used conceptualization of disability was the International Classification of Functioning (ICF) (World Health Organization, 2001), which offers more detailed thinking to consider the interaction between a person and their environment. It also demonstrates how those factors impact function and participation,

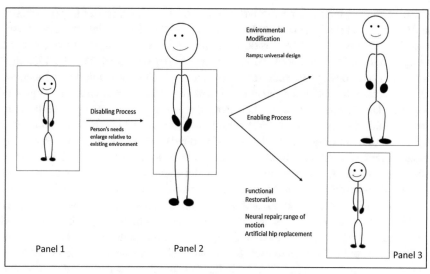

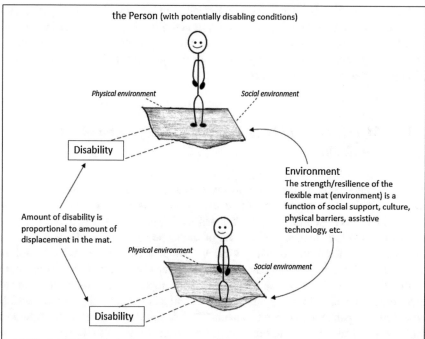

Fig. 3.2 Conceptual model of person-environment fit after onset of disabling condition (top); Depiction of how the environment can be viewed as a mat (bottom). Adapted from Chap. 3, Models of Disability and Rehabilitation. Institute of Medicine. 1997. Enabling America; Assessing the Role of Rehabilitation Science and Engineering. https://doi.org/10.17226/5779. Adapted and reproduced with permission from the National Academy of Sciences, Courtesy of the National Academies Press. Washington, DC

either serving to facilitate performance and/or health or as a barrier to performance and/or health. This approach merges concepts from the Nagi model, the IOM model, and the social ecological framework. The model is depicted in the Environmental Chapter (Chap. 5) of this book, where it is more fully described. The ICF identifies reciprocal relationships as occurring between the health condition, body functions and structures, activities the person performs (e.g., learning, communicating, performing daily tasks), as well as their participation (e.g., performing these tasks in social contexts such as school, work, or the community), all of which are influenced by environmental (physical, social, and attitudinal) and personal factors. While the model offers substantially greater detail at all levels, for the purposes of illuminating social determinants, we focus on how the model enhanced thinking about contextual factors. The two components of context are personal factors, which include sex, age, race, lifestyle, habits, education, and profession, and environmental factors. The six ICF environmental categories are (a) products and technology (such as food and medicine) for personal use in daily living, for mobility and transportation, and in buildings for public or private use; (b) the natural environment and human changes to the environment, such as climate, light, and sound; (c) social relationships that include family, friends, peers and acquaintances, neighbors and community members, healthcare professionals, and people in authority; (d) attitudes of individuals with whom people are in relationship; (e) services, systems, and policies of education, employment, housing, transportation, health services, legal services, etc.; and (f) any other environmental factors.

3.3.2   Merging Social Determinants of Health and the ICF: An Example

The following example illustrates how the various personal and environment factors identified in the ICF operate at multiple levels of influence to affect the participation and health status of people living with disability. We present a scenario in which Joe and Mike, two hypothetical individuals of the same sex, race, and age but vastly different social determinants, both experience car accidents. The accidents result in the same level of injury and impairments, as both incur an injury to their spinal cord at the sixth thoracic vertebrae that results in complete paralysis of their lower extremities as well as loss of voluntary bowel and bladder control. The table details how different personal and environmental factors could influence the trajectory of their lives and health over the subsequent 5 years post-injury (Table 3.1).

The example depicts how personal, social, and physical environmental factors at the time of injury influence the resources both men have as they transition back home and navigate issues of adjusting to life with functional limitations. Their educational backgrounds impact what each does for work, the income they earn, and financial resources available to modify their home, so they can live in the house. The impairments the men experience prevent Joe from returning to his roofing job due to the physical labor involved, whereas Mike's work as an attorney is less impacted

Table 3.1 Table illustrating impact of contextual factors on participation and health of individuals with disability

Contextual factors	Joe (30 year-old, non-Hispanic white male)			Mike (30 year-old, non-Hispanic white male)		
	Injury onset	Discharge rehab	5 years post-injury	Injury onset	Discharge rehab	5 years post-injury
Personal						
Education	High school graduate	High school graduate	High school graduate	bachelor's and law degrees	bachelor's and law degrees	bachelor's and law degrees
Employment	Full time as a roofer	Unable return job in roofing	Receiving federal disability benefits (SSDI, Medicaid)	Attorney at a large firm	Able to take extended paid medical leave, employer holds position while continuing outpatient	Returned to law firm, made partner, received salary increase
Marital & family status	Married, 2 kids ages 7 & 4 years	Wife committed to marriage	Divorced	Never married & single	Single	Met a woman 2 years post-injury, dated for a year.
Lifestyle	Family-oriented, active in church, hobbies include coaching son's tag football team & watching Sunday pro football with friends	Friends visit & together watch sports on TV	Fewer friends visit, occasionally attends kids sporting events	Works 65–80 hrs a week, enjoys waterskiing, member of wine tasting club, volunteers with big brothers, avid reader	Attends outpatient rehabilitation therapy	Works long hours, he & wife enjoy cooking together, he tried accessible waterskiing

(continued)

Table 3.1 (continued)

Contextual factors	Joe (30 year-old, non-Hispanic white male)			Mike (30 year-old, non-Hispanic white male)		
	Injury onset	Discharge rehab	5 years post-injury	Injury onset	Discharge rehab	5 years post-injury
Habits	Physically demanding job, inactive outside of work since HS football days, periodically takes kids to park, coaches kids team once a week for 4 months, heavy drinker on the weekends, eats high fat diet	Sedentary & continues to eat diet high fat diet & drink beer	Remains sedentary, diet quality remains poor, & drinks heavily on a regular basis	Long-distance runner since running cross-country in HS, eats a healthy diet, drinks wine in moderation only on weekends	Becomes member of an accessible gym to work on strength & endurance outside of therapy, learns about a wheelchair racing, continues following a healthy diet & rarely drinks	Purchased accessible gym equipment for home use, involved in wheelchair racing, drinks wine on holidays or celebrations
Environmental						
Social-Family structure						
Development phase	Parents divorced when he was 15, has 1 brother, father died 10 years ago, mother lives in another state	Mother comes for 2 weeks to assist family with transition home, returns to job & home in another state, brother lives locally & provides financial & emotional support		Parents married for 35 years, has 1 sister, all family live in town & have close relationship	moves in with parents while his home renovated, parents have accessible space for him to live for several months & he is independent	Enjoys family gatherings a couple of times a month with his & wife's families
Current	Married 8 years with 2 kids, wife stays home with kids	Wife takes on hourly wage job	Wife files for divorce & full custody of the kids	Single, no kids	Single, no kids	Married, discussing starting a family

Contextual factors	Joe (30 year-old, non-Hispanic white male)			Mike (30 year-old, non-Hispanic white male)		
	Injury onset	Discharge rehab	5 years post-injury	Injury onset	Discharge rehab	5 years post-injury
Friends	Several close friends from HS, brother in-law, & son's team	Family & friends provide help with kids	Spends time with his brother & HS friends plus fathers' of son's sports teams	Close friends from college, law school, running group, & work	College/law school friends provide emotional support, running group shares info about wheelchair racing, work friends keep in touch	Close friends from college-law school, work, gym, & wheelchair racing group
Acquaintances	From the church, work, neighbors, & son's school	Work friends & neighbors provide meals & provide maintenance services to the yard and entrance to home	Neighbors, church, paratransit system, SCI support group	Neighbors, running club, work, wine club	Neighbors from his & parents neighborhood, peer mentor from rehabilitation,	Church, other wheelchair racers
Physical						
Home	Owns older, small 2 story home & drives a 10-year old truck	no bedroom on main floor, bathroom modifications costly, bathroom configuration requires needing assistance with bathing, & cannot transfer into truck & cannot drive	Moved to subsidized, accessible public housing (Section 8 housing)	Owns newer home located near his work	Home undergoing renovations to the entryway, bathroom, & kitchen	Added square footage to home for another bedroom & family room, all accessible

(continued)

Table 3.1 (continued)

Contextual factors	Joe (30 year-old, non-Hispanic white male)			Mike (30 year-old, non-Hispanic white male)		
	Injury onset	Discharge rehab	5 years post-injury	Injury onset	Discharge rehab	5 years post-injury
Neighborhood	Sub-burb in a mid-sized southern city, sidewalks lack curb cuts, school & stores 2.5 miles away	Difficult & unsafe to wheel in the neighborhood as sidewalks without curb cuts require wheeling in the street	New neighborhood located in more mixed use area, with grocery store nearby & close to the bus line, sidewalks all have curb cuts, crime is a concern	Large, urban area in the northeast with sidewalks, mixed used space with residential, stores, & business in proximity	Sidewalks with curb cuts in his & parents neighborhood, with easy access to stores, theaters, restaurant	Sidewalks in good repair, access to stores, theaters, restaurants within a 1 mile radius of the home
Community	Numerous parks & lakes, no metro system, poorly funded bus system	Unable to locate affordable transportation to get to/from church or take kids school	City offers reduced fares for riders with a disability, bus lines are limited, but have routes to public park venues where his kids play sports	Well-funded public transit system, parks across the city	Able to use public transit system, visit parks, strong sense of cohesion across regions of the city, active neighborhood watch programs, low crime	Roads & public transit well maintained, parks busy with community events, crime remains low, good social cohesion
State	Low tax rate & state agencies, including education, transportation, health care are underfunded, & state opted not to expand Medicaid	Low funding for disability services (e.g., vocational rehabilitation, home & community-based waiver plans), long wait-times for disability determination	Eligibility redetermination for disability programs required every 1–6 years	High tax rate, provides strong funding for education, transportation, health, & parks	Using services of transportation system & parks	Tax rate remains high & state continues adequate funding of government programs
Federal	Section 8 of the Housing Act of 1937, Americans with Disabilities Act, Affordable Care Act					

Contextual factors	Joe (30 year-old, non-Hispanic white male)			Mike (30 year-old, non-Hispanic white male)		
	Injury onset	Discharge rehab	5 years post-injury	Injury onset	Discharge rehab	5 years post-injury
Services/ Systems/ Policies	Unaware of any benefit programs	Applies for Social Security Disability Insurance & Medicaid	After 26 months, approved for SSDI, Medicaid, & supplemental nutrition program (SNAP)	State expanded. Medicaid	Expanded. Medicaid present, but not plan to apply	Not need to apply for any disability benefits, but has advocated for better access at one location, travels by air for vacation, enjoys renting accessible vehicles in other cities

by his paralysis. Thus, one loses his job, while the other is allowed a longer medical leave, offering continued access to health benefits and a salary, while he is away. Both face the physical and emotional stressors of the traumatic accident and permanent changes in function, yet Mike has greater emotional and financial support from family and friends plus insurance coverage that allows him to continue rehabilitation in an outpatient setting to maximize functional gains and strength. Whereas Joe loses not only his job and health insurance, preventing him from receiving further rehabilitation services, but as the primary breadwinner, he loses a stable income source to support his young family. While he and his family receive emotional and tangible support in the early weeks and months from family and friends who help with the kids, provide home maintenance, and minor modifications, there is growing stress by both spouses over the need for the wife to return to the workforce and bring in money to cover monthly bills. The stress persists with needing to move to a more accessible home that may also result in sending their children to a new school, plus identifying how to apply and then wait for disability benefits. These occur simultaneous to adjusting emotionally to new routines and less independence for the husband and greater daily burdens for the wife, who is now working managing all home chores, while also raising the kids. This cumulative stress increases friction between the spouses, negatively impacting their relationship.

The changes observed by 5 years post-injury in both men's lives reflect the resources they each had available that could mitigate or exacerbate the issues they needed to navigate. Given what is known about the context of Joe's life, he is at increased risk for weight gain and chronic conditions based on his diet, sedentary lifestyle, and heavy drinking. As a result of fewer accessible transportation routes, he may also be more socially isolated. Whereas Mike was able to rely on social support and financial resources that provided access to greater healthcare services, better housing, disposable income to purchase home exercise equipment, and eat a healthy diet. Other assets Mike experienced were his ability to return to a high-paying job with prestige and living in a neighborhood with well-maintained sidewalks that he could navigate in his wheelchair. The neighborhood also had less crime, more parks, and better public transportation systems. The cumulative effects of these factors and with getting married, which expanded his social network, serve as protective factors as Mike ages with a spinal cord injury.

3.4   Empirical Evidence of Social Determinants Effects upon Health

This section is organized by the Healthy People 2020 objectives on social determinants (U.S. Department of Health and Human Services & Office of Disease Prevention and Health Promotion, 2020). The 2020 Healthy People initiative encompasses 1200 objectives across 42 topic areas and establishes Leading Health Indicators to serve as high priority issues that act as measures of the Nation's Health. The 2020 Leading Health Indicators were specifically selected to focus on individual and social determinants that affect people's health and contribute to health disparities and were organized around the following domains: (1) economic stability, (2) early childhood and educational attainment, (3) access to health care, (4) neighborhood and built environment, and (5) social and community context. A summary of findings is presented for both the general population and people with disabilities.

1. Economic Stability.

Economic stability impacts health through several pathways and can be defined at a micro or macro-level. Greater economic stability generally relates to better health outcomes. At an individual level, income can impact an individual's ability to access healthcare services and resources, and *employment* predicts individual-level health outcomes. Meta-analyses of largely cross-sectional data consistently indicate an association between unemployment and poorer physical and mental health outcomes, including a 63% higher mortality risk after controlling for several covariates (Hollederer, 2015). Nationally representative and longitudinal survey data show that respondents who experienced job loss were 54% more likely to rate their health as "fair" or "poor" and that job loss was associated with cardiovascular disease and arthritis, even when the individual was not at fault for the job loss (Strully, 2009).

Employment improves health and community participation for those with disabilities (Goodman, 2015). Beyond providing financial independence and stability, employment provides an important source of community participation and social relationships (Waddell & Burton, 2006). Though the magnitude of effect on physical and mental well-being is unclear (Goodman, 2015), employment is also related to reduced mental health-related spending among people with disabilities and may increase quality of life (Turner & Turner, 2004). However, systemic and attitudinal barriers make it more difficult for people with disabilities to obtain employment. Across economically developed countries, employment rates among those with disability are only slightly more than 40% compared to almost 80% of those without disabilities (Organisation for Economic, Development Directorate for Employment, & Social, 2009). This is true despite evidence that shows integrating people with disabilities into the labor force would reduce healthcare spending and improve the economy by growing the workforce. Employers have cited perceived lack of skills and possible legal issues as barriers to hiring people with disabilities, particularly for those with intellectual disabilities. These barriers could be mitigated through staff education and policy changes to incentivize hiring people with disabilities (Kocman, Fischer, & Weber, 2018). Young people with developmental and psychiatric disabilities reported encountering numerous barriers to employment such as lack of work experience, transportation, cognitive difficulties, and social skills (Hammel et al., 2015). Facilitators to employment for people with disabilities include jobs that offer flexibility with scheduling and modified work duties (Organisation for Economic et al., 2009).

Lack of employment opportunities puts people with disabilities at greater financial risk plus decreases their community participation and social isolation. Additionally, policies in the USA and other developed countries may result in people completely or partially losing disability income/government support if they have a job, which may further disincentivize people with disabilities from working (Organisation for Economic et al., 2009). This issue is further addressed in the Chap. 14.

Given low employment rates for people with disabilities, it is not surprising to learn that in the USA and worldwide, people with disabilities are more likely to live in poverty (Chan & Zoellick, 2011). In 2016, 21% of US adults with a disability lived at or below the federal poverty level, compared to 13% of US adults without a disability (Kraus, Lauer, Coleman, & Houtenville, 2018). Additional data show an association between lower SES and poorer mental health among people with disabilities (Aitken, Simpson, Bentley, & Kavanagh, 2017). It is likely that poverty operates in direct and indirect ways to negatively impact the physical and mental health status of people with disabilities. People with disability who live in poverty lack financial resources that may otherwise buffer the negative impacts of inaccessible physical environments of housing, neighborhoods, and transportation or allow for purchasing equipment to help them engage in healthy behaviors.

Employment and job instability impact other determinants of health, such as food insecurity and housing instability in the general population and people with disabilities. Seniors with *food insecurity*, or a lack of consistent access to affordable, healthy food, were more likely to report limitations in activities of daily living, lower nutrient intake, poorer health, higher rates of chronic diseases (such as diabetes and hypertension), and poorer sleep (Gundersen & Ziliak, 2015). Food insecurity is also related to race/ethnicity, income, education (Seligman, Bindman, Vittinghoff, Kanaya, & Kushel, 2007), greater healthcare use, and higher healthcare costs (Berkowitz, Seligman, Meigs, & Basu, 2018). Approximately 32% of food insecure US households include someone with a disability (Heflin, Altman, & Rodriguez, 2019). However, a scoping review (Schwartz, Buliung, & Wilson, 2019) noted that underlying social and environmental barriers to food access have not been adequately addressed or studied. Another study reported households that have a member with a disability who were food insecure had a higher odds of reporting lower perceived physical and mental health and had more frequent emergency department visits (Brucker, 2017).

Individuals with *housing instability* (i.e., difficulty paying rent, mortgage, or utilities) are more likely to lack a usual source of health care or postpone necessary health care and medications (Kushel, Gupta, Gee, & Haas, 2006). Housing instability has been associated with other social determinants that include lower educational attainment, earning less than $50,000 annually, being a woman, being of Hispanic ethnicity, being unmarried, living in a household with children, and reporting adverse childhood experiences (Stahre, VanEenwyk, Siegel, & Njai, 2015). Individuals who are housing insecure are also more likely to be smokers, delay doctor's visits because of costs, report fair or poor health status, and have poorer mental health (Stahre et al., 2015). Further, analysis of National Health Interview Survey (NHIS) and Housing and Urban Development (HUD) data found that individuals who currently received housing assistance had reduced odds of reporting fair or poor health (versus good, very good, or excellent) compared to individuals not yet receiving assistance but who would within a 2-year timeframe (Fenelon et al., 2017).

One potential contributing factor to housing instability for people with disabilities is limited affordable and accessible housing stock. A large study that included over 5000 working-age Australians found that approximately 8% of men and women with disability experienced housing instability vs. 3.5% of all men and 6.1% of all women (Kavanagh et al., 2015). In the USA, a review of housing units found less than 1% of available housing to be fully accessible for wheelchair users and less than 5% to be accessible for people with moderate mobility limitations (Bo'sher, Chan, Ellen, Karfunkel, & Liao, 2015). Further analyses indicated that accessible housing units were mostly built after 1990 and were disproportionately located in newly developed regions of the country (e.g., large cities in the west and south). The issue of housing instability for people with disabilities is impacted not only by limited accessible housing stock but also by the shortage of affordable housing facing many US cities (Florida & Schneider, 2018). Several lawsuits have been filed against US cities for their lack of affordable accessible housing (Office of Public Affairs, 2018; Serafini, 2018). A 2012 lawsuit filed in Los Angeles was settled in 2016 with a judgment requiring that the city of LA commit to spending at least $200 million over 10 years to ensure at least 4000 affordable housing units meet architectural accessibility standards (Reyes & Zahniser, 2016).

2. *Early Childhood and Educational Attainment.*

Increasing evidence points to individuals who experience adverse childhood experiences (ACEs) having worse health outcomes. ACEs include events that can cause harm to children such as physical or sexual abuse or being in difficult living situations such as with familial conflict or substance abuse (Hughes et al., 2012; Schüssler-Fiorenza Rose, Xie, & Stineman, 2014). One study reported that people with four ACEs, compared to those with no ACEs, had greater mental health issues, poorer self-rated health, higher rates of cancer, heart disease, and respiratory disease and were more likely to engage in risky health behaviors including smoking, heavy/problematic alcohol use, sexual risk-taking, and problematic substance use (Hughes et al., 2017). One European study found that a greater number of ACEs predicted higher rates of general practice healthcare use, emergency care, and hospitalization (Bellis et al., 2017).

ACEs have also been found to be associated with developing disability later in life (Bowen & González, 2010; Schüssler-Fiorenza Rose et al., 2014), although personal factors such as educational attainment and degree of upward mobility in the surrounding area reduced the odds of developing a disability. While evidence has not identified the mechanisms by which ACEs lead to disability, it is likely due to complex interactions between the person and the environment. One potential mechanism may be that engaging in significantly more risky health behaviors could predispose these individuals to incurring a disabling condition (Campbell, Walker, & Egede, 2016). Research is also investigating the effects of ACEs on biological systems (e.g., by affecting telomere length and epigenetics), which may interact with other factors for acquiring disability (Lang et al., 2019).

Lower educational attainment is related to poorer health, higher probability of major depression, risk for chronic health conditions, and poorer self-reported health status even after adjusting for other variables (Lee et al., 2016). One study reported that less education led to a 67% increased likelihood of earlier death, even after controlling for socioeconomic status and economic resources (Baker, Leon, Smith Greenaway, Collins, & Movit, 2011). Similar to the overall SES trends, there is a graduated effect of education on health, with incrementally improved health outcomes associated with higher levels of education. Results from one nationally representative study showed that those with fewer than 12 years of education had a 21% higher mortality rate, whereas lower mortality was associated with every subsequent degree level, from associates (20% lower) to bachelors (30% lower), masters (40% lower), or professional degree (45% lower) (Rogers, Everett, Zajacova, & Hummer, 2010).

Several mediating variables proposed to explain these associations include individual health or risk behaviors (Delva, O'Malley, & Johnston, 2006; Hahn & Truman, 2015; Lee et al., 2016), insurance coverage (Lee et al., 2016), and higher wages (Hahn & Truman, 2015). One other education-related mechanism that may impact the relationship is health literacy, or the "capacity to obtain, process, and understand basic health information and services" (U.S. Department of Health and Human Services & Office of Disease Prevention and Health Promotion, 2010, p. iii). Lower *health literacy* rates are related to lower use of preventive services, greater use of emergency services, poorer interpretation of dosing, labels, and health messages and subsequently increased hospitalization (Berkman, Sheridan, Donahue, Halpern, & Crotty, 2011; DeWalt, Berkman, Sheridan, Lohr, & Pignone, 2004).

Education and disability are correlated in the USA and worldwide, with lower levels of education corresponding with higher likelihood of having a disability (Hosseinpoor et al., 2012; Montez, Zajacova, & Hayward, 2017). The data indicate that educational attainment is lower for those born with or who acquire disability during the developmental period and it was suggested that the strongest social influence was lower expectations (Chatzitheochari & Platt, 2019). Education is also a consistent predictor of disability across the life span, with lower educational attainment associated with higher probability of acquiring disability later in life (Montez et al., 2017). However, having attained more education may promote better adjustment to disability (Bengtsson & Datta Gupta, 2017). Some research suggests that education alone, independent of its socioeconomic effects, is the driving force behind better adjustment to disability (Bengtsson & Datta Gupta, 2017).

3. *Access to Health Care.*

Access is a broad term which may reference multiple aspects of health care including the physical availability of services, convenience of services, adequacy of services, opportunity for services, and resources which enable use of these services (Gulliford et al., 2002; U.S. Department of Health and Human Services, n.d.). The US conversation around healthcare access has predominantly focused on assuring access to healthcare insurance and the cost of health care. The US health insurance system is structured in such a way that most Americans receive health care through their employer and publicly funded health insurance (Medicaid and Medicare) is available for a segment of the population who are low income, have a disability, or are older. Yet, due to the high cost of insurance, tens of millions of Americans are uninsured. Policymakers at the state and federal levels have argued for decades about how to implement changes to our healthcare system to improve healthcare access. Notably, the Institute of Medicine (2009) advocated for increasing health insurance access based on data that demonstrates lack of adequate healthcare insurance is linked to poor health outcomes.

In 2010 President Obama was able to pass the Patient Protection and Affordable Care Act (ACA), and by 2013 provisions were enacted to increase the number of insured Americans, which included expanding Medicaid across numerous states, creating health insurance exchanges, and adopting the individual mandate. This has allowed for studying the effects of increasing health insurance coverage on receipt of healthcare services. Several studies that analyzed data collected from national datasets after ACA was enacted indicate that the number of uninsured Americans decreased significantly, they reported greater access to health care, including being able to afford care, and fewer Americans reported having fair/health (Sommers, Gunja, Finegold, & Musco, 2015). Trends in emergency department (ED) visits, and hospital discharges have also been examined over the period before and after the ACA, which reveal that although ED visits have increased, hospital discharges have remained stable. Yet, increased ED use has increased among Medicaid recipients but decreased for those who are uninsured, thus shifting the payor mix for these visits (Singer, Thode, & Pines, 2019). In a separate national study that compared outcomes between Medicaid expansion and non-expansion states, the results showed significantly higher insurance rates for both private insurance and under Medicaid, higher healthcare use (hospital stays and physician visits, but not ED visits), and a significant increase in chronic condition diagnoses (diabetes and high cholesterol) in the expansion states, but no significant differences in self-rated health status (Wherry & Miller, 2016).

The current political environment is threatening provisions of the ACA, and policy changes enacted by the Trump administration may be contributing a rise in the uninsurance rate (Keith, 2019), which remains lower than pre-ACA levels (13% or about 42 million Americans) but has increased from 7.9% in 2017 to 8.5% (27.5 million Americans) in 2018. Currently, most Americans are covered by private health insurance (67.3%), which they receive through their employer (55%) and some (3.3%) obtain private coverage through a marketplace. About one-third (34.4%) of Americans receive public insurance by Medicaid (17.9%), Medicare (17.9%), or the Veterans Administration (1%). Notable increases in the uninsurance rate are among children under age 19 (4.9% in 2017 to 5.5% in 2018) and people with a disability (increased from 8.4% in 2017 to 9.6% in 2018).

Health insurance access intersects with other social factors. Uninsured individuals are more likely to have lower education, earn less income, be unemployed, Hispanic, or Black (Berchick, Hood, & Barnett, 2018). Healthcare access is also related geographic access; five southern states (TX, OK, MS, GA, and FL) have the highest rates of uninsured Americans, with the highest rate in Texas (17.7%,) and

Oklahoma trails by 3.5% (14.2%), while four states (RI, HI, VT, MA) and the District of Columbia have uninsured rates of less than 5% with Massachusetts (2.8%) having the lowest rate. MA achieved this low uninsurance rate after passing healthcare reform legislation in 2006 under Governor Mitt Romney that was intended to assure that nearly all MA residents receive health insurance coverage. The law had an individual mandate and provided subsidized and free healthcare insurance for residents at 150% and 300% of the federal poverty level (Gabel et al., 2008; Haislmaier & Owcharenko, 2006). Healthcare access is also related to population size, with different factors impacting rural residents (Kindig & Movassaghi, 1989; Richman, Pearson, Beasley, & Stanifer, 2019) than urban residents (Luo & Wang, 2003). A study of geospatial access to primary care clinics was conducted in Philadelphia, a city with one of the highest poverty rates and is racially diverse, yet where racial groups tends to be concentrated in geographically different areas. The authors reported the vast differences across neighborhoods in terms of demographic characteristics, especially in racial composition which led to wide variation in the spatial accessibility to primary care providers. Thus, even after adjusting for income, age, population density, and insurance coverage, African Americans and Hispanics had the lowest spatial access to primary care clinics (Brown, Polsky, Barbu, Seymour, & Grande, 2016).

People with disabilities have a higher rate of insurance (90.8%) than those without a disability (88%), yet the insurance source differs significantly between these groups. Individuals with a disability have higher rates of public insurance (53.9% vs. 16.6%) and lower rates of private insurance (44.7% vs. 74.9%) than individuals without a disability (Berchick et al., 2018). This difference in coverage source is due to employers serving as the largest source of private insurance and the low employment rate for people with disabilities. People with disabilities have an employment rate of 18.7%, which is higher for those aged 16–64 years old (30.4%) as compared to rates of 65.9% and 74.0%, respectively, for those without a disability (Bureau of Labor Statistics, 2019). Nevertheless, higher insurance rates do not translate into better access for those with disabilities.

People with disabilities are more likely to report dissatisfaction with the quality of health care, access to specialists, and ease of getting to the doctor (Fouts, Andersen, & Hagglund, 2000; Iezzoni, Davis, Soukup, & O'Day, 2002; Jha, Patrick, MacLehose, Doctor, & Chan, 2002). They are more likely to have unmet need for medical care (Beatty et al., 2003), delay medical care due to cost (Centers for Disease Control and Prevention, n.d.), have lower rates of preventive screening services (Armour, Thierry, & Wolf, 2009; Henning-Smith, McAlpine, Shippee, & Priebe, 2013; Horner-Johnson, Dobbertin, & Iezzoni, 2015; Iezzoni et al., 2000), and be less likely to access primary care than their counterparts without disability (Marrocco & Krouse, 2017). Individuals with disability also face unique barriers to accessing health care that include lack of accessible facilities and equipment (Donnelly et al., 2007; Peacock, Iezzoni, & Harkin, 2015; Story, Schwier, & Kailes, 2009), transportation problems (Bezyak, Sabella, & Gattis, 2017; National Council on Disability, 2015), and implicit discrimination or bias from healthcare providers such as ignorance of how to address health concerns of people with disabilities

Social Determinants of Health in Action: Breast Cancer Screening and Outcomes

Women with disabilities experience disparities in breast cancer mortality. In a national retrospective cohort study of women with invasive breast cancer, women with disabilities were 1.31 more times likely to die from breast cancer than women without disability, with poorer disease-specific survival at every stage of diagnosis (McCarthy et al., 2006). Thus, regular mammography is crucial for women with disabilities, as disparities are most pronounced with a late stage of diagnosis. Yet women with disabilities are 30–50% less likely than other women to receive breast cancer screening at recommended intervals (Iezzoni, Kurtz, & Rao, 2015; Wei, Findley, & Sambamoorthi, 2006). Disparities in mammography uptake and breast cancer mortality among women with disabilities may be improved by addressing social determinants at multiple levels, including provider behavior, staffing, and physical access to facilities and adaptive equipment.

Despite worse breast cancer outcomes, women with disabilities have reported lack of provider counseling and referral as reasons for not receiving mammography (Edwards, Sakellariou, & Anstey, 2020; Nosek & Howland, 1997). Increasing provider recommendation of mammography—considered one of the most important modifiable factors in improving screening adherence (Institute of Medicine, 2001; Peterson et al., 2016; Steinwachs et al., 2010)—is a key objective of the Healthy People 2020 cancer goals (Office of Disease Prevention and Health Promotion, 2017). Several randomized controlled trials have found that interventions to increase provider recommendation of mammography significantly improve patient screening rates (Peterson et al., 2016). In the context of disability, any such intervention must address negative provider attitudes, which women with disabilities have identified as a barrier to attending mammography (Mele, Archer, & Pusch, 2005). Notably, Verger et al. (2005) found that "discomfort with disability" was significantly associated with less frequent recommendation of screening or performance of breast exams for women with disabilities. Other factors associated with differential screening recommendation or performance of breast exams in women with disabilities included male gender, lack of time, lack of assistance during consultations, and communication difficulties with patients.

Women with disabilities who are motivated to attain mammography, whether upon a provider's recommendation or on their own initiative, need to be able to physically access it. In addition to financial issues, people with disabilities consistently report transportation as a barrier to accessing cancer services including mammography (Edwards et al., 2020). Concerns include difficulties with arranging services, unreliability, and entering and exiting vehicles. Furthermore, facilities must be accessible—with not only reserved parking, ramps, handrails, and automatic doors, but also adaptive equipment such as mammography machines that can be used at wheelchair height and assistive tools to assist with positioning (Edwards et al., 2020; Iezzoni, 2011). Women with disabilities have also suggested that having an additional technician to assist with difficulties in positioning would facilitate greater uptake of mammography (Edwards et al., 2020).

Healthy People 2020 includes an explicit objective of decreasing barriers to health care for people with disabilities, and the Affordable Care Act of 2010 included specific provisions for improving access to health care and adaptive equipment (Office of Disease Prevention and Health Promotion, 2017). These include provisions for the manufacture of accessible equipment, including mammography machines, as well as provisions to prohibit discrimination by health insurers and to generate educational opportunities to improve the quality of care for people with disabilities (Iezzoni, 2011). The current evidence supports policies that facilitate necessary environmental change, yet changes in related institutional and individual behaviors (e.g., purchasing the adaptive equipment, recommending mammography) may, as Iezzoni notes, require targeted intervention (Iezzoni, 2011) in order to reduce healthcare disparities among this population.

(Marrocco & Krouse, 2017). Mandates in the ACA have targeted standards for medical diagnostic equipment to meet regarding accessibility (Sect. 4203), yet one study reported that only 8% of CA primary care facilities had height-adjustable exam tables that could accommodate wheelchair users or others unable to step up and get on the standard exam table (Mudrick, Breslin, Liang, & Yee, 2012). The evidence demonstrates there are numerous levels where efforts can target to improve access to and the quality of health care for individuals with disabilities, which include physical access, insurance coverage, and cost concerns, as well as attitudinal factors.

4. *Neighborhood and Built Environment*

As research on social determinants has shifted away from microlevel factors, greater emphasis has focused on macro-level environments which shape health. Living in a disadvantaged neighborhood is typically associated with limited access to medical care, proximity to environmental pollutants, poorly maintained infrastructure, and higher levels of violent crime (Ellen, Mijanovich, & Dillman, 2001). Subsequently, individuals living in these disadvantaged neighborhoods report having poorer health, more chronic health conditions, and impaired physical functioning (Ross & Mirowsky, 2001). Poorer mental health is also commonly reported among these individuals and is believed to be partially impacted by greater exposure to trauma (Ellen et al., 2001).

Disadvantaged neighborhoods have also been shown to impact health-promoting behaviors. Low-income neighborhoods with poor access to supermarkets may have higher rates of obesity due to low-price stores actively marketing more junk foods even when store availability of healthy foods is comparable (Ghosh-Dastidar et al., 2014). Additionally, predominately Black and lower-income neighborhoods (as compared to predominately white and higher-income neighborhoods) have less healthy food availability in urban areas. Even within similar types of stores, e.g., supermarkets versus convenience stores, there remains variability in the availability of healthy foods based on neighborhood types (Franco, Roux, Glass, Caballero, & Brancati, 2008). Related factors, like housing affordability, which also tend to cluster by neighborhood, may result in decisional trade-offs between healthcare costs and other costs, which may negatively impact health (Pollack, Griffin, & Lynch, 2010).

The built environment shapes opportunity and health for all people, yet environmental obstacles that are unique to people with disabilities impact their access to health services, health behaviors, and health outcomes. A review asserted that while the ICF provides a useful framework for understanding the biopsychosocial elements of disability, the field still lacks direct measures and knowledge of how environmental factors affect health outcomes and participation among people with disability and limits our target corrective actions (Hammel et al., 2015). Environmental factors can cut across multiple levels of influence—individual, community, and societal—which make it difficult to discern the true effects of environment on opportunities for health and health-promoting activities (Magasi et al., 2015). For example, a wheelchair ramp may be available to someone with the appropriate funds, but they may not be safe to use if it's raining or snowing. Even with a ramp, lack of usable sidewalks, or transportation then limit ability to participate in the community and access health services. Current methods of measuring accessibility and resources among those with disability would not capture this nuance.

5. *Social and Community Context*

Social ties and social support are related to mental health, physical health, and longevity (Ertel, Glymour, & Berkman, 2009; Umberson & Karas Montez, 2010) with research showing that social support serves to buffer the negative effects of stress on individuals (Uchino, 2006, 2009). Several mechanisms have been proposed through which social ties and support may promote better health outcomes (Thoits, 2011). Some examples include providing people with emotional, information, and instrumental support; giving individuals a "role" identity (e.g., husband-wife, parent-child); providing a sense of belonging and companionship; and providing social control to monitor, encourage, remind, or persuade someone to follow positive health practices.

The relationship between social connectivity and positive health outcomes is also observed among people living with disability. Higher social support was associated with fewer depressive symptoms among older adults who experienced disability, with older men identified as the least likely to report adequate social support (Jensen et al., 2014). Higher social support has also been associated with lower perceived discrimination (Brown, 2010; Itzick, Kagan, & Tal-Katz, 2018). Although a systematic review reported equivocal evidence demonstrating a relationship between social support and lower levels of anxiety and depression, however the authors note that the nature of the support may have negative effects if the social interactions are unwelcome or stressful (Tough, Siegrist, & Fekete, 2017). Other published evidence indicated that those who acquire disability and have low social support or those who face declines in support after disability onset may experience worse mental health than those with consistently high social support (Aitken, Krnjacki, Kavanagh, LaMontagne, & Milner, 2017). These results were supported by another study that found adults with physical disabilities who experience reduced social support show an increase in depressive symptoms (de la Vega, Molton, Miró, Smith, & Jensen, 2019).

Factors in the macro-level social context, such as *discrimination* and *racism*, have been consistently shown to be associated with increased morbidity and mortality (Martinez et al., 2015). More specifically, a systematic meta-analysis found that racism was associated with poorer mental health, poorer general health, and poorer physical health, and these effects were not moderated by age, sex, birthplace, or education levels (Paradies et al., 2015). Some evidence suggests that institutional racism can impact health directly through stigma, stereotype threats, and prejudice of healthcare providers which can increase risk for chronic diseases through physiologic pathways (i.e., cardiovascular reactivity) or poorer quality of health care and treatment from providers with greater implicit biases. Racism can also indirectly impact health through systematic routes based on restricted socioeconomic mobility, poorer quality education, fewer employment opportunities, segregation into poor-quality housing, higher risk of exposure to environmental toxins, and higher rates of violent crime (Williams & Mohammed, 2013).

Discrimination based on disability may have similar negative effects on health. An Australian study found that people with disabilities who reported discrimination were more likely to experience psychological distress (Temple & Kelaher, 2018) and poorer self-reported health (Krnjacki et al., 2018). Perceived disability-related discrimination can result in people avoiding situations, with evidence showing that avoiding perceived discrimination limits participation in activities known to influence health—health care, education, employment, etc. (Temple, Kelaher, & Williams, 2018). Additional evidence demonstrates that disability-related discrimination is associated with worse sleep quality, which can result in poorer health outcomes (Vaghela & Sutin, 2016). People with disabilities also face greater risk of being victims of violence, due to factors such as lack of access to education and employment and dependence on others for care (Hughes et al., 2012). Those with more severe and/or apparent physical or mental disabilities are more likely to report being discriminated against in employment or education and to more often being humiliated or a victim of violence (Dammeyer & Chapman, 2018). Notably, the types of violence and discrimination differ between men and women (Daley, Phipps, & Branscombe, 2018).

Another social context illustrating the intersectionality of multiple social determinants is *incarceration*. Racial/ethnic minorities and individuals with lower educational attainment are often incarcerated at disproportionately higher rates (Freudenberg, 2002; The Pew Charitable Trusts, 2010; National Research Council, 2014). Incarceration has been shown to result in a negative change in health status and a greater number of health problems (Schnittker & John, 2007), higher rates of chronic disease, and greater substance abuse and mental illness as compared to the general population (Dumont, Brockmann, Dickman, Alexander, & Rich, 2012). One possible mechanism for this relationship could be the observed increase in body mass index associated with incarceration, which was also found to have a stronger effect for Black individuals and those with less education (Houle, 2014).

There is a higher prevalence of disability among the incarcerated population in the USA than the general population, with approximately 32% of prisoners and 40% of jail inmates having some form of hearing, vision, cognitive, ambulatory, and/or independent living disability (Reingle Gonzalez, Cannell, Jetelina, & Froehlich-Grobe, 2016; Vallas, 2016). Intellectual disability is particularly overrepresented among the

Addressing Multiple Determinants of Health: Targeting Obesity
Research to address the obesity epidemic, which has led to policy action, offers a useful example of how a social-ecological approach can be applied to a complex, multilevel health problem. A shift in obesity research occurred between 1995 and 2010 when studies moved from investigating person-level approaches for reducing obesity toward environmental or policy-level approaches (Sallis, Carlson, Mignano, Lemes, & Wagner, 2012). This was spurred by emerging evidence regarding the measurable impacts of social and environmental factors on obesity. Specifically, data revealed associations between SES-related factors of educational level (Molarius, Seidell, Sans, Tuomilehto, & Kuulasmaa, 2000), income inequality, environmental-level factors of neighborhood deprivation (Reidpath, Burns, Garrard, Mahoney, & Townsend, 2002), food cost, distance to grocery stores (Ghosh-Dastidar et al., 2014), walkability of neighborhood, and social support (Carlson et al., 2012) with increased likelihood of obesity and obesity-related illness. These findings led to research efforts focused on investigating upstream and macro-level factors. Such research also resulted in the term "obesogenic environment" (Egger & Swinburn, 1997), which refers to environmental changes such as pervasive availability of calorically dense foods and lack of physical activity opportunities, now accepted as a significant contributor to rising obesity rates (Lakerveld, Mackenbach, Rutter, & Brug, 2018).

This shift was also reflected in the WHO's Obesity Policy Action (OPA) model, which outlined upstream, midstream, and downstream targets for policy, research, and intervention (Sacks, Swinburn, & Lawrence, 2009). This and similar initiatives spurred additional research in policy and intervention approaches to understand how social and environmental factors impact obesity. Examples of two policy-level changes to influence dietary intake are the excise tax on sugar-sweetened beverages (SSBs) (Chriqui, Eidson, Bates, Kowalczyk, & Chaloupka, 2008; Smith, 2010) and restaurant menu-labeling with calorie information (Krieger et al., 2013; Radwan, Faroukh, & Obaid, 2017). A 2013 meta-analysis showed that SSBs are associated with a lower demand for SSBs and a decrease in BMI (Escobar, Veerman, Tollman, Bertram, & Hofman, 2013), yet menu labeling has yielded mixed results (Bollinger, Leslie, & Sorensen, 2011; Finkelstein, Strombotne, Chan, & Krieger, 2011).

Importantly, conducting interventions across multiple levels of influence allow for investigating the relative efficacy of macro-level versus microlevel interventions.

Successful interventions often target specific communities such as schools where there is more control over options available in the environment and where policy changes can impact the availability of food options (e.g., increase availability of fruit, vegetables, and milk or limiting higher fat foods or restricting sugar-sweetened beverages) (Craddock et al., 2011; Cullen, Watson, Zakeri, & Ralston, 2006; Mayne, Auchincloss, & Michael, 2015). These place-based interventions have yielded significant improvements in outcomes such as reduced caloric intake (Mendoza, Watson, & Cullen, 2010), reduced intake of SSB (Craddock et al., 2011; Cullen et al., 2006), and increased fruit and vegetable consumption (Hendy, Williams, & Camise, 2005). These macro-level targeted interventions may also be more effective across time if policy changes alter the underlying mechanisms related to health disparities (Rummo et al., 2019; Vo, Albrecht, & Kershaw, 2019).

incarcerated population, with a large systematic review concluding that internationally, about 0.5–1.5% of prisoners have an intellectual disability (Fazel, Xenitidis, & Powell, 2008; Young et al., 2017). Public health concerns include a lack of appropriate treatment and facilities for inmates with disabilities and lack of connection with needed resources post-release, resulting in recidivism and unaddressed health issues (Reingle Gonzalez et al., 2016; Vallas, 2016; Young et al., 2017).

This example shows the evolution of obesity research, which moved from focusing exclusively on individual-level factors (i.e., responsibility for making health behavior change) to a multilevel approach that includes studying factors that may influence dietary intake across different environments. Public health researchers in disability can learn from this body of research to target multiple levels of influence related to an array of health outcomes in disability such as physical activity, dietary intake, or cancer screening.

3.5   Conclusions

The evidence demonstrates that individuals who are socially disadvantaged have poorer health. Further, like the original SES research shows, increases in the number of social disadvantages results in a gradient-like increase in poorer health outcomes. As reported in various chapters in this book, the evidence reveals that individuals with disabilities have poorer health as measured across numerous outcomes than those in the general population. The information presented in this chapter demonstrates that relationships between social determinants and health are complex. Nevertheless, to fully address and reverse the health disparities facing the 53 (Courtney-Long et al., 2015) to 85 (Taylor, 2018) million Americans living with disability, it will be important to examine how these complex personal, social, and environmental factors influence the function, participation, and health status of individuals with disabilities. We need to investigate how upstream factors individually and collectively contribute to poorer health across a myriad of measured domains for people living with disabilities. The evidence presented in this chapter can offer a road map to those in public health in addressing macro-level systems and factors, bulleted here:

- Low employment rates.
- Lack of affordable and accessible housing and transportation.
- Unmet medical needs; high costs of medical supplies and prescription medications.
- Inadequate access to durable medical equipment and assistive technology.
- Inaccessible built environments that include sidewalks, parking lots, building entrances and bathrooms, and parks; fewer community-based recreation options.
- Higher rates of violence and discrimination.

In summary, the data reveal there are many leverage points that can be targeted to improve the health status of those with disabilities. While living with a disabling condition may impair one's daily functioning and necessitate use of adaptive equipment, many barriers a person faces to enjoying an active, rich, and healthy life reside in the social and physical environments. Now that we have more national data sources that include disability identifiers that can be analyzed to reveal the extent of disparities confronting individuals with disabilities, it is time to explore the fundamental causes of these disparities and target macro-level approaches to address these inequities. Public health professionals should ensure that people with disabilities have a seat and voice at the table to define the issues and identify solutions. This is a matter of social justice, as the World Health Organization states, "the development of a society, rich or poor, can be judged by the quality of its population's health, how fairly health is distributed across the social spectrum, and the degree of protection provided from disadvantage as a result of ill-health" (preface). We urge public health professionals beyond the fields of disability and rehabilitation to recognize that disability does not equal poor health, but rather that most health disparities can be prevented through addressing inaccessible environments and discrimination and targeting changes in services, systems, and policies can help to reduce the inequities.

References

Adler, N. E., Boyce, T., Chesney, M. A., Cohen, S., Folkman, S., Kahn, R. L., & Syme, S. L. (1994). Socioeconomic status and health: The challenge of the gradient. *American Psychologist, 49*(1), 15.

Adler, N. E., & Newman, K. (2002). Socioeconomic disparities in health: Pathways and policies. *Health Affairs, 21*(2), 60–76.

Aitken, Z., Krnjacki, L., Kavanagh, A. M., LaMontagne, A. D., & Milner, A. (2017). Does social support modify the effect of disability acquisition on mental health? A longitudinal study of

Australian adults. *Social Psychiatry and Psychiatric Epidemiology, 52*(10), 1247–1255. https://doi.org/10.1007/s00127-017-1418-5

Aitken, Z., Simpson, J. A., Bentley, R., & Kavanagh, A. M. (2017). Disability acquisition and mental health: Effect modification by demographic and socioeconomic characteristics using data from an Australian longitudinal study. *BMJ Open, 7*(9), e016953. https://doi.org/10.1136/bmjopen-2017-016953

Armour, B. S., Thierry, J. M., & Wolf, L. A. (2009). State-level differences in breast and cervical cancer screening by disability status, United States, 2008. *Women's Health Issues, 19*, 406–414. https://doi.org/10.1016/j.whi.2009.08.006

Baker, D. P., Leon, J., Smith Greenaway, E. G., Collins, J., & Movit, M. (2011). The education effect on population health: A reassessment. *Population and Development Review, 37*(2), 307–332.

Beatty, P. W., Hagglund, K. J., Neri, M. T., Dhont, K. R., Clark, M. J., & Hilton, S. A. (2003). Access to health care services among people with chronic or disabling conditions: Patterns and predictors. *Archives of Physical Medicine and Rehabilitation, 84*(10), 1417–1425.

Bellis, M., Hughes, K., Hardcastle, K., Ashton, K., Ford, K., Quigg, Z., & Davies, A. (2017). The impact of adverse childhood experiences on health service use across the life course using a retrospective cohort study. *Journal of Health Services Research and Policy, 22*(3), 168–177.

Bengtsson, S., & Datta Gupta, N. (2017). Identifying the effects of education on the ability to cope with a disability among individuals with disabilities. *PLoS One, 12*(3), e0173659. https://doi.org/10.1371/journal.pone.0173659

Berchick, E. R., Hood, E., & Barnett, J. C. (2018). *Health insurance coverage in the United States: 2017. Current population reports.* Washington, DC: US Government Printing Office.

Berkman, N. D., Sheridan, S. L., Donahue, K. E., Halpern, D. J., & Crotty, K. (2011). Low health literacy and health outcomes: An updated systematic review. *Annals of Internal Medicine, 155*(2), 97–107. https://doi.org/10.7326/0003-4819-155-2-201107190-00005

Berkowitz, S. A., Seligman, H. K., Meigs, J. B., & Basu, S. (2018). Food insecurity, healthcare utilization, and high cost: A longitudinal cohort study. *The American Journal of Managed Care, 24*(9), 399–404. Retrieved from https://www.ncbi.nlm.nih.gov/pubmed/30222918, https://www.ncbi.nlm.nih.gov/pmc/articles/PMC6426124/

Berthelot, J.-M., Wilkins, R., & Ng, E. (2002). Trends in mortality by neighbourhood income in urban Canada from 1971 to 1996 [Canadian Community Health Survey-2002 Annual Report]. *Health Reports, 13*, 45.

Bezyak, J. L., Sabella, S. A., & Gattis, R. H. (2017). Public transportation: An investigation of barriers for people with disabilities. *Journal of Disability Policy Studies, 28*(1), 52–60. https://doi.org/10.1177/1044207317702070

Billete, A., & Hill, G. B. (1978). The relative risk of mortality amongst males by social class in Canada 1974. *Union Medicale du Canada, 107*(6), 583–590. Retrieved from https://www.scopus.com/inward/record.uri?eid=2-s2.0-0018124260&partnerID=40&md5=1052639b529630af917bfab5933bc953

Bo'sher, L., Chan, S., Ellen, I. G., Karfunkel, B., & Liao, H.-L. (2015). Accessibility of America's housing stock: Analysis of the 2011 American Housing Survey (AHS). Available at *SSRN 3055191.*

Bollinger, B., Leslie, P., & Sorensen, A. (2011). Calorie posting in chain restaurants. *American Economic Journal: Economic Policy, 3*(1), 91–128.

Bowen, M. E., & González, H. M. (2010). Childhood socioeconomic position and disability in later life: Results of the health and retirement study. *American Journal of Public Health, 100*(S1), S197–S203. https://doi.org/10.2105/AJPH.2009.160986

Brandt, E. N., Jr., & Pope, A. M. (1997). Models of disability and rehabilitation. In E. N. Brandt Jr. & A. M. Pope (Eds.), *Enabling America: Assessing the role of rehabilitation science and engineering.* Washington, DC: National Academies Press.

Braveman, P., Egerter, S., & Williams, D. R. (2011). The social determinants of health: Coming of age. *Annual Review of Public Health, 32*, 381–398. https://doi.org/10.1146/annurev-publhealth-031210-101218

Braveman, P. A., Cubbin, C., Egerter, S., Williams, D. R., & Pamuk, E. (2010). Socioeconomic disparities in health in the United States: What the patterns tell us. *American Journal of Public Health, 100*(S1), S186–S196.

Braveman, P. A., Egerter, S. A., & Mockenhaupt, R. E. (2011). Broadening the focus: The need to address the social determinants of health. *American Journal of Preventive Medicine, 40*(1 Suppl 1), S4–S18. https://doi.org/10.1016/j.amepre.2010.10.002

Bronfenbrenner, U. (1977). Toward an experimental ecology of human development. *American Psychologist, 32*(7), 513–531. https://doi.org/10.1037/0003-066X.32.7.513

Bronfenbrenner, U. (1979). *The ecology of human development: Experiments by nature and design.* Cambridge, MA: Harvard University Press.

Brown, E. J., Polsky, D., Barbu, C. M., Seymour, J. W., & Grande, D. (2016). Racial disparities in geographic access to primary care in Philadelphia. *Health Affairs, 35*(8), 1374–1381. https://doi.org/10.1377/hlthaff.2015.1612

Brown, R. (2010). Physical disability and quality of life: The stress process and experience of stigma in a chronically-strained population.

Brucker, D. L. (2017). The association of food insecurity with health outcomes for adults with disabilities. *Disability and Health Journal, 10*(2), 286–293. https://doi.org/10.1016/j.dhjo.2016.12.006

Bureau of Labor Statistics. (2019). Persons with a disability: Labor force characteristics summary—2018. *Economics News Release.* Retrieved from https://www.bls.gov/news.release/pdf/disabl.pdf

Campbell, J. A., Walker, R. J., & Egede, L. E. (2016). Associations between adverse childhood experiences, high-risk behaviors, and morbidity in adulthood. *American Journal of Preventive Medicine, 50*(3), 344–352. https://doi.org/10.1016/j.amepre.2015.07.022

Carlson, J. A., Sallis, J. F., Conway, T. L., Saelens, B. E., Frank, L. D., Kerr, J., … King, A. C. (2012). Interactions between psychosocial and built environment factors in explaining older adults' physical activity. *Preventive Medicine, 54*(1), 68–73.

Centers for Disease Control and Prevention. (n.d.). *Disability and Health Data System (DHDS) data [online].* Retrieved from https://dhds.cdc.gov. from National Center on Birth Defects and Developmental Disabilities, Division of Human Development and Disability. https://dhds.cdc.gov

Chan, D. M., & Zoellick, M. R. B. (2011). *World report on disability* (p. 24). Geneva: WHO.

Charlton, J. I. (2000). *Nothing about us without us: Disability oppression and empowerment.* Berkeley, CA: Univ of California Press.

Chatzitheochari, S., & Platt, L. (2019). Disability differentials in educational attainment in England: Primary and secondary effects. *The British Journal of Sociology, 70*(2), 502–525. https://doi.org/10.1111/1468-4446.12372

Chriqui, J. F., Eidson, S. S., Bates, H., Kowalczyk, S., & Chaloupka, F. J. (2008). State sales tax rates for soft drinks and snacks sold through grocery stores and vending machines, 2007. *Journal of Public Health Policy, 29*(2), 226–249.

Commission on Social Determinants of Health. (2008). *Closing the gap in a generation: Health equity through action on the social determinants of health. Final report of the Commission on Social Determinants of Health.* Geneva: World Health Organization.

Courtney-Long, E. A., Carroll, D. D., Zhang, Q. C., Stevens, A. C., Griffin-Blake, S., & Armour, B. S. (2015). Prevalence of disability and disability types among adults—United States, 2013. *MMWR. Morbidity and Mortality Weekly Report, 64*(29), 777–783.

Craddock, A. L., McHugh, A., Mont-Ferguson, H., Grant, L., Barrett, J. L., & Wang, C. (2011). Effect of school district policy change on consumption of sugar-sweetened beverages among high school students, Boston, Massachusetts, 2004–2006. *Preventing Chronic Disease, 8*(4), A74.

Cullen, K. W., Watson, K., Zakeri, I., & Ralston, K. (2006). Exploring changes in middle-school student lunch consumption after local school food service policy modifications. *Public Health Nutrition, 9*(6), 814–820.

Daley, A., Phipps, S., & Branscombe, N. R. (2018). The social complexities of disability: Discrimination, belonging and life satisfaction among Canadian youth. *SSM - Population Health, 5*, 55–63. https://doi.org/10.1016/j.ssmph.2018.05.003

Dammeyer, J., & Chapman, M. (2018). A national survey on violence and discrimination among people with disabilities. *BMC Public Health, 18*(1), 355. https://doi.org/10.1186/s12889-018-5277-0

de la Vega, R., Molton, I. R., Miró, J., Smith, A. E., & Jensen, M. P. (2019). Changes in perceived social support predict changes in depressive symptoms in adults with physical disability. *Disability and Health Journal, 12*(2), 214–219. https://doi.org/10.1016/j.dhjo.2018.09.005

Delva, J., O'Malley, P. M., & Johnston, L. D. (2006). Racial/ethnic and socioeconomic status differences in overweight and health-related behaviors among American students: National trends 1986–2003. *Journal of Adolescent Health, 39*(4), 536–545. https://doi.org/10.1016/j.jadohealth.2006.02.013

DeWalt, D. A., Berkman, N. D., Sheridan, S., Lohr, K. N., & Pignone, M. P. (2004). Literacy and health outcomes. *Journal of General Internal Medicine, 19*(12), 1228–1239. https://doi.org/10.1111/j.1525-1497.2004.40153.x

Donnelly, C., McColl, M., Charlifue, S., Glass, C., O'Brien, P., Savic, G., & Smith, K. (2007). Utilization, access and satisfaction with primary care among people with spinal cord injuries: A comparison of three countries. *Spinal Cord, 45*(1), 25–36.

Dumont, D. M., Brockmann, B., Dickman, S., Alexander, N., & Rich, J. D. (2012). Public health and the epidemic of incarceration. *Annual Review of Public Health, 33*, 325–339.

Dwyer-Lindgren, L., Bertozzi-Villa, A., Stubbs, R. W., Morozoff, C., Mackenbach, J. P., Van Lenthe, F. J., … Murray, C. J. L. (2017). Inequalities in life expectancy among US counties, 1980 to 2014: Temporal trends and key drivers. *JAMA Internal Medicine, 177*(7), 1003–1011. https://doi.org/10.1001/jamainternmed.2017.0918

Edwards, D. J., Sakellariou, D., & Anstey, S. (2020). Barriers to, and facilitators of, access to cancer services and experiences of cancer care for adults with a physical disability: A mixed methods systematic review. *Disability and Health Journal, 13*(1), 100844.

Egger, G., & Swinburn, B. (1997). An "ecological" approach to the obesity pandemic. *British Medical Journal, 315*(7106), 477–480.

Ellen, I. G., Mijanovich, T., & Dillman, K.-N. (2001). Neighborhood effects on health: Exploring the links and assessing the evidence. *Journal of Urban Affairs, 23*(3–4), 391–408. https://doi.org/10.1111/0735-2166.00096

Ertel, K. A., Glymour, M. M., & Berkman, L. F. (2009). Social networks and health: A life course perspective integrating observational and experimental evidence. *Journal of Social and Personal Relationships, 26*(1), 73–92.

Escobar, M. A. C., Veerman, J. L., Tollman, S. M., Bertram, M. Y., & Hofman, K. J. (2013). Evidence that a tax on sugar sweetened beverages reduces the obesity rate: A meta-analysis. *BMC Public Health, 13*(1), 1072.

Fazel, S., Xenitidis, K., & Powell, J. (2008). The prevalence of intellectual disabilities among 12000 prisoners—A systematic review. *International Journal of Law and Psychiatry, 31*(4), 369–373. https://doi.org/10.1016/j.ijlp.2008.06.001

Fenelon, A., Mayne, P., Simon, A. E., Rossen, L. M., Helms, V., Lloyd, P., … Steffen, B. L. (2017). Housing assistance programs and adult health in the United States. *American Journal of Public Health, 107*(4), 571–578. https://doi.org/10.2105/AJPH.2016.303649

Finkelstein, E. A., Strombotne, K. L., Chan, N. L., & Krieger, J. (2011). Mandatory menu labeling in one fast-food chain in King County, Washington. *American Journal of Preventive Medicine, 40*(2), 122–127. https://doi.org/10.1016/j.amepre.2010.10.019

Florida, R., & Schneider, B. (2018). The global housing crisis. *CityLab*. Retrieved from https://www.citylab.com/equity/2018/04/the-global-housing-crisis/557639/

Fouts, B. S., Andersen, E., & Hagglund, K. (2000). Disability and satisfaction with access to health care. *Journal of Epidemiology and Community Health, 54*(10), 770–771.

Franco, M., Roux, A. V. D., Glass, T. A., Caballero, B., & Brancati, F. L. (2008). Neighborhood characteristics and availability of healthy foods in Baltimore. *American Journal of Preventive Medicine, 35*(6), 561–567.

Freudenberg, N. (2002). Adverse effects of US jail and prison policies on the health and well-being of women of color. *American Journal of Public Health, 92*(12), 1895–1899.

Gabel, J. R., Whitmore, H., Pickreign, J., Sellheim, W., Kc, S., & Bassett, V. (2008). After the mandates: Massachusetts employers continue to support health reform as more firms offer coverage: Bay State employers have fewer reservations about the reform than they did last year, shortly after the reform took effect. *Health Affairs, 27*(Suppl1), w566–w575.

Ghosh-Dastidar, B., Cohen, D., Hunter, G., Zenk, S. N., Huang, C., Beckman, R., & Dubowitz, T. (2014). Distance to store, food prices, and obesity in urban food deserts. *American Journal of Preventive Medicine, 47*(5), 587–595.

Goodman, N. (2015). The impact of employment on the health status and health care costs of working-age people with disabilities. *Lead Center Policy Brief.*

Gregorio, D. I., Walsh, S. J., & Paturzo, D. (1997). The effects of occupation-based social position on mortality in a large American cohort. *American Journal of Public Health, 87*(9), 1472–1475. https://doi.org/10.2105/AJPH.87.9.1472

Grosse, S. D., Lollar, D. J., Campbell, V. A., & Chamie, M. (2009). Disability and disability-adjusted life years: Not the same. *Public Health Reports, 124*(2), 197–202.

Gulliford, M., Figueroa-Munoz, J., Morgan, M., Hughes, D., Gibson, B., Beech, R., & Hudson, M. (2002). What does 'access to health care' mean? *Journal of Health Services Research and Policy, 7*(3), 186–188. https://doi.org/10.1258/135581902760082517

Gundersen, C., & Ziliak, J. P. (2015). Food insecurity and health outcomes. *Health Affairs, 34*(11), 1830–1839. https://doi.org/10.1377/hlthaff.2015.0645

Hahn, R. A., & Truman, B. I. (2015). Education improves public health and promotes health equity. *International Journal of Health Services: Planning, Administration, Evaluation, 45*(4), 657–678. https://doi.org/10.1177/0020731415585986

Haislmaier, E. F., & Owcharenko, N. (2006). The Massachusetts approach: A new way to restructure state health insurance markets and public programs. *Health Affairs, 25*(6), 1580–1590.

Hammel, J., Magasi, S., Heinemann, A., Gray, D. B., Stark, S., Kisala, P., … Hahn, E. A. (2015). Environmental barriers and supports to everyday participation: A qualitative insider perspective from people with disabilities. *Archives of Physical Medicine and Rehabilitation, 96*(4), 578–588. https://doi.org/10.1016/j.apmr.2014.12.008

Hardin, M. M., & Hardin, B. (2004). The supercrip; in sport media: Wheelchair athletes discuss hegemony's disabled hero. *Sociology of Sport Online-SOSOL, 7*(1).

Heflin, C. M., Altman, C. E., & Rodriguez, L. L. (2019). Food insecurity and disability in the United States. *Disability and Health Journal, 12*(2), 220–226. https://doi.org/10.1016/j.dhjo.2018.09.006

Hendy, H. M., Williams, K. E., & Camise, T. S. (2005). "Kids Choice" school lunch program increases children's fruit and vegetable acceptance. *Appetite, 45*(3), 250–263.

Henning-Smith, C., McAlpine, D., Shippee, T., & Priebe, M. (2013). Delayed and unmet need for medical care among publicly insured adults with disabilities. *Medical Care, 51*, 1015–1019.

Hollederer, A. (2015). Unemployment, health and moderating factors: The need for targeted health promotion. *Journal of Public Health, 23*(6), 319–325.

Horner-Johnson, W., Dobbertin, K., & Iezzoni, L. I. (2015). Disparities in receipt of breast and cervical cancer screening for rural women age 18 to 64 with disabilities. *Women's Health Issues, 25*(3), 246–253. https://doi.org/10.1016/j.whi.2015.02.004

Hosseinpoor, A., Stewart Williams, J., Jann, B., Kowal, P., Officer, A., Posarac, A., & Chatterji, S. (2012). Social determinants of sex differences in disability among older adults: A multi-country decomposition analysis using the World Health Survey. *International Journal for Equity in Health, 11*(1), 52. https://doi.org/10.1186/1475-9276-11-52

Houle, B. (2014). The effect of incarceration on adult male BMI trajectories, USA, 1981–2006. *Journal of Racial and Ethnic Health Disparities, 1*(1), 21–28.

Hughes, K., Bellis, M. A., Hardcastle, K. A., Sethi, D., Butchart, A., Mikton, C., … Dunne, M. P. (2017). The effect of multiple adverse childhood experiences on health: A systematic review and meta-analysis. *The Lancet Public Health, 2*(8), e356–e366.

Hughes, K., Bellis, M. A., Jones, L., Wood, S., Bates, G., Eckley, L., … Officer, A. (2012). Prevalence and risk of violence against adults with disabilities: A systematic review and meta-analysis of observational studies. *The Lancet, 379*(9826), 1621–1629. https://doi.org/10.1016/S0140-6736(11)61851-5

Iezzoni, L. I. (2011). Eliminating health and health care disparities among the growing population of people with disabilities. *Health Affairs, 30*(10), 1947–1954. https://doi.org/10.1377/hlthaff.2011.0613

Iezzoni, L. I., Davis, R. B., Soukup, J., & O'Day, B. (2002). Satisfaction with quality and access to health care among people with disabling conditions. *International Journal for Quality in Health Care, 14*(5), 369–381.

Iezzoni, L. I., Kurtz, S. G., & Rao, S. R. (2015). Trends in mammography over time for women with and without chronic disability. *Journal of Women's Health, 24*(7), 593–601.

Iezzoni, L. I., McCarthy, E. P., Davis, R. B., & Siebens, H. (2000). Mobility impairments and use of screening and preventive services. *The American Journal of Public Health, 90*(6), 955–961.

Institute of Medicine. (2001). *Health and behavior: The interplay of biological, behavioral, and societal influences*. Washington, DC: The National Academies Press.

Institute of Medicine. (2009). *In America's uninsured crisis: Consequences for health and health care*. Washington, DC: National Academies Press.

Itzick, M., Kagan, M., & Tal-Katz, P. (2018). Perceived social support as a moderator between perceived discrimination and subjective well-being among people with physical disabilities in Israel. *Disability and Rehabilitation, 40*(18), 2208–2216. https://doi.org/10.1080/09638288.2017.1331380

Jensen, M. P., Smith, A. E., Bombardier, C. H., Yorkston, K. M., Miró, J., & Molton, I. R. (2014). Social support, depression, and physical disability: Age and diagnostic group effects. *Disability and Health Journal, 7*(2), 164–172. https://doi.org/10.1016/j.dhjo.2013.11.001

Jha, A., Patrick, D. L., MacLehose, R. F., Doctor, J. N., & Chan, L. (2002). Dissatisfaction with medical services among Medicare beneficiaries with disabilities. *Archives of Physical Medicine and Rehabilitation, 83*(10), 1335–1341.

Kavanagh, A. M., Krnjacki, L., Aitken, Z., LaMontagne, A. D., Beer, A., Baker, E., & Bentley, R. (2015). Intersections between disability, type of impairment, gender and socio-economic disadvantage in a nationally representative sample of 33,101 working-aged Australians. *Disability and Health Journal, 8*(2), 191–199. https://doi.org/10.1016/j.dhjo.2014.08.008

Keith, K. (2019). *Uninsured rate rose in 2018, says Census Bureau report*. Retrieved from https://www.healthaffairs.org/do/10.1377/hblog20190911.805983/full/

Kindig, D. A., & Movassaghi, H. (1989). The adequacy of physician supply in small rural counties. *Health Affairs, 8*(2), 63–76.

Kocman, A., Fischer, L., & Weber, G. (2018). The Employers' perspective on barriers and facilitators to employment of people with intellectual disability: A differential mixed-method approach. *Journal of Applied Research in Intellectual Disabilities, 31*(1), 120–131. https://doi.org/10.1111/jar.12375

Kraus, L., Lauer, E., Coleman, R., & Houtenville, A. (2018). Disability statistics annual report. *University of New Hampshire*, 48.

Krieger, J. W., Chan, N. L., Saelens, B. E., Ta, M. L., Solet, D., & Fleming, D. W. (2013). Menu labeling regulations and calories purchased at chain restaurants. *American Journal of Preventive Medicine, 44*(6), 595–604. https://doi.org/10.1016/j.amepre.2013.01.031

Krnjacki, L., Priest, N., Aitken, Z., Emerson, E., Llewellyn, G., King, T., & Kavanagh, A. (2018). Disability-based discrimination and health: Findings from an Australian-based population study. *Australian and New Zealand Journal of Public Health, 42*(2), 172–174. https://doi.org/10.1111/1753-6405.12735

Kushel, M. B., Gupta, R., Gee, L., & Haas, J. S. (2006). Housing instability and food insecurity as barriers to health care among low-income Americans. *Journal of General Internal Medicine, 21*(1), 71–77. https://doi.org/10.1111/j.1525-1497.2005.00278.x

Lakerveld, J., Mackenbach, J. D., Rutter, H., & Brug, J. (2018). Obesogenic environment and obesogenic behaviours. In C. Hankey & K. Whelan (Eds.), *Advanced nutrition and dietetics in obesity* (p. 132). Hoboken, NJ: Wiley.

Lang, J., McKie, J., Smith, H., McLaughlin, A., Gillberg, C., Shiels, P. G., & Minnis, H. (2019). Adverse childhood experiences, epigenetics and telomere length variation in childhood and beyond: A systematic review of the literature. *European Child & Adolescent Psychiatry.* https://doi.org/10.1007/s00787-019-01329-1

Lantz, P. M., House, J. S., Lepkowski, J. M., Williams, D. R., Mero, R. P., & Chen, J. (1998). Socioeconomic factors, health behaviors, and mortality: Results from a nationally representative prospective study of US adults. *Journal of the American Medical Association, 279*(21), 1703–1708. https://doi.org/10.1001/jama.279.21.1703

Lee, J. O., Kosterman, R., Jones, T. M., Herrenkohl, T. I., Rhew, I. C., Catalano, R. F., & Hawkins, J. D. (2016). Mechanisms linking high school graduation to health disparities in young adulthood: A longitudinal analysis of the role of health behaviours, psychosocial stressors, and health insurance. *Public Health, 139*, 61–69.

Link, B. G., & Phelan, J. (1995). Social conditions as fundamental causes of disease. *Journal of Health and Social Behavior*, 80–94.

Luo, W., & Wang, F. (2003). Measures of spatial accessibility to health care in a GIS environment: Synthesis and a case study in the Chicago region. *Environment and Planning B: Planning and Design, 30*(6), 865–884.

Mackenbach, J. P., Bopp, M., Deboosere, P., Kovacs, K., Leinsalu, M., Martikainen, P., … de Gelder, R. (2017). Determinants of the magnitude of socioeconomic inequalities in mortality: A study of 17 European countries. *Health & Place, 47*, 44–53. https://doi.org/10.1016/j.healthplace.2017.07.005

Magasi, S., Wong, A., Gray, D. B., Hammel, J., Baum, C., Wang, C.-C., & Heinemann, A. W. (2015). Theoretical foundations for the measurement of environmental factors and their impact on participation among people with disabilities. *Archives of Physical Medicine and Rehabilitation, 96*(4), 569–577. https://doi.org/10.1016/j.apmr.2014.12.002

Marmot, M. G., Rose, G., Shipley, M., & Hamilton, P. J. S. (1978). Employment grade and coronary heart disease in British civil servants. *Journal of Epidemiology and Community Health, 32*(4), 244–249. https://doi.org/10.1136/jech.32.4.244

Marmot, M. G., Shipley, M. J., & Rose, G. (1984). Inequalities in death-specific explanations of a general pattern? *The Lancet, 323*(8384), 1003–1006. https://doi.org/10.1016/S0140-6736(84)92337-7

Marmot, M. G., Stansfeld, S., Patel, C., North, F., Head, J., White, I., … Smith, G. D. (1991). Health inequalities among British civil servants: The Whitehall II study. *The Lancet, 337*(8754), 1387–1393.

Marrocco, A., & Krouse, H. J. (2017). Obstacles to preventive care for individuals with disability: Implications for nurse practitioners. *Journal of the American Association of Nurse Practitioners, 29*(5), 282–293. https://doi.org/10.1002/2327-6924.12449

Martinez, O., Wu, E., Sandfort, T., Dodge, B., Carballo-Dieguez, A., Pinto, R., … Chavez-Baray, S. (2015). Evaluating the impact of immigration policies on health status among undocumented immigrants: A systematic review. *Journal of Immigrant and Minority Health, 17*(3), 947–970. https://doi.org/10.1007/s10903-013-9968-4

Martz, E., Livneh, H., Priebe, M., Wuermser, L. A., & Ottomanelli, L. (2005). Predictors of psychosocial adaptation among people with spinal cord injury or disorder. *Archives of Physical Medicine and Rehabilitation, 86*(6), 1182–1192.

Mayne, S. L., Auchincloss, A. H., & Michael, Y. L. (2015). Impact of policy and built environment changes on obesity-related outcomes: A systematic review of naturally occurring experiments. *Obesity Reviews, 16*(5), 362–375.

McCarthy, E. P., Ngo, L. H., Roetzheim, R. G., Chirikos, T. N., Li, D., Drews, R. E., & Iezzoni, L. I. (2006). Disparities in breast cancer treatment and survival for women with disabilities. *Annals of Internal Medicine, 145*(9), 637–645.

McEwen, B. S. (1998). Protective and damaging effects of stress mediators. *New England Journal of Medicine, 338*(3), 171–179.

Mele, N., Archer, J., & Pusch, B. D. (2005). Access to breast cancer screening services for women with disabilities. *Journal of Obstetric, Gynecologic, and Neonatal Nursing, 34*(4), 453–464. https://doi.org/10.1177/0884217505276158

Mendoza, J. A., Watson, K., & Cullen, K. W. (2010). Change in dietary energy density after implementation of the Texas Public School Nutrition Policy. *Journal of the American Dietetic Association, 110*(3), 434–440.

Molarius, A., Seidell, J. C., Sans, S., Tuomilehto, J., & Kuulasmaa, K. (2000). Educational level, relative body weight, and changes in their association over 10 years: An international perspective from the WHO MONICA Project. *American Journal of Public Health, 90*(8), 1260.

Montez, J. K., Zajacova, A., & Hayward, M. D. (2017). Disparities in disability by educational attainment across US states. *American Journal of Public Health, 107*(7), 1101–1108. https://doi.org/10.2105/AJPH.2017.303768

Mudrick, N. R., Breslin, M. L., Liang, M. H., & Yee, S. (2012). Physical accessibility in primary health care settings: Results from California on-site reviews. *Disability and Health Journal, 5*(3), 159–167. https://doi.org/10.1016/j.dhjo.2012.02.002

Nagi, S. Z. (1964). A study in the evaluation of disability and rehabilitation potential: Concepts, methods, and procedures. *American Journal of Public Health and the Nations Health, 54*(9), 1568–1579.

Nagi, S. Z. (1965). Some conceptual issues in disability and rehabilitation. In M. Sussman (Ed.), *Sociology and rehabilitation*. Washington, DC: American Sociological Society.

Nagi, S. Z. (1969). Disability and rehabilitation: Legal, clinical, and self-concepts and measurement. Columbus, OH: Ohio State University Press

National Center on Injury Prevention and Control. (n.d.). *The social-ecological model: A framework for prevention*. Retrieved from https://www.cdc.gov/violenceprevention/publichealthissue/social-ecologicalmodel.html

National Research Council (2014). The Growth of Incarceration in the United States: Exploring Causes and Consequences. Committee on Causes and Consequences of High Rates of Incarceration, J. Travis, B. Western, and S. Redburn, Editors. Committee on Law and Justice, Division of Behavioral and Social Sciences and Education. Washington, DC: The National Academies Press.

National Council on Disability. (2015). *Transportation Update: Where we've gone and what we've learned*. Washington DC: National Council on Disability.

Nosek, M. A., & Howland, C. A. (1997). Breast and cervical cancer screening among women with physical disabilities. *Archives of Physical Medicine and Rehabilitation, 78*(12 Suppl 5), S39–S44.

Office of Disease Prevention and Health Promotion. (2017). *HealthyPeople.gov: Cancer objectives*. Retrieved from https://www.healthypeople.gov/2020/topics-objectives/topic/cancer/objectives

Office of Public Affairs. (2018, November 21). *Justice Department obtains $11.3 million settlement of disability-based housing discrimination lawsuit in District of Columbia. 18-450*. Retrieved from https://www.justice.gov/opa/pr/justice-department-obtains-113-million-settlement-disability-based-housing-discrimination

Organisation for Economic, C.-o., Development Directorate for Employment, L., & Social, A. (2009). Sickness, disability and work. *Background Paper, 44*.

Paradies, Y., Ben, J., Denson, N., Elias, A., Priest, N., Pieterse, A., … Gee, G. (2015). Racism as a determinant of health: A systematic review and meta-analysis. *PLoS One, 10*(9), e0138511.

Peacock, G., Iezzoni, L. I., & Harkin, T. R. (2015). Health care for Americans with disabilities—25 years after the ADA. *New England Journal of Medicine, 373*(10), 892–893. https://doi.org/10.1056/NEJMp1508854

Peterson, E. B., Ostroff, J. S., DuHamel, K. N., D'Agostino, T. A., Hernandez, M., Canzona, M. R., & Bylund, C. L. (2016). Impact of provider-patient communication on cancer screening adherence: A systematic review. *Preventive Medicine, 93*, 96–105. https://doi.org/10.1016/j.ypmed.2016.09.034

Pickett, K. E., & Pearl, M. (2001). Multilevel analyses of neighbourhood socioeconomic context and health outcomes: A critical review. *Journal of Epidemiology and Community Health, 55*(2), 111–122.

Pollack, C. E., Griffin, B. A., & Lynch, J. (2010). Housing affordability and health among homeowners and renters. *American Journal of Preventive Medicine, 39*(6), 515–521. https://doi.org/10.1016/j.amepre.2010.08.002

Radwan, H., Faroukh, E. M., & Obaid, R. S. (2017). Menu labeling implementation in dine-in restaurants: The Public's knowledge, attitude and practices. *Archives of Public Health, 75*(1), 8.

Reidpath, D. D., Burns, C., Garrard, J., Mahoney, M., & Townsend, M. (2002). An ecological study of the relationship between social and environmental determinants of obesity. *Health & Place, 8*(2), 141–145.

Reingle Gonzalez, J. M., Cannell, M. B., Jetelina, K. K., & Froehlich-Grobe, K. (2016). Disproportionate prevalence rate of prisoners with disabilities: Evidence from a nationally representative sample. *Journal of Disability Policy Studies, 27*(2), 106–115. https://doi.org/10.1177/1044207315616809

Reyes, E. A., & Zahniser, D. (2016, August 30). L.A. to spend more the $200 million to settle suit on housing for disabled. *Los Angeles Times.* Retrieved from https://www.latimes.com/local/lanow/la-me-ln-housing-settlement-disabled-20160828-snap-story.html

Richman, L., Pearson, J., Beasley, C., & Stanifer, J. (2019). Addressing health inequalities in diverse, rural communities: An unmet need. *SSM-Population Health, 7*, 100398.

Rock, M. (2000). Discounted lives? Weighing disability when measuring health and ruling on "compassionate" murder. *Social Science & Medicine, 51*(3), 407–417.

Rogers, R. G., Everett, B. G., Zajacova, A., & Hummer, R. A. (2010). Educational degrees and adult mortality risk in the United States. *Biodemography and Social Biology, 56*(1), 80–99.

Ross, C., & Mirowsky, J. (2001). Neighborhood disadvantage, disorder, and health. *Journal of Health and Social Behavior, 42*, 258–276.

Ross, N. A., Garner, R., Bernier, J., Feeny, D. H., Kaplan, M. S., McFarland, B., … Oderkirk, J. (2012). Trajectories of health-related quality of life by socio-economic status in a nationally representative Canadian cohort. *Journal of Epidemiology and Community Health, 66*(7), 593–598.

Rummo, P. E., Feldman, J. M., Lopez, P., Lee, D., Thorpe, L. E., & Elbel, B. (2019). Impact of changes in the food, built, and socioeconomic environment on BMI in US counties, BRFSS 2003-2012. *Obesity.*

Sacks, G., Swinburn, B., & Lawrence, M. (2009). Obesity Policy Action framework and analysis grids for a comprehensive policy approach to reducing obesity. *Obesity Reviews, 10*(1), 76–86.

Sallis, J. F., Carlson, J. A., Mignano, A. M., Lemes, A., & Wagner, N. (2012). Trends in presentations of environmental and policy studies related to physical activity, nutrition, and obesity at society of behavioral medicine, 1995–2010: A commentary to accompany the active living research supplement to annals of behavioral medicine. *Annals of Behavioral Medicine, 45*(suppl_1), S14–S17.

Schnittker, J., & John, A. (2007). Enduring stigma: The long-term effects of incarceration on health. *Journal of Health and Social Behavior, 48*(2), 115–130.

Schüssler-Fiorenza Rose, S. M., Xie, D., & Stineman, M. (2014). Adverse childhood experiences and disability in U.S. adults. *PM&R, 6*(8), 670–680. https://doi.org/10.1016/j.pmrj.2014.01.013

Schwartz, N., Buliung, R., & Wilson, K. (2019). Disability and food access and insecurity: A scoping review of the literature. *Health & Place, 57*, 107–121. https://doi.org/10.1016/j.healthplace.2019.03.011

Seeman, T., Epel, E., Gruenewald, T., Karlamangla, A., & McEwen, B. S. (2010). Socio-economic differentials in peripheral biology: Cumulative allostatic load. *Annals of the New York Academy of Sciences, 1186*, 223–239. https://doi.org/10.1111/j.1749-6632.2009.05341.x

Seeman, T. E., McEwen, B. S., Rowe, J. W., & Singer, B. H. (2001). Allostatic load as a marker of cumulative biological risk: MacArthur studies of successful aging. *Proceedings of the National Academy of Sciences, 98*(8), 4770–4775.

Seligman, H. K., Bindman, A. B., Vittinghoff, E., Kanaya, A. M., & Kushel, M. B. (2007). Food insecurity is associated with diabetes mellitus: Results from the National Health Examination and Nutrition Examination Survey (NHANES) 1999–2002. *Journal of General Internal Medicine, 22*(7), 1018–1023. https://doi.org/10.1007/s11606-007-0192-6

Serafini, M. W. (2018). For people with disabilities, a fight for access to housing. *Health Affairs, 37*(3), 346–348. https://doi.org/10.1377/hlthaff.2018.0050

Silva, C. F., & Howe, P. D. (2012). The (In)validity of supercrip representation of para-lympian athletes. *Journal of Sport and Social Issues, 36*(2), 174–194. https://doi.org/10.1177/0193723511433865

Singer, A. J., Thode, H. C., & Pines, J. M. (2019). US emergency department visits and hospital discharges among uninsured patients before and after implementation of the Affordable Care Act. *JAMA Network Open, 2*(4), e192662–e192662.

Smith, T. A. (2010). *Taxing caloric sweetened beverages: Potential effects on beverage consumption, calorie intake, and obesity.* Darby, PA: Economic Research Service, USDA: DIANE publishing.

Sommers, B. D., Gunja, M. Z., Finegold, K., & Musco, T. (2015). Changes in self-reported insurance coverage, access to care, and health under the Affordable Care Act. *JAMA, 314*(4), 366–374. https://doi.org/10.1001/jama.2015.8421

Stahre, M., VanEenwyk, J., Siegel, P., & Njai, R. (2015). Housing insecurity and the association with health outcomes and unhealthy behaviors, Washington State, 2011. *Preventing Chronic Disease, 12*, E109–E109. https://doi.org/10.5888/pcd12.140511

Steinwachs, D., Allen, J. D., Barlow, W. E., Duncan, R. P., Egede, L. E., Friedman, L. S., … LaVeist, T. A. (2010). NIH state-of-the-science conference statement: Enhancing use and quality of colorectal cancer screening. *NIH Consensus and State-of-the-Science Statements, 27*(1), 1–31.

Steptoe, A., & Feldman, P. J. (2001). Neighborhood problems as sources of chronic stress: Development of a measure of neighborhood problems, and associations with socioeconomic status and health. *Annals of Behavioral Medicine, 23*(3), 177–185.

Story, M. F., Schwier, E., & Kailes, J. I. (2009). Perspectives of patients with disabilities on the accessibility of medical equipment: Examination tables, imaging equipment, medical chairs, and weight scales. *Disability and Health Journal, 2*(4), 169–179.e161.

Strully, K. W. (2009). Job loss and health in the U.S. labor market. *Demography, 46*(2), 221–246. https://doi.org/10.1353/dem.0.0050

Taylor, D. (2018). Americans with disabilities: 2014. *Curr Popul Rep* P70-152, U.S. Census Bureau, Washington, DC

Temple, J. B., & Kelaher, M. (2018). Is disability exclusion associated with psychological distress? Australian evidence from a national cross-sectional survey. *BMJ Open, 8*(5), e020829. https://doi.org/10.1136/bmjopen-2017-020829

Temple, J. B., Kelaher, M., & Williams, R. (2018). Discrimination and avoidance due to disability in Australia: Evidence from a National Cross Sectional Survey. *BMC Public Health, 18*(1), 1347. https://doi.org/10.1186/s12889-018-6234-7

The Pew Charitable Trusts (2010) Collateral Costs: Incarceration's Effect on Economic Mobility. Washington, DC: The Pew Charitable Trusts.

Thoits, P. A. (2011). Mechanisms linking social ties and support to physical and mental health. *Journal of Health and Social Behavior, 52*(2), 145–161.

Tough, H., Siegrist, J., & Fekete, C. (2017). Social relationships, mental health and wellbeing in physical disability: A systematic review. *BMC Public Health, 17*(1), 414. https://doi.org/10.1186/s12889-017-4308-6

Turner, J. B., & Turner, R. J. (2004). Physical disability, unemployment, and mental health. *Rehabilitation Psychology, 49*(3), 241.

U.S. Department of Health and Human Services. (n.d.). *Healthy people 2020.* Retrieved from http://www.healthypeople.gov/2020/topicsobjectives2020/objectiveslist.aspx?topicId=33

U.S. Department of Health and Human Services, & Office of Disease Prevention and Health Promotion. (2010). *National action plan to improve health literacy*. Washington, DC: U.S. Department of Health and Human Services.

U.S. Department of Health and Human Services, & Office of Disease Prevention and Health Promotion. (2020). *Healthy people 2020: Social determinants of health*. Internet.

U.S. Department of Health and Human Services and U.S. Department of Agriculture. (2015). *2015–2020 Dietary guidelines for Americans*. Washington, DC: U.S. Government Printing Office. Retrieved from http://health.gov/dietaryguidelines/2015/guidelines/

Uchino, B. N. (2006). Social support and health: A review of physiological processes potentially underlying links to disease outcomes. *Journal of Behavioral Medicine, 29*(4), 377–387.

Uchino, B. N. (2009). Understanding the links between social support and physical health: A life-span perspective with emphasis on the separability of perceived and received support. *Perspectives on Psychological Science, 4*(3), 236–255.

Umberson, D., & Karas Montez, J. (2010). Social relationships and health: A flashpoint for health policy. *Journal of Health and Social Behavior, 51*(1_suppl), S54–S66.

Vaghela, P., & Sutin, A. R. (2016). Discrimination and sleep quality among older US adults: The mediating role of psychological distress. *Sleep Health, 2*(2), 100–108. https://doi.org/10.1016/j.sleh.2016.02.003

Vallas, R. (2016). The mass incarceration of people with disabilities in America's jails and prisons. *Center for American Progress, 34*.

Verger, P., Aulagnier, M., Souville, M., Ravaud, J. F., Lussault, P. Y., Garnier, J. P., & Paraponaris, A. (2005). Women with disabilities: General practitioners and breast cancer screening. *American Journal of Preventive Medicine, 28*(2), 215–220. https://doi.org/10.1016/j.amepre.2004.10.010

Vo, L., Albrecht, S. S., & Kershaw, K. N. (2019). Multilevel interventions to prevent and reduce obesity. *Current Opinion in Endocrine and Metabolic Research, 4*, 62–69.

Waddell, G., & Burton, A. K. (2006). *Is work good for your health and well-being?* The Stationery Office.

Wei, W., Findley, P. A., & Sambamoorthi, U. (2006). Disability and receipt of clinical preventive services among women. *Women's Health Issues, 16*(6), 286–296.

Wherry, L. R., & Miller, S. (2016). Early coverage, access, utilization, and health effects associated with the affordable care act medicaid expansions: A quasi-experimental study. *Annals of Internal Medicine, 164*(12), 795–803. https://doi.org/10.7326/M15-2234

Wilkins, R., Tjepkema, M., Mustard, C., & Choinière, R. (2008). The Canadian census mortality follow-up study, 1991 through 2001. *Health Reports, 19*(3), 25.

Williams, D. R. (1999). Race, socioeconomic status, and health the added effects of racism and discrimination ESN - 1749-6632. *Annals of the New York Academy of Sciences, 896*(1), 173–188. https://doi.org/10.1111/j.1749-6632.1999.tb08114.x

Williams, D. R., & Mohammed, S. A. (2013). Racism and health I: Pathways and scientific evidence. *American Behavioral Scientist, 57*(8), 1152–1173.

Williams, D. R., Mohammed, S. A., Leavell, J., & Collins, C. (2010). Race, socioeconomic status, and health: Complexities, ongoing challenges, and research opportunities. *Annals of the New York Academy of Sciences, 1186*, 69–101. https://doi.org/10.1111/j.1749-6632.2009.05339.x

Wing, S., Casper, M., Hayes, C., Dargent-Molina, P., Riggan, W., & Tyroler, H. A. (1987). Changing association between community occupational structure and ischaemic heart disease mortality in the United States. *The Lancet, 330*(8567), 1067–1070. https://doi.org/10.1016/S0140-6736(87)91490-5

World Health Organization. (2001). *International Classification of functioning, disability, and health*. Geneva: World Health Organization.

Yen, I. H., & Syme, S. L. (1999). The social environment and health: A discussion of the epidemiologic literature. *Annual Review of Public Health, 20*(1), 287–308.

Young, J. T., Cumming, C., van Dooren, K., Lennox, N. G., Alati, R., Spittal, M. J., … Kinner, S. A. (2017). Intellectual disability and patient activation after release from prison: A prospective cohort study: Intellectual disability and patient activation. *Journal of Intellectual Disability Research, 61*(10), 939–956. https://doi.org/10.1111/jir.12349

Chapter 4
Disability, Intersectionality, and Inequity: Life at the Margins

Willi Horner-Johnson

4.1 Introduction

As a whole, the population of people with disabilities experiences substantial health inequities in comparison to people without disabilities. Those disparities can be magnified when disability intersects with other marginalized sociodemographic characteristics. This chapter briefly summarizes some of the inequities experienced by people with disabilities, broadly speaking. It then presents evidence of even greater inequities among people with disabilities in historically minority racial and ethnic groups, women with disabilities, sexual and gender diverse individuals with disabilities, and people with disabilities living in rural areas. The chapter closes with a discussion of the need for targeted efforts to address inequities at these intersections and promote health across the full diversity of the disability population.

4.2 Key Concepts

4.2.1 Inequality, Inequity, and Disparity

The words inequality, inequity, and disparity are easily confused. The term health disparity is primarily used in the United States, while other countries more commonly use the terms health inequality and health inequity (Carter-Pokras & Baquet, 2002). Inequality simply describes differences between groups. Such differences

W. Horner-Johnson (✉)
Institute on Development and Disability, Oregon Health & Science University,
Portland, OR, USA

OHSU-PSU School of Public Health, Portland, OR, USA
e-mail: hornerjo@ohsu.edu

© Springer Science+Business Media, LLC, part of Springer Nature 2021
D. J. Lollar et al. (eds.), *Public Health Perspectives on Disability*,
https://doi.org/10.1007/978-1-0716-0888-3_4

could occur for any number of reasons; the existence of inequality does not necessarily indicate a need for intervention. In contrast, inequity refers specifically to a difference that is unjust or unfair. Thus, the term inequity carries an ethical judgement regarding the cause of the difference (Carter-Pokras & Baquet, 2002). The interpretation of the word disparity has shifted somewhat over time. Disparity has often been defined as a synonym of inequality: a difference without a value judgment. However, in recent decades and especially in public health contexts, the concepts of injustice and lack of fairness have been attached to the term disparity (Carter-Pokras & Baquet, 2002). Healthy People 2020 defined health disparities specifically as differences linked to economic, social, or environmental disadvantage. Based on this definition, Braveman (2014, p.7) asserted that "health disparities are inequitable, even when we do not know the causes, because they put an already economically/socially disadvantaged group at further disadvantage with respect to their health."

Distinctions between inequality and inequity also apply to decisions about how to distribute resources. Should public health resources be distributed evenly to all (equality), or should more resources be allocated to those with greater need (equity)? If we are to reduce disparities between population groups, then groups that have historically been disadvantaged should receive more intensive and targeted public health resources to help overcome the disproportionate burden of poor health experienced by these groups. Similarly, different population groups have different levels of need for healthcare resources. People with disabilities often need more frequent and more specialized care than is the case for people without disabilities. Equitable distribution of healthcare resources would recognize those greater needs and provide care according to need. Distinguishing between equal and equitable access to health care is important when analyzing public health data. For example, if we simply look at receipt of a minimum basic level of health care, people with disabilities appear to be faring well: 71% of adults with disabilities have had a routine checkup in the past year compared to 68% of adults without disabilities (CDC, 2019). However, adults with disabilities are more than twice as likely as adults without disabilities to have unmet healthcare needs due to cost (26% versus 10%). Clearly, people with disabilities need more health care than they are able to obtain. The inability to afford that care is in indicator of inequity.

4.2.2 Disability Versus Poor Health

In the public health field, disability is commonly seen as a health problem that public health interventions are intended to prevent. In essence, disability is assumed to be equivalent to poor health. From this perspective, poor health among people with disabilities is simply to be expected rather than being considered inequitable. Conversely, researchers and practitioners who focus on the health of people with disabilities perceive disability and health as separate concepts. The latter view, which is the one underlying this book, acknowledges that people can both have a disability *and* be healthy. In fact, a consistent finding in national surveys is that more than half of adults with disabilities describe their health as excellent, very good, or good (CDC, 2019; Wolf, Armour, & Campbell, 2008). While that is substantially lower than the proportion of people without disabilities who describe their health in such terms, it does indicate that it is entirely possible to have a disability and enjoy positive health. The challenge for public health is to ensure that people with disabilities have equitable access to the means and opportunities for living healthy lives.

4.3   Health Inequities Experienced by People with Disabilities

There is ample evidence of health differences between people with and without disabilities. What has proven more difficult is convincing public health professionals and agencies that at least some of these differences represent inequities rather than being an inherent component of the disability experience (Krahn, Klein Walker, & Correa-De-Araujo, 2015). Indeed, there are some conditions for which people with disabilities are at greater risk specifically because of their underlying disabilities; these are called secondary conditions (Turk, 2006). Examples include urinary tract infections and pressure ulcers among people with spinal cord injuries and aspiration pneumonia among people with cerebral palsy. We expect such conditions to be more common among people with disabilities than among people without disabilities, because they typically would not exist in the absence of the primary disability (Turk, 2006). Thus, differences between people with and without disabilities in the occurrence of these conditions are not necessarily unfair. At the same time—because there are certain known risks for people with certain types of disabling conditions—we expect medical care for people with those primary disabling conditions to be more intensely directed toward preventing secondary conditions to the maximum extent possible and providing early treatment of those that occur (Turk, 2006). Within the population of people with disabilities, some groups receive less preventive medical care than others, have insurance plans that more aggressively limit coverage for preventive items such as durable medical equipment and sufficient catheter supplies, and have fewer resources available to help advocate for their health needs. These differences are linked to uneven access to social determinants of health and may result in inequitable distribution of secondary conditions among people with disabilities.

Importantly, it is not only secondary conditions that are more common among people with disabilities than among people without disabilities. Many chronic conditions that affect people both with and without disabilities are markedly more prevalent among people with disabilities. For example, age-adjusted analyses of data from the US adult population indicate that people with disabilities are significantly more likely to have cancer (8.8% vs. 5.1%), chronic obstructive pulmonary disease (13.7% vs. 3.0%), hypertension (41.9% vs. 25.9%), obesity (39.5% vs. 26.3%), and diabetes (16.2% vs. 7.1%) than their counterparts without disabilities (CDC, 2019).

If we accept Braveman's (2014) premise that health differences between socially advantaged and socially disadvantaged groups are inherently inequitable, then the differences between people with and without disabilities should be seen as evidence of inequity. People with disabilities are demonstrably disadvantaged in our society. For much of the nineteenth and twentieth centuries, many people with disabilities were excluded from society entirely and isolated in institutions. It was not until 1974 that legislation was passed to guarantee a free and appropriate public education to children with disabilities. The Americans with Disabilities Act—the first comprehensive legislation prohibiting discrimination against people with disabilities—was signed in 1990. As noted in the chapter on Social Determinants of Health (Chap. 3), people with disabilities are more than twice as likely to live in poverty as people without disabilities. For any other population group, the presence of such disadvantages would lead to the conclusion that health differences between the disadvantaged group and those with more economic and social advantages are inequitable, regardless of whether or not we can determine the precise cause of the health differences (Braveman, 2014). Conversely, the same conclusion has not consistently been applied to people with disabilities because disability and poor health are commonly viewed as inextricably (i.e., biologically) linked (Krahn et al., 2015).

When discussing chronic conditions among people with disabilities, a question often arises as to which is the chicken and which is the egg (Krahn et al., 2015). Because much of the data we rely on are cross-sectional in nature, we cannot always be certain whether disability preceded the onset of chronic conditions or emerged from them. In some cases, disability does result from chronic health conditions. For instance, if diabetes is not controlled, it can lead to blindness and limb loss. However, there is also evidence that people with preexisting disabilities are at greater risk of developing chronic conditions, compared to people without disabilities. A study using data from the National Health Interview Survey found that people with life-long disabilities were substantially more likely than people with no disabilities to have heart disease, cancer, diabetes, obesity, and hypertension (Dixon-Ibarra & Horner-Johnson, 2014). The study focused specifically on people whose disabilities were diagnosed by the age of 6 years, and it excluded people who reported lifelong conditions similar to the health problems studied (e.g., heart conditions, cancer, diabetes). Therefore, it is highly likely that the health problems developed after the onset of disability and were not directly related to the disability. In other words, they were comorbid conditions that could potentially be prevented if people with disabilities had equitable access to health promotion opportunities and other social determinants of health.

The high prevalence of poverty among people with disabilities results in substantially curtailed access to opportunities to engage in behavioral determinants of positive health, such as healthy eating and exercise. The reduction in opportunities for healthy living associated with low-socioeconomic status may be magnified by attitudes and environments that are not welcoming to people with disabilities. For example, as outlined in the Environmental Contexts chapter (Chap. 5) of this volume, people with disabilities often encounter physical barriers to community-based health venues. Few fitness centers offer adapted exercise equipment such as hand cycles. Health promotion classes and other events are sometimes held in locations that do not meet accessibility requirements as specified by the Americans with Disabilities Act. Health promotion materials further exclude people with disabilities if the materials are not available in formats that can be read and understood by people with sensory or cognitive disabilities. Moreover, health promotion materials rarely include images of people with disabilities, resulting in a more subtle form of exclusion by creating the impression that such materials are not applicable to individuals with disabilities.

While inequitable access to opportunities to live a healthy lifestyle places people with disabilities at risk for chronic conditions, disparities are further exacerbated by inequitable access to and receipt of health care. People with disabilities face a barrage of negative attitudes, structural barriers, and communication problems in healthcare settings. For example, people with physical disabilities often encounter narrow doorways, restricted maneuvering space, and a lack of accessible medical equipment (e.g., wheelchair accessible scales and adjustable height exam tables). People with intellectual disabilities may have particular difficulty understanding complex medical language and instructions. People who are deaf or hard of hearing frequently face challenges with obtaining appropriate and timely sign language interpreter services. People who are blind or have low vision may have difficulty navigating to and within clinics and obtaining information in accessible formats such as large print or screen-readable electronic documents. These barriers contribute to disparities in prevention, diagnosis, and management of chronic conditions and life-threatening diseases. For example, numerous studies have found that women with disabilities are less likely than those without disabilities to receive breast and cervical cancer screening as often as recommended (e.g., Armour, Thierry, & Wolf, 2009; Steele, Townsend, Courtney-Long, & Young, 2017). Delays in screening can result in delays in diagnosis and treatment, which increase the likelihood that women with disabilities will die of cancer. In fact, research has found that women with disabilities tend to have their cancers diagnosed at later stages, receive less aggressive cancer treatment, and have higher cancer mortality than women without disabilities (Iezzoni et al., 2008; McCarthy et al., 2006; Roetzheim & Chirikos, 2002).

The many barriers and stressors people with disabilities face likely contribute to observed disparities in mental health. Depression is highly prevalent, with 43.3% of adults with disabilities reporting depression versus 12.1% of adults without disabilities (CDC, 2019). Moreover, adults with disabilities are significantly and substantially less likely to receive adequate social and emotional support than is the case for adults without disabilities (Krahn et al., 2015). People with disabilities are also disproportionately affected by health risks that are even more clearly socially mediated: individuals with disabilities are 2.5 more likely than people without disabilities to be victims of violent crime (Harrell, 2017). People with disabilities are at especially high risk of sexual assault and intimate partner violence (Breiding & Armour, 2015; CDC, 2008; Harrell, 2017). It is difficult to see how such differences could be interpreted as anything other than inequities. Disability does not cause the health threats associated with experiences of violence; rather, those threats emerge directly from the way people with disabilities are treated by others.

4.4 Intersections of Disability with Other Marginalized Identities: Compounded Inequities

Although health inequities are widespread in the disability population as a whole, some subsets of the population are especially vulnerable. Further, while disability cuts across all population groups, some groups are more affected than others. Disability is more common in certain historically minority racial and ethnic groups, in rural areas, among women, and among people who identify as lesbian, gay, bisexual, transgender, nonbinary, queer, and/or other gender identity (LGBTQ+), as will be detailed below. There are well-established literatures on the significant health disparities and inequities experienced by each of these other populations. When individuals in these population groups also experience disability, the inequities may be compounded. Below are some examples of evidence indicating greater inequity for people living at these intersections.

4.4.1 Race and Ethnicity

In estimates adjusted for age differences between racial and ethnic groups, disability prevalence is significantly higher among American Indians and Alaska Natives (41% with a disability), multiracial adults (34%), Blacks (29%), and Hispanics (29%) than it is among non-Hispanic White adults (24%) (CDC, 2019). Racial and ethnic minorities have been described as doubly burdened by inequities associated with both their disability status and their race or ethnicity (ACMH, 2011). They experience the many covert and overt forms of bias and discrimination associated with each of these characteristics (Yee et al., 2018). As such, their health is often worse than that of non-Hispanic Whites with disabilities, as well as members of their own racial or ethnic groups who do not have disabilities.

Adults with disabilities in historically minority racial and ethnic groups are more likely to report fair/poor health, and that their health has worsened in the past year, compared to people without disabilities in the same racial/ethnic groups and compared to non-Hispanic Whites with disabilities (Gulley, Rasch, & Chan, 2014; Jones & Sinclair, 2008; Magaña, Parish, Morales, Li, & Fujiura, 2016; Wolf et al., 2008). Minorities with disabilities also have substantially less access to social determinants of health. For example, 21% to 34% of American Indian or Alaska Native, Black, multiracial, and Hispanic adults with disabilities live below the federal poverty level, compared with 14% of non-Hispanic Whites with disabilities and 6% of non-Hispanic Whites without disabilities (Horner-Johnson & Dobbertin, 2013).

Income disparities often contribute directly to unmet healthcare needs. Blacks and Hispanics with disabilities are significantly more likely to say there was a time in the past year when they needed to see a doctor but could not due to cost (27% and 31%, respectively) compared to non-Hispanic Whites with disabilities (24%) (CDC, 2019). In a study using data from the Medical Expenditure Panel Survey, working-age adults with disabilities who were American Indian or Alaska Native, Black, or multiracial had significantly elevated odds of having less than one dental checkup per year (odds ratios of 2.51, 2.99, and 2.43, respectively), compared to the reference group of non-Hispanic Whites without disabilities (Horner-Johnson, Dobbertin, & Beilstein-Wedel, 2015). Furthermore, odds ratios for these groups were significantly higher than those for people without disabilities in the same racial groups and for non-Hispanic Whites with disabilities (Horner-Johnson, Dobbertin, & Beilstein-Wedel, 2015). Significant differences remained but were markedly attenuated when taking poverty and presence of dental insurance into account (Horner-Johnson, Dobbertin, & Beilstein-Wedel, 2015). Similar patterns have been found specifically among adults with intellectual and developmental disabilities (IDD). An analysis of National Core Indicators data for adults with IDD showed that Blacks had significantly lower odds of visiting a dentist in the past year (OR = 0.60) or receiving a flu vaccine in the past year (OR = 0.68) compared to non-Hispanic White adults with IDD (Bershadsky, Hiersteiner, Fay, & Bradley, 2014).

As noted earlier, a substantial body of research has documented lower rates of breast and cervical cancer screening among women with disabilities overall compared to women without disabilities. A few studies have delved further and examined racial and ethnic differences in screening among women with disabilities. In reviewing medical records of women with IDD, Parish and colleagues found that 51% of eligible Black women had received a mammogram during a 2-year period compared to 76% of White women (Parish, Swaine, Son, & Luken, 2013). A study of deaf women found that 44% of Black or Hispanic women in the sample had received a mammogram in the past 2 years versus 70% of non-Hispanic White women (Berman, Jo, Cumberland, et al., 2013). The proportion of each racial/ethnic group that had received a mammogram in the deaf sample was also substantially lower than proportions reported for the same racial/ethnic groups in the general population, supporting the premise that there are compounded disparities for women who are both deaf and members of a disadvantaged racial or ethnic group (Berman et al., 2013).

Chronic health conditions and health risk factors are also unevenly distributed by race and ethnicity within the disability population. National-level data from the Behavioral Risk Factor Surveillance System (CDC, 2019) provide several examples:

- Blacks and Hispanics with disabilities are less likely to engage in aerobic physical activity (35% of each group do so, versus 41% of non-Hispanic Whites with disabilities).
- Nearly 46% of Blacks with disabilities are obese, compared to 39% of non-Hispanic Whites with disabilities.

- High blood pressure is significantly more prevalent among Blacks with disabilities than among non-Hispanic Whites with disabilities (52% vs. 41%),
- Diabetes is significantly more common among Blacks, Hispanics, and other/multiracial groups than among non-Hispanic Whites with disabilities (21%, 20%, and 20%, respectively, vs. 14%).

The fact that such racial and ethnic variations are apparent within the population of adults with disabilities suggests that these conditions are not part and parcel of the disability experience. Rather, they are potentially avoidable health problems that inequitably impact members of oppressed racial and ethnic groups in a way that mirrors disparities in income, access to health care, and other social determinants of health.

4.4.2 Gender

Women in the United States live longer than men and thus have more opportunity to experience disability. Yet, even in age-adjusted analyses, women are significantly more likely than men to have one or more disabilities (27% versus 24%) (CDC, 2019). Women with disabilities have historically had limited participation in the workforce and low income, compared both to women without disabilities and to men with disabilities. In one of the first studies to focus specifically on women with disabilities, Hanna and Rogovsky (1991) found that the employment and income differences between women with disabilities and men without disabilities were greater than what would result if the disparities associated with gender alone and disability alone were simply added together. The authors noted that there appeared to be a "plus factor" specific to the combination of being a woman and having a disability that resulted in exacerbated disparities.

More recently, Parish, Rose, and Andrews (2009) found that US women with disabilities were more than twice as likely to be living in poverty as women without disabilities. Moreover, even among women with incomes above the federal poverty level, women with disabilities were significantly more likely than women without disabilities to experience other indicators of material hardship, including food insecurity and difficulty making rent payments (Parish et al., 2009). Inadequate nutrition and housing – and worries about being able to afford such basic necessities as food and shelter—leave women with disabilities disproportionately vulnerable to chronic physical and mental health conditions.

Women with disabilities continue to be disadvantaged relative to women without disabilities and to men with disabilities. In 2018 women with disabilities who were employed full-time earned an average of 80 cents for each dollar earned by men with disabilities (National Women's Law Center, 2019). Further, women with disabilities are significantly more likely than men with disabilities to say there was a time in the past 12 months when they needed to see a doctor but could not due to cost (28.2% vs. 23.5%) (CDC, 2019). Compared to men with disabilities, women with disabilities also are significantly more likely to (CDC, 2019):

- Be obese (42% vs. 36%).
- Have asthma (21% vs. 12%), chronic obstructive pulmonary disease (15% vs. 12%), cancer (11% vs. 7%), or arthritis (46% vs. 35%).
- Have had at least 1 day in the past 30 days when their physical health was not good (64% vs. 55%).
- Have had at least 1 day in the past 30 days when their mental health was not good (63% vs. 52%).
- Experience depression (50% vs. 35%).

Given these differences, perhaps it is not surprising that women with disabilities are significantly more likely than men with disabilities to describe their general health as fair or poor (43% versus 39%) (CDC, 2019).

4.4.3   Sexual Orientation

Several studies have described an overlap between disability and sexual orientation and/or gender identity. Disability prevalence is higher among lesbian, gay, or bisexual (LGB) adults than among heterosexual adults (Fredriksen, Kim, & Barkan, 2012). Youth with disabilities are more likely than those without disabilities to report same-sex or both-sex attraction or identify as LGB (Blum, Kelly, & Ireland, 2001; Cheng & Udry, 2002; Cheng & Udry, 2005; Higgins Tejera, Horner-Johnson, & Andresen, 2019; Kahn & Halpern, 2018). People with disabilities, particularly those who are autistic, are also more likely than people without disabilities to be gender nonconforming (George & Stokes, 2018).

Despite this overlap, few analyses have examined the health of people with disabilities who have a minority sexual orientation (LGB) and/or gender identity (e.g., transgender, nonbinary, or genderqueer [TQ+]). A national survey of adults with disabilities found that LGBTQ+ respondents were significantly more likely than non-LGBTQ+ respondents to report fair or poor health and have unmet healthcare needs (Hall, Batza, & Kurth, 2019). Further, those who identified as LGBTQ+ were more than twice as likely as non-LGBT+ respondents to say that a healthcare provider had refused to provide services to them (Hall et al., 2019). LGBTQ+ adults also were significantly more likely to report social isolation (28% versus 17%) (Hall et al., 2019). The stigma and social isolation experienced by individuals experiencing both disability and a minority sexual identity can have profound health consequences. In a survey of high school students in Oregon, more than half of LGB teens with disabilities (56%) said they had seriously considered suicide during the past 12 months, compared to 27% of LGB teens without disabilities, 28% of heterosexual teens with disabilities, and 9% of heterosexual teens without disabilities (Higgins Tejera et al., 2019).

4.4.4 Rurality

Across the USA, 17.7% percent of people ages 5 and up living in noncore counties (those with an urban core population of less than 10,000) have a disability, compared to 11.7% of the population in metropolitan areas (Myers, Greiman, von Reichert, & Seekins, 2016). The difference in disability prevalence is not simply due to the higher average age of rural residents; in every age group, disability is more common in rural areas than it is in metropolitan areas (Myers et al., 2016). Complexity of disability also appears to vary with rurality. Among adults ages 18 and older, those living in the most rural areas are significantly more likely than those in metropolitan areas to have three or more disabilities (Zhao, Okoro, Hsia, Garvin, & Town, 2019).

People with disabilities living in rural areas experience disparities in socioeconomic determinants of health that are even greater than those experienced by people with disabilities in metropolitan areas (Myers et al., 2016). Rural residents with disabilities also appear to be more vulnerable to the long-term effects of economic downturns. While overall employment rates for people with disabilities in the USA increased slightly in the first several years after the 2008–2011 recession, employment of people with disabilities in rural areas decreased (RTC: Rural, 2019a). These socioeconomic disparities may exacerbate the effects of geographic isolation, leaving people with disabilities in rural areas at high risk for poor outcomes.

People with disabilities living in rural areas face substantial barriers to obtaining needed health care. Barriers include long travel distances to healthcare facilities, lack of transportation, limited availability of specialized care and knowledgeable care providers, clinic sites that are not sufficiently accessible to people with disabilities, and difficulty affording co-payments and medications (Davidsson & Södergård, 2016; Iezzoni, Killeen, & O'Day, 2006; Walker, Alfonso, Colquitt, Weeks, & Telfair, 2016). These barriers are likely contributors to the disparities that have been observed in receipt of preventive cancer screenings for adults with disabilities in rural areas compared to their urban counterparts (Horner-Johnson, Dobbertin, & Iezzoni, 2015; Horner-Johnson, Dobbertin, Lee, & Andresen, 2014). In short, people with disabilities in rural areas are more likely to be living in circumstances that contribute to poor health and less likely to be able to obtain the care and services needed to prevent or treat poor health.

4.5 Addressing Compounded Inequities

In order to address inequities, we must first be aware that they exist. Thus, data collection and analysis plays a key role. The Patient Protection and Affordable Care Act (ACA), passed in 2010, not only recognized people with disabilities as a health disparity population, it also mandated collection of data on disability status to ensure that disability-related health disparities will be measured and monitored.

That mandate has spurred the addition of a set of six disability questions to population-based health surveys, as detailed in the chapters on Epidemiology (Chap. 2) and Global Disability (Chap. 7). Consistent and ongoing data collection will help clarify the nature and extent of the health problems experienced by people with disabilities compared to those with no disabilities. However, it is also important to analyze those data in combination with information about other sociodemographic characteristics in order to better understand how disability interacts with other marginalized identities. Analyzing data from smaller subgroups of people with disabilities often will require pooling multiple years of data. Thus, data collection systems should continue to use consistent measures and methods from year to year, to the maximum extent possible (Yee et al., 2018). Reports generated from these data should include comparisons between people with and without disabilities and address how disparities may differ as disability intersects with other characteristics such as race and ethnicity (Yee et al., 2018). Such analyses will enable public health professionals to identify population subgroups most impacted by specific disparities and will inform efforts to address inequities experienced by the most vulnerable members of the disability population. Ongoing data collection and analysis also will contribute to evaluation and improvement of targeted intervention efforts.

As disparities continue to be identified, public health professionals have a responsibility to develop programs and policies to address these disparities. Federal policy changes already have resulted in substantial improvements in health equity. For example, many more Americans with disabilities now have health insurance because of the Affordable Care Act (Kennedy, Wood, & Frieden, 2017). In Medicaid expansion states, gains in insurance coverage have been particularly strong for people with disabilities living in rural areas (RTC: Rural, 2019b), reducing one barrier to equitable health care. While these gains are impressive, there remains a considerable need to develop additional policies and programs and advocate for the societal and institutional changes needed to support health equity. A key issue is that some federal funding agencies do not yet recognize people with disabilities as a population that experiences disparities. Nor are people with disabilities or subgroups of people with disabilities designated as Medically Underserved Populations (MUPs). Addressing these gaps would facilitate more extensive research on health disparities within disability populations. Moreover, MUP designation would allow health professionals interested in providing care to people with disabilities to qualify for federal loan repayment programs, which would help increase the number of professionals qualified to provide care to people with disabilities (ACMH, 2011). Incentives are also needed to encourage providers of specialty care needed by people with disabilities to serve in rural areas and communities of color. Other policy initiatives could include increasing Medicaid reimbursement rates. Some doctors are reluctant to accept patients on Medicaid, which is a challenge for people with disabilities in general, and especially so for racial and ethnic minorities and rural residents with disabilities who disproportionately rely on Medicaid coverage (Gulley et al., 2014; RTC: Rural, 2019b). Policies and programs are also needed at state, local, and organizational levels to ensure inclusion of diverse people with disabilities in health equity efforts.

Another crucial component of addressing inequities is assuring that health professionals are equipped to address the needs of diverse people with disabilities. A well-trained and culturally competent workforce is essential for providing inclusive health promotion and high-quality health care. Achieving health equity requires competency in meeting the needs of all population demographic groups, including those with disabilities. In a 2011 report, the Advisory Committee on Minority Health (ACMH) highlighted the lack of professional training and disability competence among healthcare providers as among the "most significant and fundamental barriers preventing people with disabilities from receiving quality health care" (ACMH, 2011, p. 10). Limited disability competency can result in poor patient-provider communication, inappropriate diagnoses and treatment, and distrust of providers (ACMH, 2011). Moreover, it is important to consider cultural differences within the disability population and understand that beliefs, values, and practices may vary among subgroups of people with disabilities (ACMH, 2011).

The chapter on Preparing a Disability Competnet Workforce (Chap. 16) in this volume presents disability competencies and strategies to guide training. Competencies include accommodating and addressing the specific needs of individuals with disabilities, but also understanding the many ways in which people with and without disabilities are alike. The competency frameworks emphasize the need to recognize disability as a demographic characteristic similar to and intersecting with age, gender, sexual identity, race, ethnicity, and language. Now that these competencies have been developed, the next crucial step is for entities such as the Association of American Medical Colleges and the Liaison Committee on Medical Education to mandate that these competencies be adopted as core curriculum components and licensing requirements, as was recommended by the ACMH several years ago (ACMH, 2011). The ACMH further recommended that demonstration of disability competency be required for accreditation and receipt of federal funding by healthcare training institutions and hospitals (ACMH, 2011). Such a requirement would provide a strong financial incentive for improving disability competency and advancing health equity.

In addition to promoting inclusion of disability in health equity efforts, we must ensure attention to equity in disability programs, services, and research. Too often, disability and diversity are seen as separate issues to be addressed in separate silos (Goode, Carter-Pokras, Horner-Johnson, & Yee, 2014). Yet disability is present in all sociodemographic categories and in all spheres of life. We cannot logically talk about population health or health equity without addressing the health of people with disabilities. Likewise, we cannot effectively address the health of people with disabilities without attention to the diversity of the disability population and the range of sociocultural factors that influence the health of this heterogeneous, cross-cutting demographic. As stated in a recent report commissioned by the National Academies of Science: "Disability is only one of multiple cultural identities. It is essential to recognize and respond to the myriad within group differences among people with disabilities and their lived experience" (Yee et al., 2018, p. 60).

4.6 Discussion Questions

1. Define the terms health inequality, health inequity, and health disparity. Describe some of the different ways the term disparity has been defined.
2. How is disability similar to or different from other sociodemographic characteristics associated with health disparities?
3. What are some of the ways in which disability and health can be associated? In what ways does evidence indicate that disability and health are conceptually distinct?
4. What best practices can you incorporate into your work to ensure inclusion of people with disabilities in public health efforts?
5. What programmatic and policy steps can you take to decrease barriers to quality health care for people with disabilities?
6. What are some additional strategies that may be necessary to fully address the needs of people with disabilities who also belong to other marginalized and underserved population groups?

References

Advisory Committee on Minority Health. (2011). *Assuring health equity for minority persons with disabilities: A statement of principles and recommendations.* Submitted to the U.S. Department of Health and Human Services, Office of Minority Health.

Armour, B. S., Thierry, J. M., & Wolf, L. A. (2009). State-level differences in breast and cervical cancer screening by disability status: United States, 2008. *Women's Health Issues, 19*(6), 406–414.

Berman, B. A., Jo, A., Cumberland, W. G., et al. (2013). Breast cancer knowledge and practices among D/deaf women. *Disability and Health Journal, 6*(4), 303–316.

Bershadsky, J., Hiersteiner, D., Fay, M. L., & Bradley, V. (2014). Race/ethnicity and the use of preventive health care among adults with intellectual and developmental disabilities. *Medical Care, 52*(10 Suppl 3), S25–S31.

Blum, R. W., Kelly, A., & Ireland, M. (2001). Health-risk behaviors and protective factors among adolescents with mobility impairments and learning and emotional disabilities. *The Journal of Adolescent Health, 28*(6), 481–490.

Braveman, P. (2014). What are health disparities and health equity? We need to be clear. *Public Health Reports, 129*(Suppl 2), 5–8.

Breiding, M. H., & Armour, B. S. (2015). The association between disability and intimate partner violence in the United States. *Annals of Epidemiology, 25*, 455–457.

Carter-Pokras, O., & Baquet, C. (2002). What is a "health disparity"? *Public Health Reports, 117*, 426–434.

Centers for Disease Control and Prevention. (2008). Adverse health conditions and health risk behaviors associated with intimate partner violence—United States, 2005. *MMWR. Morbidity and Mortality Weekly Report, 57*(5), 113–117.

Centers for Disease Control and Prevention, National Center on Birth Defects and Developmental Disabilities, Division of Human Development and Disability. (2019). *Disability and Health Data System (DHDS) Data [online].* Retrieved November 22, 2019, from https://dhds.cdc.gov

Cheng, M. M., & Udry, J. R. (2002). Sexual behaviors of physically disabled adolescents in the United States. *The Journal of Adolescent Health, 31*(1), 48–58.

Cheng, M. M., & Udry, J. R. (2005). Sexual experiences of adolescents with low cognitive abilities in the U.S. *Journal of Developmental and Physical Disabilities, 17*(2), 155–172.

Davidsson, N., & Södergård, B. (2016). Access to healthcare among people with physical disabilities in rural Louisiana. *Social Work in Public Health, 31*(3), 188–195.

Dixon-Ibarra, A., & Horner-Johnson, W. (2014). Disability status as an antecedent to chronic disease: National Health Interview Survey 2006-2012. *Preventing Chronic Disease, 11*, 130251.

Fredriksen, K. I., Kim, H. J., & Barkan, S. E. (2012). Disability among lesbian, gay, and bisexual adults: Disparities in prevalence and risk. *American Journal of Public Health, 102*, e16–e21.

George, R., & Stokes, M. A. (2018). Gender identify and sexual orientation in autism spectrum disorder. *Autism, 22*(8), 970–982.

Goode, T. D., Carter-Pokras, O. D., Horner-Johnson, W., & Yee, S. (2014). Parallel tracks: Reflections on the need for collaborative health disparities research on race/ethnicity and disability. *Medical Care, 52*(Suppl 3), S3–S8.

Gulley, S. P., Rasch, E. K., & Chan, L. (2014). Difference, disparity, and disability: A comparison of health, insurance coverage, and health service use on the basis of race/ethnicity among US adults with disabilities, 2006-2008. *Medical Care, 52*(10 Suppl 3), S9–S16.

Hall, J. P., Batza, K., & Kurth, N. (2019). *Intersectionality of disability and LGBTQ: Historical context and current health disparities*. American Public Health Association Annual Meeting, November 5, 2020, Philadelphia, PA.

Hanna, W. J., & Rogovsky, B. (1991). Women with disabilities: Two handicaps plus. *Disability, Handicap & Society, 6*(1), 49–63.

Harrell, E. (2017). Crime against persons with disabilities, 2009-2015—Statistical tables. *Bureau of Justice Statistical Tables*. NCJ250632.

Higgins Tejera, C., Horner-Johnson, W., & Andresen, E. M. (2019). Application of an intersectional framework to understanding the association of disability and sexual orientation with suicidal ideation among Oregon Teens. *Disability and Health Journal, 12*, 557–663.

Horner-Johnson, W., & Dobbertin, K. (2013). *Healthcare access at the intersection of race, ethnicity, and disability*. Health Disparities Research at the Intersection of Race, Ethnicity, and Disability: A National Conference; April 2013; Washington, DC.

Horner-Johnson, W., Dobbertin, K., & Beilstein-Wedel, E. (2015). Disparities in dental care associated with disability and race and ethnicity. *Journal of the American Dental Association (1939), 146*(6), 366–374.

Horner-Johnson, W., Dobbertin, K., & Iezzoni, L. I. (2015). Disparities in receipt of breast and cervical cancer screening for rural women age 18-64 with disabilities. *Women's Health Issues, 25*(3), 246–253.

Horner-Johnson, W., Dobbertin, K., Lee, J. C., & Andresen, E. M. (2014). Rural disparities in receipt of colorectal cancer screening among adults ages 50-64 with disabilities. *Disability and Health Journal, 7*(4), 394–401.

Iezzoni, L. I., Killeen, M. B., & O'Day, B. L. (2006). Rural residents with disabilities confront substantial barriers to obtaining primary care. *Health Services Research, 41*(4, part I), 1258–1275.

Iezzoni, L. I., Ngo, L. H., Dongline, I., Roetzheim, R. G., Drews, R. E., & McCarthy, E. P. (2008). Early stage breast cancer treatments for younger Medicare beneficiaries with different disabilities. *Health Services Research, 43*(5 pt I), 1752–1767.

Jones, G. C., & Sinclair, L. B. (2008). Multiple health disparities among minority adults with mobility limitations: San application of the ICF framework and codes. *Disability and Rehabilitation, 30*(12–13), 901–915.

Kahn, N. F., & Halpern, C. T. (2018). The relationship between cognitive ability and experiences of vaginal, oral, and anal sex in the United States. *Journal of Sex Research, 55*(1), 99–105.

Kennedy, J., Wood, E. G., & Frieden, L. (2017). Disparities in insurance coverage, health services use, and access following implementation of the Affordable Care Act: A comparison of disabled and nondisabled working-age adults. *Inquiry: The Journal of Health Care Organization, Provision, and Financing, 54*, 1–10.

Krahn, G. L., Klein Walker, D., & Correa-de-Araujo, R. (2015). Persons with disabilities as an unrecognized health disparity population. *American Journal of Public Health, 105*(S2), S198–S206.

Magaña, S., Parish, S., Morales, M. A., Li, H., & Fujiura, G. (2016). Racial and ethnic health disparities among people with intellectual and developmental disabilities. *Intellectual and Developmental Disabilities, 54*(3), 161–172.

McCarthy, E. P., Long, H. N., Roetzheim, R. G., Chirikos, T. N., Li, D., Drews, R. E., & Iezzoni, L. I. (2006). Disparities in breast cancer treatment and survival for women with disabilities. *Annals of Internal Medicine, 145*(9), 637–645.

Myers, A., Greiman, L., von Reichert, C., & Seekins, T. (2016, July). *Rural matters: The geography of disability in rural America.* Missoula, MT: The University of Montana Rural Institute for Inclusive Communities. Retrieved from http://rtc.ruralinstitute.umt.edu/research-findings/geography/

National Women's Law Center. (2019). *Workplace justice: The wage gap: The who, how, why, and what to do. National Women's Law Center fact sheet.* Washington, DC: National Women's Law Center.

Parish, S. L., Rose, R. A., & Andrews, M. E. (2009). Income poverty and material hardship among US women with disabilities. *The Social Service Review, 83*(1), 33–52.

Parish, S. L., Swaine, J. G., Son, E., & Luken, K. (2013). Receipt of mammography among women with intellectual disabilities: Medical record data indicate substantial disparities for African American women. *Disability and Health Journal, 6*(1), 36–42.

Research and Training Center on Disability in Rural Communities. (2019a). *Employment disparity grows for rural Americans with disability.* Missoula, MT: The University of Montana, Rural Institute for Inclusive Communities.

Research and Training Center on Disability in Rural Communities. (2019b). *ACA and Medicaid expansion associated with increased insurance coverage for rural Americans with disabilities.* Missoula, MT: The University of Montana, Rural Institute for Inclusive Communities.

Roetzheim, R. G., & Chirikos, T. N. (2002). Breast cancer detection and outcomes in a disability beneficiary population. *Journal of Health Care for the Poor and Underserved, 13*(4), 461–476.

Steele, C. B., Townsend, J. S., Courtney-Long, E. A., & Young, M. (2017). Prevalence of cancer screening among adults with disabilities, United States, 2013. *Preventing Chronic Disease, 14,* 160312. https://doi.org/10.5888/pcd14.160312

Turk, M. (2006). Secondary conditions and disability. In M. J. Field, A. M. Jette, & L. Martin (Eds.), *Workshop on disability in America: A new look: Summary and background papers* (pp. 185–193). Washington, DC: The National Academies Press.

Walker, A., Alfonso, M. L., Colquitt, G., Weeks, K., & Telfair, J. (2016). "When everything changes": Parent perspectives on the challenges of accessing care for a child with a disability. *Disability and Health Journal, 9,* 157–161.

Wolf, L. A., Armour, B. S., & Campbell, V. A. (2008). Racial/ethnic disparities in self-rated health status among adults with and without disabilities—United States, 2004-2006. *MMWR. Morbidity and Mortality Weekly Report, 57*(39), 1069–1073.

Yee, S., Breslin, M. L., Goode, T. D., Havercamp, S. M., Horner-Johnson, W., Iezzoni, L. I., & Krahn, G. (2018). *Compounded disparities: Health equity at the intersection of disability, race, and ethnicity.* Washington, DC: National Academies of Science, Engineering, and Medicine.

Zhao, G., Okoro, C. A., Hsia, J., Garvin, W. S., & Town, M. (2019). Prevalence of disability and disability types by urban-rural county classification—U.S., 2016. *American Journal of Preventive Medicine, 57*(6), 749–756.

Chapter 5
Environmental Contexts Shaping Disability and Health

Yochai Eisenberg and Jordana Maisel

5.1 Introduction

The environment's impact on health is embedded in the history of public health. Various elements of the environment have been known to affect human health as far back as John Snow and the London cholera outbreak in 1854, in which he removed the handle of a water pump that was allowing the disease to spread, thus eliminating access to deadly infectious water. The built environment's impact on health was recognized almost as long ago. Frederick Law Olmsted, a landscape architect, designed Central Park as an ecological refuge in the city supporting urban residents' physical and mental health (Kochtitzky et al., 2006). In the early twentieth century, the US Supreme Court also took an environmental stance when it validated zoning codes due to their "aiding the health and safety of the community by excluding from residential areas the confusion and danger of fire, contagion and disorder" (Taft & Supreme Court of the United States, 1926).

The environment's importance is apparent in several national and international health organizations. The World Health Organization (WHO) considers health promotion to be the process of enabling people to increase control over and to improve their health, through actions directed toward changing social, economic, and *environmental* conditions (World Health Organization, 1998). Government agencies, including the Environmental Protection Agency, the National Institute of Environmental Health Sciences from the National Institutes of Health, and the

Y. Eisenberg (✉)
Department of Disability and Human Development, University of Illinois at Chicago,
Chicago, IL, USA
e-mail: yeisen2@uic.edu

J. Maisel
Center for Inclusive Design and Environmental Access, School of Architecture and Planning,
University at Buffalo, Buffalo, NY, USA
e-mail: jlmaisel@buffalo.edu

© Springer Science+Business Media, LLC, part of Springer Nature 2021   107
D. J. Lollar et al. (eds.), *Public Health Perspectives on Disability*,
https://doi.org/10.1007/978-1-0716-0888-3_5

National Center for Environmental Health from the Centers for Disease Control and Prevention, represent the enormous governmental commitment to protecting the environment and promoting health through environmental policies, programs, and science.

For people with disabilities, the environment's impact on health is even stronger than for people without disabilities. This difference has much to do with environmental barriers. Specifically, barriers exist in the physical and social environment that prevent people with disabilities from accessing places, systems, and services in their community, including healthcare sites, and environments for accessing food or participating in physical activity. Restricted access leads to reduced participation, which can both limit the benefits of health-promoting environments (e.g., parks, fitness centers, farmers markets) and strengthen the effect of harmful environments (e.g., areas abundant with only unhealthy/junk foods). Further, the relationship between a person and their environment varies by their type of disability. People who use wheelchairs as an assistive device for community-based mobility have a different relationship with their community's environment than individuals with hearing loss or low vision and therefore require a different set of accommodations (changes to the environment) to support participation. Understanding the complexities of these relationships with the environment, the reasons why they exist, and the approaches shown to improve the relationship between people with disabilities and their environment is critical for public health professionals and students.

5.2 Learning Objectives

The learning objectives of this chapter are to explain: (1) the role of various environments, at multiple scales, in contributing toward or detracting from the health of people with disabilities and (2) the roles that the public health sector can play in promoting the health of this population via environmental activities and interventions particularly in partnership with other sectors (e.g., transportation, community planning, housing, and health care).

5.3 Background

Environmental health comprises the aspects of human health, disease, and injury that are determined or influenced by factors in the environment. Environmental health includes the study of both the direct pathological effects of various chemical, physical, and biological agents and the effects on health of the broad physical and social environment, which includes housing, urban development, land use, and transportation (United States Department of Health and Human Services, 2010). Direct and indirect environmental factors have been found to contribute to more than 10% of deaths based on examinations of actual causes of death (McGinnis &

Foege, 1993). Successful health promotion efforts therefore need to address the various environments that affect heath (ecological, built, and social) at every scale (micro, meso, and macro) (Schulz & Northridge, 2004).

The ecological environment makes up the air, water, and soil all around us and can be of importance, for instance, to those whose disability might include a greater sensitivity to environmental contaminants, such as air pollution (Weuve et al., 2016). The built environment includes our homes, schools, workplaces, parks/recreation areas, business areas, and roads. The built environment encompasses all buildings, spaces, and products that are created or modified by people. It impacts indoor and outdoor physical environments (e.g., climatic conditions), as well as social environments (e.g., civic participation) and subsequently our health and quality of life (Srinivasan, O'Fallon, & Dearry, 2003). "Social environment" refers to broad objective socio-physical structures (people and institutions) with unidirectional influences on people, whereas "social context" refers to the subjective experience of individuals regarding the places, activities, people, and objects where the person-environment interaction occurs. Reciprocal influences are therefore possible for individuals and environments (Batorowicz, King, Mishra, & Missiuna, 2016).

People experience these types of environments at a variety of scales (Schulz & Northridge, 2004). These scales include microlevel environments such as individual home, school, or worksite conditions. At a higher scale, there are meso-level environments such as community land uses or transportation systems. Finally, there are macro-level environmental conditions such as climate, topography, and availability of natural resources.

The specific recognition of the built environment's potential impact on the lives of persons with a disability gained momentum after World War II, when returning veterans with newly acquired injuries and functional limitations helped launch the Barrier Free Movement. The acknowledgment of environmental significance led to passage of various laws to ensure civil rights for individuals with disabilities, including the Architectural Barriers Act of 1968, the Rehabilitation Act of 1973, and the Education of the Handicapped Act of 1975. At the same time, Ed Roberts and others in Berkeley, California, founded the Berkeley Center for Independent Living, helping to create the Independent Living Movement, which emphasizes consumer control and the idea that people with disabilities have a right to decide how to live, work, and take part in their communities. Their efforts led to the passage of the Americans with Disabilities Act (ADA) in 1990, which continues to serve as the primary civil rights law used to ensure equal access for people with disabilities. Under the ADA, public entities and most private entities are required to remove barriers that restrict access for people with disabilities.

5.3.1 Theoretical/Conceptual Models

The relationship between the environment and health for people with disabilities has been described and conceptually organized through various models of disability, most notably the International Classification of Functioning, Disability and

Health (ICF). The ICF is a biopsychosocial model of health and function that serves as a conceptual framework and important tool for studying environmental public health and disability (see Fig. 5.1).

In the ICF, human functioning is expressed across three domains of body function/structure, activities, and participation. Individuals can experience limitations in any one of these domains or across multiple domains. Functioning is moderated by environmental and personal factors and health conditions (World Health Organization, 2002). The arrows in the ICF model are bidirectional to show how the domains, health conditions, and contextual factors can influence each other.

Based on the ICF, the barriers that people experience in the environment limit access and degrade the environmental appropriateness for that person or their person-environment fit. The term person-environment fit fully embodies the concepts of the ICF by emphasizing the dual role of examining and addressing the needs and capabilities of the person and the barriers or supports found in their environment. Access and inclusion can only be achieved by ensuring the balancing of and integration between these two factors.

The domains and subdomains of the ICF tell a full story of person-environment fit only when they are looked at in an integrated fashion. The environmental factors make up the physical, social, and attitudinal environment in which people live and conduct their lives. In close consultation with the individual(s) with a disability, professionals can deploy ICF codes as an assessment tool. The type and amount of impact the various environmental factors have on the functioning of the individual are rated across a 5-point "barrier" scale and a 5-point "facilitator" scale. Including positive codes, "facilitators" is a major breakthrough in classification systems. It is

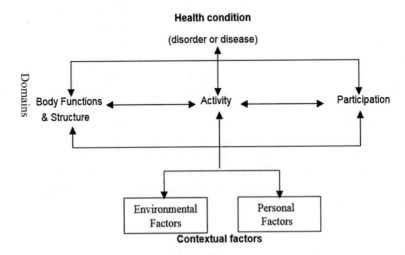

Fig. 5.1 The WHO International Classification of Functioning, Disability and Health (ICF) (Reproduced with permission from Towards a Common Language for Functioning, Disability and Health: ICF, The International Classification of Functioning, Disability and Health, the World Health Organization, page 9, Copyright 2002, URL: www.who.int/classifications/icf/icfbeginners-guide.pdf?ua=1) (World Health Organization, 2002)

particularly important for public health professionals to be able to code positive characteristics of the environment for assessment, policy, and assurance purposes. The subdomains within the environmental factors domain include:

- Products and technology (e.g., design, construction and building products and technology of buildings for public use, etc.)
- Natural environment and human-made changes to environments (e.g., climate, light, sound, etc.)
- Support and relationships (e.g., neighbors and community members, people in position of authority, health professionals, other related professionals, etc.)
- Attitudes (e.g., societal attitudes, attitudes of health professionals, attitudes of related professionals, social norms, practices and ideologies, etc.)
- Services, systems, and policies (e.g., housing services, systems and policies, transportation services, systems and policies, etc.)

Within the ICF context, the environment has elements of the physical and social environments and elements of the societal policies, systems, and services that cause the environment to be either a barrier or a facilitator. ICF is currently primarily deployed in clinical settings, but has also been used by public health practitioners, as well as referenced by other sectors such as city planning, housing, and transportation. Within the clinical setting, it has been used as a classification and a healthcare coding tool. Within public health, it is often used as a surveillance and research tool. Finally, within both public health and the other sectors, it is used to design, prioritize, evaluate, and/or justify interventions such as zero step entries or modified transit equipment or station design (Seekins, Traci, Cummings, Oreskovich, & Ravesloot, 2008).

More recent and somewhat more expansive models, such as the Framework for Assessing Factors that Impact Vulnerable Populations (Kochtitzky, Freeland, & Yen, 2011), have drawn heavily from the ICF while also including elements from other models such as Glass and Balfour (2003) and Lawton and Nahemow (1973) that address person-environment fit issues across a (1) wider variety of scales, (2) wider varieties of environmental change, and (3) include consideration of the individuals responses—adaptive or otherwise—to the environmental circumstances they encounter. These newer models also include perspectives outside of the health and medical sector.

5.3.2 Environment Disability Mismatch

Based on the ICF, disability results from a mismatch between the goals and abilities of an individual and the demands of both the social and physical environment. Barriers across the environment, in health care, housing, streetscapes, and transportation, create additional challenges for people with disabilities, which further impede their ability to participate in the community (Nary, Froehlich, & White, 2000). Reports from several national institutions emphasize the importance of accessible housing, transportation, and healthcare environments for improving the health and quality of life of people with a disability (Institute of Medicine, 2007; National Council on Disability, 2006; Office of the United States Surgeon General, 2005).

Reduced access to health care disproportionately affects members of marginalized groups, including people with disabilities (Nelson, 2002; United States Department of Health and Human Services, 2010; Peterson-Besse, Walsh, Horner-Johnson, Goode, & Wheeler, 2014). Barriers include limited appointment availability and inconvenient office hours; lack of accessible and timely transportation; substantial cost and insurance barriers; poor physician-patient communication; and discrimination, negative attitudes, and lack of respect (Peterson-Besse et al., 2014). Unique to people with disabilities are architectural barriers associated with physical access to and navigation in healthcare facilities. For individuals who rely on wheeled-mobility devices and/or have limited stamina, an insufficient number of medical exam tables that raise/lower, medical diagnostic machines that require standing (e.g., mammography), and inaccessible scales create significant challenges for both the individuals and clinician. These barriers to health care are associated with worse health outcomes for people with disabilities, such as lower rates of preventive screening (Krahn, Walker, & Correa-De-Araujo, 2015).

While the benefits of physical activity on health are universal, physical activity and exercise are an extremely important means for health promotion and prevention of secondary conditions (Rimmer & Lai, 2017). Unfortunately, recent data from the US National Health Interview Survey (NHIS) reported that 47.1% of US adults with a disability, aged 18–64 years, are physically inactive (reporting no periods of aerobic physical activity lasting 10 min or more per week) compared to only 26.1% of adults without disabilities (Carroll et al., 2014). Opportunities for recreation, leisure, and fitness participation are often impeded by a community that is underprepared to support health and wellness needs of people with disabilities (Vasudevan, 2016). In 2011, 76.8% of adults with disabilities reported that barriers limited or prevented them from accessing community health and wellness programs (United States Department of Health and Human Services, 2010). Several barriers to exercise have been identified, including inaccessible fitness and recreation centers, knowledge of accessible facilities, inexperienced staff, and insufficient resources to pay for program and transportation costs (Rimmer & Lai, 2017).

In addition to healthcare and recreation facilities, researchers and policymakers expect the need for accessible housing in the USA and other developed countries, to increase substantially in the next few decades as the population ages. According to Smith, Rayer, and Smith (2008), in 2050, 21% of households will have at least one resident with a physical limitation, and 7% of households will have at least one resident with a self-care limitation. They estimate that there is a 60% probability that a newly built single-family detached unit will house at least one resident with a physical limitation during its expected lifetime and a 25% probability of a resident with a self-care limitation. When disabled visitors are accounted for, the probabilities rise to 91% and 53%, respectively.

Approximately 70% of Americans, for example, live in single-family homes (US Census Bureau, 2011), and the overwhelming majority of these housing units have barriers that make it difficult or impossible for someone with disabilities to enter/exit or live independently. Many houses have steps at all entrances and hallways and doorways too narrow for users of wheelchairs or walkers to pass through easily, if at all. Furthermore, architectural barriers make it difficult for other households to accommodate visits from friends and relatives who need basic accessibility. These barriers often result in significant consequences. In addition to social isolation and dependence, many people with severe mobility impairments may be unable to exit their homes independently in an emergency, and risk injury from falling. Barriers within a home can also increase the work and stress of the caretakers who assist older adults and people with disabilities. Many family caregivers report that they suffer physical injuries because of lifting and handling their relatives, as well as psychological health problems such as fatigue, anxiety, and depression (Brown & Mulley, 1997). Young people with disabilities who live in inaccessible housing have little chance of leading independent lives or seeking employment.

Housing accessibility barriers can make it difficult for older people to remain in their homes as they encounter age-related physical limitations. According to a survey conducted for the American Association of Retired Persons (AARP), a non-profit, nonpartisan membership organization that seeks to address the needs and interests of the 50+ population in the USA, 87% of adults aged 65+ want to stay in their current residence for as long as possible (Harrell, Lynott, Guzman, & Lampkin, 2014). Aging in place offers numerous social and financial benefits. Research shows that independent living promotes life satisfaction, health, and self-esteem, three keys to successful aging. Unfortunately, a number of barriers, including inaccessible housing (e.g., steps, bathtubs, high-pile carpets), hinder aging in place, pushing frail older people toward less desirable and more restrictive settings, such as nursing homes (Pynoos, Nishita, Cicero, & Caraviello, 2008). Compounding the barrier is the fact that home modifications are expensive and home modification programs face budget limitations and unstable sources of funding. Moreover, the public and private sources of financing are far from comprehensive and have confusing eligibility requirements (Pynoos & Nishita, 2003).

Infrastructure for pedestrians is important for aging in place as well as for livability for people with disabilities. In a recent Call to Action by the Surgeon General on increasing walking and walkable communities, inclusion of people with disabilities in walking initiatives and improving access to walkable places for people with disabilities was highlighted as important interventions that could address the low levels of physical activity among this group (United States Department of Health and Human Services, 2015). The pedestrian infrastructure encompasses the areas that people walk/roll on in the community, including sidewalks and other off-street paths, curb ramps, crosswalks, and traffic signals. Neighborhoods are needed that have conveniently located community services, opportunities for recreation and work nearby, a vibrant street life, and pedestrian environments that are usable for all.

There are important design challenges associated with the pedestrian infrastructure, including steep slopes, rough and slippery surface materials, irregular pavement, and lack of curb ramps. Many injuries are related to outdoor ramps used by wheeled mobility users (Xiang, Chany, & Smith, 2006). In a national poll of people over 50 years old, 47% said it was unsafe to cross the street near their home. Almost 40% said their neighborhood lacks adequate sidewalks (Lynott et al., 2009), creating a disincentive to walking. The oldest pedestrians (75+ years) incur fatality rates nearly twice the national average for those under 65 years of age (Ernst & Shoup, 2009). People with disabilities report encountering pedestrian environmental barriers to neighborhood walking, including broken or uneven sidewalks, intersections that have poor walking signals, crosswalks that are unsafe to cross, curb ramps that are too steep, and fast-moving traffic being too close (Gell, Rosenberg, Carlson, Kerr, & Belza, 2015; Haselwandter et al., 2015). Since residents with disabilities drive less frequently and already feel more isolated from their communities (BTS, 2003), any barrier to outdoor mobility further impedes their ability to function independently and participate in the community (Clarke, Ailshire, & Lantz, 2009; Glass & Balfour, 2003).

Transportation is critical for ensuring community engagement, productivity, and social participation for individuals with disabilities (Sundar, Brucker, Pollack, & Chang, 2016). Millions of Americans, however, experience transportation barriers, including lack of personal vehicles, cost of transportation, and lack of available public transportation (NCD, 2015; Rosso, Auchincloss, & Michael, 2011; Syed, Gerber, & Sharp, 2013). These barriers are exponentially worse for people with disabilities, who have a more frequent need for health care, require greater accessibility to transportation, and often have lower incomes than the general population (Syed et al., 2013). Approximately 3.6 million people with disabilities cannot leave their homes because of transportation problems (BTS, 2018). Without access to transportation, older adults and people with disabilities are more likely to be excluded from services and social contact and become stuck in a disability-poverty cycle (Roberts & Babinard, 2004; Venter et al., 2004), which in turn can lead to social isolation, depression, and health deterioration (Steptoe, Shankar, Demakakos, & Wardle, 2013; Sundar et al., 2016).

The Transportation Cooperative Research Program (TCRP) reported that nationally there has been an increase in individuals with disabilities using public transit, including large accessible transit vehicles (LATVs) and paratransit services (Thatcher et al., 2013). Current LATVs do not adequately address the accessibility needs of all riders and lead to challenges and frustrations for riders with disabilities, bus operators, and transit agencies. Although LATVs are generally thought to be a safe means of transportation (Shaw, 2000; Shaw & Gillispie, 2003), research demonstrates that public transit may present unique safety challenges for wheeled mobility device users (Shaw & Gillispie, 2003; Songer, Fitzgerald, & Rotko, 2004). Individuals who use wheeled mobility devices specifically cite securement while riding LATVs as an important concern relating to safety, independence, and dignity (Frost, Bertocci, & Salipur, 2013).

A more recent TCRP study revealed that individuals with different disabilities experience different barriers in the environment, which in turn impacts their mobility decision-making (Thatcher, 2015). For example, individuals with a mobility disability rated two built environment-related factors, barriers in the pedestrian environment and distances to or from stops/stations, as very important as to whether or not they use fixed-route transit, and they rated these variables as significantly more important than scheduling-related factors. In contrast, individuals with an intellectual and/or cognitive disability rated complex/multiple transfers as very important to their fixed-route usage.

Conventional public transportation practices are currently being challenged by the disruptive technologies of ride hailing, ride sharing, and crowdsourcing used by companies like Uber and Lyft. The disruption offers flexibility to traditional transportation systems, whose structure can be limiting, such as the need to schedule a ride 48 h in advance. However, there are major controversies about whether these new forms of public transportation are covered by existing accessibility regulations (Said, 2018). Are they a public service, which clearly is regulated by laws such as the Americans with Disabilities Act, or are they a private transaction between two individuals not covered by the laws? Even though ride-hailing companies take the position that they are not covered by the ADA, in negotiating with local municipalities, they agree to offer services to riders with disabilities to gain access to a market and promote goodwill in the community. Despite this, these ride-hailing fleets have a shortage of wheelchair-accessible vehicles (WAVs), which forces people with disabilities to resort to less flexible transportation services.

Because of the environmental barriers outlined in this section, there is a tendency for public and/or private agencies to offer segregated services specific to people with disabilities. In health care, there are a limited number of medical specialists with experience caring for individuals with intellectual disabilities (Ward, Nichols, & Freedman, 2010). As a result, there are often only a few specialists that treat individuals with intellectual disabilities. Thus, the number of potential locations in a community for health/dental care is much smaller than for individuals without disabilities. Fitness and recreation departments develop separate adaptive programming that offer important opportunities for physical activity where none exist but also segregate people with disabilities from their peers (Rimmer et al., 2014). Housing agencies create group homes specifically for people with disabilities, which might lend themselves to residing only in certain parts of a community that are also not spatially integrated with their neighbors. Transportation agencies use separate private vehicles to transport individuals door-to-door. It is important for public health professionals to understand that this segregation of services across many aspects of community living results in spatial and social segregation and less participation with peers and contributes to stigma/attitudes about disability (Keith, Bennetto, & Rogge, 2015). Because of the environmental barriers discussed and segregation they facilitate, there is a need for public health professionals to understand and implement inclusive approaches and strategies that impact all populations.

5.4   The Universal Design Approach

Universal design (UD) is an ideal framework to address barriers in the built environment related to public health. Unlike accessibility, which views design narrowly as a reaction to disablement by removing barriers, UD (or inclusive design) can also support health and wellness through positive action to reduce the incidence of disablement and improve quality of life for all. Due to rising healthcare costs, seeking design solutions to health issues is not only a socially responsible goal but also a financial necessity. UD seeks to bring the benefits of more usable, healthier, and friendlier settings to the entire population, recognizing that everyone encounters disablement at some time in their lives. It is aligned with other progressive environmental design practices like design for inclusion of minority groups, design for active living, and design for health, all of which position human needs and aspirations as the central focus of design practice.

Most developed countries and many developing countries have laws that ensure some level of physical access to the built environment for people with disabilities. For example, in the USA, the Americans with Disabilities Act (1990, 2008) requires accessibility to all types of buildings with the exception of privately financed housing. The Fair Housing Act and its amendments (1968, 1988) require accessibility to multifamily housing. In response to the limitations of current regulations, the concept of UD emerged in the mid-1980s as a new paradigm for physical access. Rooted in the disability rights movement and the social model of disability, UD does not eliminate the need for standards that define the legal baseline for minimum accessibility. Instead, UD seeks to provide more aspirational goals than minimum regulatory requirements. UD raises the bar on accessibility, to address issues not yet covered by regulations and to make access an integral part of good design. Initially defined as "the design of products and environments to be usable by all people, to the greatest extent possible, without the need for adaptation or specialized design," UD has since evolved from focusing on usability and supporting independent function to also addressing social inclusion goals (Mace, 1985; Watchorn, Larkin, Hitch, & Ang, 2014). Social inclusion is consistent with the current paradigm of disablement theory in which the outcome of interventions to ameliorate the negative impact of impairment is *both* improving function and improving social participation (World Health Organization, 2011).

To capture these new ideas of health and social participation, a new definition for universal design was coined: "Universal design is a process that enables and empowers a diverse population by improving human performance, health and wellness, and social participation" (Steinfeld & Maisel, 2012). The eight goals of universal design accompany and support the new definition.

Goal 1: Body fit—accommodating a wide range of body sizes and abilities.
Goal 2: Comfort—keeping demands within desirable limits of body function.
Goal 3: Awareness—ensuring that critical information for use is easily perceived.
Goal 4: Understanding—making methods of operation and use intuitive, clear, and
   unambiguous.

Goal 5: Wellness—contributing to health promotion, avoidance of disease, and prevention of injury.

Goal 6: Social integration—treating all groups with dignity and respect.

Goal 7: Personalization—incorporating opportunities for choice and the expression of individual preferences.

Goal 8: Cultural appropriateness—respecting and reinforcing cultural values and the social and environmental context of any design project.

The goals define the outcomes of UD practice in measurable ways and apply to all environmental design domains (i.e., housing, public buildings, streetscapes, transportation, products, etc.). Moreover, each goal is supported by an interdisciplinary knowledge base (e.g., anthropometrics, biomechanics, perception, cognition, safety and health promotion, social interaction, and cultural values and practices). Thus, the goals can be used effectively as a framework for both knowledge discovery and knowledge translation to practice in public health. Table 5.1 describes examples for each UD goal applied in public health.

5.5 Integrating Universal Design into Public Health

The Centers for Disease Control and Prevention (CDC) outlined the three core functions and ten essential services of public health that serve as a framework for all public health activities, performance standards, and accreditation (Centers for

Table 5.1 Examples of universal design goals[a] applied in public health

Universal design goal	Application of UD goal to public health
Goal 1: Body Fit—Accommodating a wide range of body sizes and abilities	Accessible weight scales that can be used by individuals who use wheelchairs as well as those without
Goal 2: Comfort—Keeping demands within desirable limits of body function	Benches for resting during walking
Goal 3: Awareness—Ensuring that critical information for use is easily perceived	Policy to have communication materials in alternative formats
Goal 4: Understanding—Making methods of operation and use intuitive, clear, and unambiguous	Wayfinding signage that can be used by all to navigate indoor and outdoor spaces
Goal 5: Wellness—Contributing to health promotion, avoidance of disease, and prevention of injury	Subsidized transportation to preventive health care
Goal 6: Social Integration—Treating all groups with dignity and respect	Disability awareness for public health staff
Goal 7: Personalization—Incorporating opportunities for choice and the expression of individual preferences	Complete streets policies to ensure usability of pedestrian environments for all ages and abilities
Goal 8: Cultural Appropriateness—Respecting and reinforcing cultural values and the social and environmental context of any design project	Customizing evidence-based guidelines to fit the local context when designing parks and playgrounds

[a]Universal Design goals as defined in Steinfeld and Maisel (2012)

Disease Control and Prevention, 2018). The ten essential services are under review, and an updated set is likely to be released in 2020 (Krisberg, 2020). Table 5.2 describes the functions and essential services, and examples of how UD can be incorporated throughout. The remaining sections of the chapter describe in greater detail how these strategies can be implemented, including several case studies that highlight impacts on people with disabilities.

Across all core functions and services, a key to making public health universally designed is to engage people with disabilities in the process. Engaging people with disabilities and disability organization representatives is vital for obtaining feedback on the data collection process, recruiting respondents, and interpreting the results of the assessment. Universally designed stakeholder engagement helps

Table 5.2 Incorporation of UD into public health core functions and ten essential services[a]

Core functions	Essential services	Incorporation of UD
Assessment	1. Monitor health status to identify and solve community health problems 2. Diagnose and investigate health problems and health hazards in the community	• Assess environmental barriers and facilitators that affect person-environment fit • Ensure engagement of disability stakeholders
Policy development	3. Inform, educate, and empower people about health issues 4. Mobilize community partnerships and action to identify and solve health problems 5. Develop policies and plans that support individual and community health efforts	• Participatory design of UD solutions • Ensure engagement of disability stakeholders
Assurance	6. Enforce laws and regulations that protect health and ensure safety 7. Link people to needed personal health services and assure the provision of health care when otherwise unavailable 8. Assure competent public and personal healthcare workforce 9. Evaluate effectiveness, accessibility, and quality of personal and population-based health services	• Work with non-health sectors, such as transportation, planning, education, and employment to move beyond compliance with the ADA toward UD goals • Ensure engagement of disability stakeholders
All	10. Research for new insights and innovative solutions to health problems	• Understanding of resource centers on disability and health

[a]Core functions and essential services as defined by Centers for Disease Control and Prevention (2018). The Public Health System and the 10 Essential Public Health Services. https://www.cdc.gov/publichealthgateway/publichealthservices/essentialhealthservices.html

ensure relevance and impact of the policy objectives and additional guidance on details for policy implementation.

5.5.1 Core Function 1: Assessment

Under the core function of assessment are two essential services of monitor health and diagnose and investigate. Public health plans and policies are developed from the data-generating process of assessment. Practitioners cannot address environmental barriers and facilitators affecting people with disabilities unless data are gathered on these characteristics affecting health and well-being. One of the common ways that local health departments address these assessment services is through their community health assessments (CHAs), which are completed every 5 years and are required to become accredited by the Public Health Accreditation Board (Stoto, 2013). The CHA is used in some communities to assess current environmental strengths and gaps as well as how the local environment affects human health.

The CHA process can incorporate UD to help ensure that the environmental problems identified by the data also reflect the environmental problems experienced by people with disabilities. As part of the CHA, local health departments can include questions about the experience of living with a disability in that community and determine what barriers derail person-environment fit. The experience of conducting an environmental audit can be very enlightening for students and professionals who have not had the opportunity to examine accessibility of the built environment. Using checklists available for Readily Achievable Barrier Removal is one way to examine accessibility that follows ADA guidelines (Adaptive Environments Center, Inc., & Barrier Free Environments, Inc., 1995).

Several useful data collection instruments have been developed that go beyond the ADA to capture aspects of usability, including the Community Health Inclusion Index (CHII) (Eisenberg, Rimmer, Mehta, & Fox, 2015), the Community Health Environment Checklist (CHEC) (Stark, Hollingsworth, Morgan, & Gray, 2007), and the Facilitators and Barriers Survey (FABS) (Gray, Hollingsworth, Stark, & Morgan, 2008). CHII is a multilevel community health assessment used to assess the extent to which communities' policies, systems, and environments support physical activity and healthful eating among people with disabilities. FABS is useful for obtaining the subjective experience of people with disabilities in regard to their supports and challenges across a variety of community settings. The CHEC has also been used to assess the usability of community sites and includes several variations that provide a fine level of detail related to specific types of disabilities (e.g., mobility, vision, hearing). Use of any of these instruments will help ensure that public health practitioner's plans and implementation will incorporate the needs of all residents, including those with disabilities.

Public health practitioners can also utilize existing data sets that may shed light on aspects of person-environment fit. Existing environmental data may be available from nontraditional health sectors, such as urban planning, transportation, and housing, who collect data on the environment in many forms. For instance, housing agencies often have data on the number of accessible housing units, park departments often have data on accessible playgrounds, and transportation agencies often have data on the number and location of accessible transit stops. This is a great opportunity to engage these stakeholders who potentially hold rich data that can help inform environmental public health planning.

5.5.1.1 Case Study: UD in Assessment

The Coalition for a Healthy Greater Worcester in Massachusetts was interested in identifying ways to improve physical activity among youth. Their approach was to focus on physical activity at school playgrounds. The Worcester school board wanted to prioritize playgrounds that were in the most need of improvement. To help in that prioritization, a team from the coalition used the CHII and assessed all the school playgrounds in Worcester. This process generated a large database of information on inclusion of playgrounds. The coalition used the CHII data and other neighborhood level criteria to select two priority schools that would be funded to build new universally designed playgrounds (National Center on Health, Physical Activity and Disability, 2019). The physical audit was enlightening for the auditors from the coalition with limited disability backgrounds as well as for the school board, who learned various ways their playgrounds could be improved.

5.5.2 Core Function 2: Policy Development

The second core function of public health is policy development, which includes three essential services: (1) inform, educate, and empower; (2) mobilize community partnerships; and (3) develop policies. These training, planning, and policy development services require use of the data organized in the assessment stage to develop strategies that are informed by scientific evidence and relevant stakeholder participation. Practitioners draft guidelines, regulations, standards, and organizational policies and work to have policies or plans adopted by local stakeholders and government officials.

An inclusive approach can be integrated into these services by engaging diverse stakeholders and end users in the policymaking process. Gathering different perspectives during decision-making, particularly from community members, is another critical UD strategy because solutions developed to address environmental barriers in one community, for a particular population, may or may not be transferable to another community and/or group. For instance, solutions to a lack of accessible housing units developed for a dense urban community may not transfer to a rural community. Utilizing a participatory design process can help ensure solutions are contextually appropriate and that policy recommendations are embraced and implemented by the local community.

Universal design in policy development is not only about engaging diverse stakeholders, including traditionally marginalized populations, in the process but also about drafting policies that address the needs of a diverse constituency. A policy that integrates UD identifies opportunities to address the needs of all users. UD in public health policy development can address the need for more accessible housing, pedestrian infrastructure, and transportation. For example, a proposed Healthy People 2030 objective is to "Increase the proportion of all occupied homes and residential buildings that have visitable features" (US Department of Health and Human Services, 2019a, b).

5.5.2.1 Case Study: UD in Policy Development

Complete Streets (CS) policy expands access to the built environment for a diverse population of citizens, including people with disabilities. The CS approach encourages right of ways (ROWs) to be "…designed for the safety and comfort of all road users, regardless of age and ability" and introduce public health and economic vitality as critical transportation goals (Lynott et al., 2009). CS policy encourages changes to planning efforts that balance the needs of pedestrians, bicyclists, public transportation users, and motorists, regardless of age, ability, income, ethnicity, or mode of travel. Over 1400 municipalities have adopted "Complete Streets" (CS) policies to date in order to address pedestrian infrastructure design challenges, including steep slopes, rough and slippery surface materials, irregular pavement, lack of curb ramps, and traffic signal timing that does not support safe crossing. Design interventions on a community scale, implemented as a result of enacted policies, can increase physical activity levels and help reduce the increasing prevalence of obesity (Saelens, Sallis, Black, & Chen, 2003). Well-connected sidewalks, designated bike paths and parking, streetlights, and aesthetically pleasing streetscapes encourage children to walk to school, employees to bike to work, and families to take afternoon strolls. Because they are designed for all users, there is improved access for walking and biking for older adults and people with disabilities (McCann & Rynne, 2010).

5.5.3   Core Function 3: Assurance

The third core function of public health is assurance and includes (1) enforce laws and regulations that protect health and ensure safety, (2) link people to needed personal health services and assure the provision of health care when otherwise unavailable, (3) assure competent public and personal healthcare workforce, and (4) evaluate effectiveness, accessibility, and quality of personal and population-based health services. These services are largely implemented by the public health and healthcare sectors with cooperation from other sectors. Addressing environmental barriers experienced by people with disabilities requires an even stronger role for non-health sectors.

Engaging organizations from non-health sectors is vital for addressing environmental barriers because the public health sector does not have authority to implement changes to most aspects of the environment. Therefore non-health sectors need to play a key role in adopting and implementing UD solutions. Across sectors of transportation, housing, and fitness and recreation, UD solutions can help address the many environmental barriers people with disabilities experience. Various public health organizations and associations such as the American Public Health Association (APHA) and the National Association of County and City Health Officials (NACCHO) have consistently called for inter-sectoral collaborations to equitably protect and improve the health, safety, and quality of life of subpopulations such as persons with a disability (National Association of County and City Health Officials, 2017).

For public health professionals, identifying key actors and sectors to collaborate with and ensuring that public health staff are knowledgeable in nontraditional areas can be a challenge (Kochtitzky et al., 2011). Architects, community planners, and transportation engineers can bolster environmental public health efforts by (1) designing in such a way as to create compact, pedestrian-friendly communities that allow residents to walk to shops, services, cultural resources, and jobs; (2) providing choices by creating variety in housing, shopping, recreation, transportation, and employment, all to accommodate residents throughout the life span; and (3) providing direct, safe, and comfortable transportation infrastructure to help people of all ages and abilities acquire the knowledge and income they need to be productive members of society. There is a need for both public health and their multi-sector collaborators to be educated about the desires and needs of individuals with disabilities in that community. The best way to gain such understanding is through including disability organizations and people with disabilities in public health essential functions. The multi-sector coalition that includes people with disabilities is poised to work collaboratively to conduct assessments, plan, implement, and evaluate universally designed solutions.

5.5.3.1 Case Study: UD in Assurance

Transportation is increasingly becoming part of public health goals and strategies as it is recognized as an important social determinant of health. For public health goals related to transportation to be successful, public health practitioners need to engage and get buy-in from the transportation sector. The Jefferson County Health Department engaged transportation partners in their health impact assessment (HIA) process to better understand the impact of transportation on healthcare access (http://design4mobility.org/rapid-health-impact-assessment/). As part of that process, the HIA included recommendations for changes to transportation that would be implemented by the transportation agencies and which address needs of a diverse group of individuals with mobility challenges, including people with disabilities, older adults, low-income individuals, etc. The broad approach to defining mobility challenges helped assure that transportation improvements could have broad impact, including on people with disabilities. By engaging the transportation sector, the recommendations were more likely to be adopted and actually implemented.

5.6 Research Innovations

The tenth essential public health service is research for new insights and innovative solutions to health problems. Researching innovations occurs across all three core public health functions and the previous nine essential services described. It highlights the importance of being up-to-date on the evidence-based and potential solutions to new problems that lack evidence. Many examples of innovative practices exist and can be accessed online to learn more about UD applications to public health-related activities. For instance, the Guidelines, Recommendations, Adaptations, Including Disability or GRAIDs were developed through an extensive adaptation process and can be used by public health practitioners to ensure that environmental policies and interventions reach people with disabilities (Rimmer et al., 2014). These can be accessed through the National Center on Health, Physical Activity and Disability (https://inclusion.nchpad.org/). Another resource is *innovative solutions for Universal Design* or isUD™ (http://www.thisisud.com/). isUD™ has higher and more inclusive goals than accessibility standards and regulations. The research-backed assessment and certification program guides users through the entire design process, from planning the project through building design, including facility operation. More than 500 solutions are based on years of extensive research and practice and guided by the goals of universal design (UD).

5.7 Future Needs

For the field of environmental public health, it will be important to monitor and document the adoption and implementation of UD goals. Although we know that improving the environmental conditions can improve access, there is a need to build the evidence for how implementation of UD affects health and participation and more importantly, how local implementation differences affect outcomes. Building the evidence base for UD within public health can begin by developing what is called practice-based evidence (Ammerman, Smith, & Calancie, 2014). Practice-based evidence comes from testing of innovative practices in the field and is considered a beginning approach to build new areas of evidence. For environmental public health to better serve people with disabilities, there is a need to document and catalog the UD practices that are successfully implemented in the field (Vanderbom et al., 2018). Further, understanding the success of these practices comes from long-term evaluation and monitoring of health behaviors and outcomes among people with disabilities.

UD is an innovative concept, not because the idea is new but because it is perceived to be new by a majority of public health students and practitioners. Research on the diffusion of innovation demonstrates that communicating the innovation better and making it meaningful to those who will implement it are two of the most important strategies for improving adoption (Rogers, 2010). "Change agents" like UD advocates and experts can help spread knowledge through their persuasive power. What can advocates do to increase adoption of UD for environmental public health efforts? The most direct way to increase demand is to make public health students and professionals at large more aware of UD through training and dissemination efforts. To engage professionals, the development of communities of practice, especially among educators in environmental public health, is a priority. Successful innovation requires compatibility with the many existing contexts of practice, such as continuing education credits or accreditation of public health departments.

Increased awareness about UD for both public health professionals and people with disabilities will increase the implementation of UD in public health services. Supporting and participating in these initiatives should be a priority for all universal design advocates and experts. Given the breadth of stakeholders described in this chapter, UD advocates can come from all backgrounds and specialties within health and non-health sectors. UD goals can be applied to public health practice to support person-environment fit, helping to improve opportunities for better health outcomes for people with disabilities.

Acknowledgments We'd like to acknowledge the significant contribution of Chris Kochtitzky, M.S.P., who passed away before the publication of this book. Chris collaborated on shaping the form and content of this chapter and contributed important ideas and substantive text. In this chapter, and as he had done throughout his career, Chris brought together different disciplines in order to advance and disseminate social justice and health equity goals.

References

Adaptive Environments Center, Inc., Barrier Free Environments, Inc. (1995). *The Americans with Disabilities Act checklist for readily achievable barrier removal.* Washington, DC: United States Department of Justice. Retrieved from https://www.ada.gov/checkweb.htm

Americans With Disabilities Act (ADA) of 1990, Pub. L. No. 101–336, § 1, 104 Stat. 328 (1990 and revised 2008).

Ammerman, A., Smith, T. W., & Calancie, L. (2014). Practice-based evidence in public health: Improving reach, relevance, and results. *Annual Review of Public Health, 35*(1), 47–63. https://doi.org/10.1146/annurev-publhealth-032013-182458

Batorowicz, B., King, G., Mishra, L., & Missiuna, C. (2016). An integrated model of social environment and social context for pediatric rehabilitation. *Disability and Rehabilitation, 38*(12), 1204–1215. https://doi.org/10.3109/09638288.2015.1076070

Brown, A. R., & Mulley, G. P. (1997). Injuries sustained by caregivers of disabled elderly people. *Age and Ageing, 26*(1), 21–23.

Bureau of Transportation Statistics, U.S. Department of Transportation. (2018). *Travel patterns of American adults with disabilities.* Retrieved from https://www.bts.gov/travel-patterns-with-disabilities

Bureau of Transportation Statistics, U.S. Department of Transportation. (2003). Transportation difficulties keep over half a million disabled at home, April 2003. *BTS Issue Brief, No. 3.* Retrieved March 6, 2008, from http://www.bts.gov/publications/issue_briefs/number_03

Carroll, D. D., Courtney-Long, E. A., Stevens, A. C., Sloan, M. L., Lullo, C., Visser, S. N., … Dorn, J. M. (2014). Vital signs: Disability and physical activity—United States, 2009–2012. *MMWR. Morbidity and Mortality Weekly Report, 63*(18), 407.

Centers for Disease Control and Prevention. (2018). *The public health system & the 10 essential public health services.* Retrieved from https://www.cdc.gov/publichealthgateway/publichealthservices/essentialhealthservices.html

Clarke, P., Ailshire, J., & Lantz, P. (2009). Urban built environments and trajectories of mobility disability: Findings from a national sample of community-dwelling American adults (1986–2001). *Social Science & Medicine, 69*(6), 964–970.

Eisenberg, Y., Rimmer, J. H., Mehta, T., & Fox, M. H. (2015). Development of a community health inclusion index: An evaluation tool for improving inclusion of people with disabilities in community health initiatives. *BMC Public Health, 15*(1), 1050. https://doi.org/10.1186/s12889-015-2381-2

Ernst, M., & Shoup, L. (2009). Dangerous by design: Solving the epidemic of preventable deaths (and making great neighborhoods).

Fair Housing Act of 1968, Pub. L. 90–284, title VIII, §801, 82 Stat. 81 (1968 and revised 1988).

Frost, K. L., Bertocci, G., & Salipur, Z. (2013). Wheelchair securement and occupant restraint system (WTORS) practices in public transit buses. *Assistive Technology, 25*(1), 16–23.

Gell, N. M., Rosenberg, D. E., Carlson, J., Kerr, J., & Belza, B. (2015). Built environment attributes related to GPS measured active trips in mid-life and older adults with mobility disabilities. *Disability and Health Journal, 8*(2), 290–295.

Glass, T. A., & Balfour, J. L. (2003). Neighborhoods, aging, and functional limitations. *Neighborhoods and Health, 1*, 303–334.

Gray, D. B., Hollingsworth, H. H., Stark, S., & Morgan, K. A. (2008). A subjective measure of environmental facilitators and barriers to participation for people with mobility limitations. *Disability and Rehabilitation, 30*(6), 434–457.

Harrell, R., Lynott, J., Guzman, S., & Lampkin, C. (2014). *What is livable? Community preferences of older adults.* Retrieved from http://www.aarp.org/research/ppi/liv-com2/policy/Other/articles/what-is-livable-AARP-ppi-liv-com/

Haselwandter, E. M., Corcoran, M. P., Folta, S. C., Hyatt, R., Fenton, M., & Nelson, M. E. (2015). The built environment, physical activity, and aging in the United States: A state of the science review. *Journal of Aging and Physical Activity, 23*(2), 323–329.

Institute of Medicine. (2007). *The future of disability in America.* Washington, DC: National Academies Press.

Keith, J. M., Bennetto, L., & Rogge, R. D. (2015). The relationship between contact and attitudes: Reducing prejudice toward individuals with intellectual and developmental disabilities. *Research in Developmental Disabilities, 47*, 14–26.

Kochtitzky, C. S., Freeland, A. L., & Yen, I. H. (2011). Ensuring mobility-supporting environments for an aging population: Critical actors and collaborations. *Journal of Aging Research, 2011*, 138931. https://doi.org/10.4061/2011/138931

Kochtitzky, C. S., Frumkin, H., Rodriguez, R., Dannenberg, A. L., Rayman, J., Rose, K., … Kanter, T. (2006). Urban planning and public health at CDC. *MMWR. Morbidity and Mortality Weekly Report, 55*(2), 34–38. Retrieved from https://www.cdc.gov/mmwr/preview/mmwrhtml/su5502a12.htm

Krahn, G. L., Walker, D. K., & Correa-De-Araujo, R. (2015). Persons with disabilities as an unrecognized health disparity population. *American Journal of Public Health, 105*(S2), S198–S206. https://doi.org/10.2105/ajph.2014.302182

Krisberg, K. (2020). *Are the 10 essential public health services out of date? Review underway.* Retrieved from http://thenationshealth.aphapublications.org/content/49/10/1.1?rss=1

Lawton, M. P., & Nahemow, L. (1973). Ecology and the aging process. In C. Eisdorfer & M. P. Lawton (Eds.), *Psychology of adult development and aging* (pp. 619–674). Washington, DC: American Psychological Association.

Lynott, J., Haase, J., Nelson, K., Taylor, A., Twaddell, H., Ulmer, J., … Stollof, E. R. (2009). *Planning complete streets for an aging America.* Retrieved from https://www.ca-ilg.org/sites/main/files/file-attachments/resources__2009-02-streets_0.pdf?1441323100

Mace, R. (1985). Universal design: Barrier free environments for everyone. *Designers West, 33*(1), 147–152.

McCann, B., & Rynne, S. (2010). *Complete streets: Best policy and implementation practices.* Chicago, IL: American Planning Association.

McGinnis, J. M., & Foege, W. H. (1993). Actual causes of death in the United States. *Journal of the American Medical Association, 270*(18), 2207–2212. https://doi.org/10.1001/jama.270.18.2207

Nary, D. E., Froehlich, A. K., & White, G. W. (2000). Accessibility of fitness facilities for persons with physical disabilities using wheelchairs. *Topics in Spinal Cord Injury Rehabilitation, 6*(1), 87–98.

National Association of County and City Health Officials. (2017). *Statement of policy on transportation and health.* Retrieved from https://www.naccho.org/uploads/downloadable-resources/17-01-Transportation-and-health.pdf

National Center on Health, Physical Activity and Disability, Quarterly Digest. (2019). Retrieved from https://conta.cc/2Y2neI1

National Council on Disability. (2015). *Transportation update: Where we've gone and what we've learned.* Washington, DC: National Council on Disability. https://ncd.gov/rawmedia_repository/862358ac_bfec_4afc_8cac_9a02122e231d.pdf

National Council on Disability. (2006). *Creating livable communities.* Washington, DC: National Council on Disability.

Nelson, A. (2002). Unequal treatment: Confronting racial and ethnic disparities in health care. *Journal of the National Medical Association, 94*(8), 666.

Office of the United States Surgeon General. (2005). *The surgeon general's call to action to improve the health and wellness of persons with disabilities.* Retrieved from https://www.ncbi.nlm.nih.gov/books/NBK44667/pdf/Bookshelf_NBK44667.pdf

Peterson-Besse, J. J., Walsh, E. S., Horner-Johnson, W., Goode, T. D., & Wheeler, B. (2014). Barriers to health care among people with disabilities who are members of underserved racial/ethnic groups: A scoping review of the literature. *Medical Care, 52*, S51–S63.

Pynoos, J., Nishita, C., Cicero, C., & Caraviello, R. (2008). Aging in place, housing, and the law. *Elder Law Journal, 16*, 77.

Pynoos, J., & Nishita, C. M. (2003). The cost and financing of home modifications in the United States. *Journal of Disability Policy Studies, 14*(2), 68–73.

Rimmer, J., & Lai, B. (2017). Framing new pathways in transformative exercise for individuals with existing and newly acquired disability. *Disability Rehabilitation, 39*(2), 173–180.

Rimmer, J. H., Vanderbom, K. A., Bandini, L. G., Drum, C. E., Luken, K., Suarez-Balcazar, Y., & Graham, I. D. (2014). GRAIDs: A framework for closing the gap in the availability of health promotion programs and interventions for people with disabilities. *Implementation Science, 9*, 100–100. https://doi.org/10.1186/s13012-014-0100-5

Roberts, P. W., & Babinard, J. (2004). Transport strategy to improve accessibility in developing countries. In *10th international conference on mobility and transport for elderly and disabled people.*

Rogers, E. M. (2010). *Diffusion of innovations.* New York, NY: Simon and Schuster.

Rosso, A. L., Auchincloss, A. H., & Michael, Y. L. (2011). The urban built environment and mobility in older adults: A comprehensive review. *Journal of Aging Research, 2011*, 816106.

Saelens, B. E., Sallis, J. F., Black, J. B., & Chen, D. (2003). Neighborhood-based differences in physical activity: An environment scale evaluation. *American Journal of Public Health, 93*(9), 1552–1558.

Said, C. (2018). *Lyft sued by disability advocates over wheelchair access. San Francisco Chronicle.* Retrieved from https://www.sfchronicle.com/business/article/Lyft-sued-by-disabled-advocates-over-lack-of-12750101.php

Schulz, A., & Northridge, M. E. (2004). Social determinants of health: Implications for environmental health promotion. *Health Education & Behavior, 31*(4), 455–471. https://doi.org/10.1177/1090198104265598

Seekins, T., Traci, M. A., Cummings, S., Oreskovich, J., & Ravesloot, C. (2008). Assessing environmental factors that affect disability: Establishing a baseline of visitability in a rural state. *Rehabilitation Psychology, 53*(1), 80.

Shaw, G. (2000). Wheelchair rider risk in motor vehicles: A technical note. *Journal of Rehabilitation Research & Development, 37*, 89–100.

Shaw, G., & Gillispie, T. (2003). Appropriate protection for wheelchair riders on public transit buses. *Journal of Rehabilitation Research and Development, 40*, 309–319.

Smith, S. K., Rayer, S., & Smith, E. A. (2008). Aging and disability: Implications for the housing industry and housing policy in the United States. *Journal of the American Planning Association, 74*(3), 289–306.

Songer, T., Fitzgerald, S., & Rotko, K. (2004). *The injury risk to wheelchair occupants using motor vehicle transportation.* In Annual proceedings/association for the advancement of automotive medicine (Vol. 48, p. 115).

Srinivasan, S., O'Fallon, L. R., & Dearry, A. (2003). Creating healthy communities, healthy homes, healthy people: Initiating a research agenda on the built environment and public health. *American Journal of Public Health, 93*(9), 1446–1450. https://doi.org/10.2105/ajph.93.9.1446

Stark, S., Hollingsworth, H. H., Morgan, K. A., & Gray, D. B. (2007). Development of a measure of receptivity of the physical environment. *Disability and Rehabilitation, 29*(2), 123–137.

Steinfeld, E., & Maisel, J. (2012). *Universal design: Creating inclusive environments.* New York, NY: John Wiley & Sons.

Steptoe, A., Shankar, A., Demakakos, P., & Wardle, J. (2013). Social isolation, loneliness, and all-cause mortality in older men and women. *Proceedings of the National Academy of Sciences, 110*(15), 5797–5801.

Stoto, M. A. (2013). *Population health in the Affordable Care Act era* (Vol. Vol. 1). Washington, DC: Academy Health.

Sundar, V., Brucker, D. L., Pollack, M. A., & Chang, H. (2016). Community and social participation among adults with mobility impairments: A mixed methods study. *Disability and Health Journal, 9*(4), 682–691.

Syed, S. T., Gerber, B. S., & Sharp, L. K. (2013). Traveling towards disease: Transportation barriers to health care access. *Journal of Community Health, 38*(5), 976–993.

Taft, W. H. & Supreme Court of the United States. (1926) *U.S. Reports: Euclid v. Ambler, 272 U.S. 365. [Periodical].* Retrieved from the Library of Congress, https://www.loc.gov/item/usrep272365/

Thatcher, R. H. (2015). *Practices for establishing ADA paratransit eligibility assessment facilities* (No. Project J-7, Topic SB-25).

Thatcher, R., Ferris, C., Chia, D., Purdy, J., Ellis, B., Hamby, B., … Golden, M. (2013). *Strategy guide to enable and promote the use of fixed-route transit by people with disabilities* (No. Project B-40).

U.S. Department of Health and Human Services. (2010). *Healthy people 2020.* Retrieved from https://www.healthypeople.gov/2020/topics-objectives/topic/disability-and-health/objectives

U.S. Census Bureau, Housing and Household Economic Statistics Division. (2011). Last revised: October 31, 2011, from https://www.census.gov/hhes/www/housing/census/historic/units.html

U.S. Department of Health and Human Services. (2015). *Step it up! The surgeon general's call to action to promote walking and walkable communities.* Retrieved from https://www.hhs.gov/sites/default/files/call-to-action-walking-and-walkable-communites.pdf

U.S. Department of Health and Human Services. (2019a). *Proposed objectives for inclusion in Health People 2030.* Retrieved from https://www.healthypeople.gov/sites/default/files/ObjectivesPublicComment508_1.17.19.pdf

U.S. Department of Health and Human Services. (2019b). *Healthy People 2030 Framework.* Retrieved from https://www.healthypeople.gov/2020/About-Healthy-People/Development-Healthy-People-2030/Framework

Vanderbom, K., Eisenberg, Y., Tubbs, A., Washington, T., Martínez, A., & Rauworth, A. (2018). Changing the paradigm in public health and disability through a knowledge translation center. *International Journal of Environmental Research and Public Health, 15*(2), 328.

Vasudevan, V. (2016). An exploration of how people with mobility disabilities rate community barriers to physical activity. *California Journal of Health Promotion, 14*(1), 37–43.

Venter, C., Mashiri, M., Rickert, T., Maunder, D., Sentinella, J., de Deus, K., …, Bogopane, H. (2004). Towards the development of comprehensive guidelines for practitioners in developing countries. In *Proceedings of the 10th international conference on mobility and transport for elderly and disabled persons (TRANSED 2004)*, Hamamatsu, (pp. 23–26).

Ward, R. L., Nichols, A. D., & Freedman, R. I. (2010). Uncovering health care inequalities among adults with intellectual and developmental disabilities. *Health & Social Work, 35*(4), 280–290.

Watchorn, V., Larkin, H., Hitch, D., & Ang, S. (2014). Promoting participation through the universal design of built environments: Making it happen. *Journal of Social Inclusion, 5*(2), 65–88.

Weuve, J., Kaufman, J. D., Szpiro, A. A., Curl, C., Puett, R. C., Beck, T., … Mendes de Leon, C. F. (2016). Exposure to traffic-related air pollution in relation to progression in physical disability among older adults. *Environmental Health Perspectives, 124*(7), 1000–1008. https://doi.org/10.1289/ehp.1510089

World Health Organization. (1998). *The WHO health promotion glossary.* Geneva: World Health Organization.

World Health Organization. (2002). *WHO | International Classification of Functioning, Disability and Health (ICF).* WHO. Retrieved from https://www.who.int/classifications/icf/en/

World Health Organization. (2011). *World Report on Disability*, 2011. http://www.who.int/disabilities/world_report/2011/report.pdf

Xiang, H., Chany, A.-M., & Smith, G. A. (2006). Wheelchair related injuries treated in US emergency departments. *Injury Prevention, 12*(1), 8–11.

Chapter 6
Public Health Ethics and Disability: Centering Disability Justice

Bill Gaventa, Devan Stahl, and Katherine McDonald

6.1 Public Health Ethics and Disability: Centering Disability Justice

Throughout history, people with disabilities and their families have faced stigma, harmful stereotypes, discrimination, abuse, inequities, and injustice in multiple arenas of public life and professional care (Carey, 2009; Charlton, 1998; Shapiro, 1994; Smith & Wehmeyer, 2012). In the last two centuries, scientific advances have both helped and harmed people with disabilities. Institutionalization and the compulsory sterilization of people with disabilities within the eugenics movement represent the extreme of harm, but more subtle—and yet equally insidious—forms of harm included the shaping of public beliefs that disability is an individual medical issue and the province of specialized health care. Disability thus became a disease, deformity, defect, or disaster.

Public health was not immune from these forces; the prevention of disease, disability, and death are long-standing, entrenched goals of public health, and health and disability have long been perceived as antonymous. The US Supreme Court's 1927 *Buck v. Bell* decision stands as an exemplar of how these widespread beliefs informed policy approaches to public health. Deciding in favor of compulsory sterilization as a way to restrict genetic threats (Carey, 2009; Smith & Wehmeyer, 2012), the ruling explained "It is better for all the world, if instead of waiting to

B. Gaventa (✉)
Collaborative on Faith and Disability, Austin, TX, USA
e-mail: bill.gaventa@gmail.com

D. Stahl
Department of Religion, Baylor University, Waco, TX, USA
e-mail: Devan_Stahl@baylor.edu

K. McDonald
Department of Public Health, Syracuse University, Syracuse, NY, USA
e-mail: kemcdona@syr.edu

© Springer Science+Business Media, LLC, part of Springer Nature 2021
D. J. Lollar et al. (eds.), *Public Health Perspectives on Disability*,
https://doi.org/10.1007/978-1-0716-0888-3_6

execute degenerate offspring for crime, or let them starve for their imbecility, society can prevent those who are manifestly unfit from continuing their kind. ... Three generations of imbeciles are enough" (*Buck v. Bell, 274 US 200, (1927), paragraph 4*), 1927, paragraph 4). Related, disability can also easily be seen as a failure of health care's capacity to fix, prevent, or control impairing conditions. When disability is first seen as a failure, mistake, or accident, rather than a part of the natural biodiversity of life, negative public attitudes about people with disabilities, and their quality of life are not far behind. Too often, those negative attitudes became embedded in public policies that further diminish their quality of life, e.g., institutionalization. As evidenced in the newly revised American Public Health Association's Public Health Code of Ethics (APHA, 2019), public health is increasingly recognizing the imperative to hear and honor the voices of multiple communities of race, ethnicity, income level, gender, and other characteristics who have been marginalized, oppressed or neglected in the past (APHA Code of Ethics, 2019, pp.7-8 and 4.4.7, p. 18).

Only as individuals with disabilities, their families, and other allies began to push for community-based services and supports did more inclusive models of disability begin to evolve. The social model of disability diagnosed society as a collection of attitudes, environmental barriers, laws, value judgments, and customs that disable people more than individual impairment. The WHO International Classification of Functioning, Disability, and Health (ICF) model of disability embraces the dynamic relationship among impairing conditions and individual and social characteristics and their resulting impact on social barriers to participation in community life (World Health Organization, 2001). Drawing from both civil rights and this multi-level model to understand where to effect structural change, campaigns for rights, justice, and equal opportunities have led to legal rights, community-based programs, inclusive education, public awareness campaigns, and much higher visibility and participation of people with disabilities in communities. Public health initiatives continue to include prevention of disability as a goal, but emerging leadership initiatives also recognize that people with disabilities are not by definition unhealthy and emphasize that disability prevention efforts should maintain dignity and respect to people with disabilities. While some people with disabilities may have specific health needs related to their disability that benefit from specialized health care, they face the same routine health needs as anyone else, including needs for preventive care, health promotion, and equal access to primary health care. The corresponding challenges of learning to cope, thrive, and even flourish with sufficient supports and opportunities are far too often heightened by unequal access to quality health care and services (Krahn, Klein, & Correa-De-Araujo, 2015). Moreover, ongoing developments in health care such as enhanced prenatal detection of disabling conditions and the growing access to euthanasia or assisted suicide reflect modern opportunities for eugenics to persist (Reinders, Stainton, & Parmenter, 2019).

If disability is not by definition antithetical to health or flourishing, then it becomes one factor of the many that contribute to vast human diversity. As we increasingly understand the social determinants of health, so do we become aware of the fact that what is good for people without disabilities is also good for people with disabilities and, often, vice versa. Both health care and public health are beginning to factor in issues of diversity and disenfranchisement as possible social determinants of health that impact equitable and just approaches to public health. Disability thus becomes one of the social realities that needs to be included in those intersections. At the center of this systems transformation work are issues of ethics and justice: how do we create a public health system that reflects a just approach to public health and thus ensure equal access to public health functions and benefits? This ethical imperative is bolstered by legal mandates in the Americans with Disabilities Act (see Chap. 12 on the law, rights, and disability).

Our goal in this chapter is not to list or explore all of the injustices or ethical violations that have impacted the lives of people with disabilities and their families and their intersections with public health. Rather, our goal is to explore how the inclusion of disability as an important and far-reaching social factor, and disability justice as part of any framework of public health ethics, advances our successful approaches to achieving the aims of public health. As we promote equal access to health for all, we create healthier people and stronger, inclusive communities. The ethical issues often raised by people with disabilities in public health are not unique to them. Infusing explicit attention to justice into ethics can light the way for everyone. We also believe that the accommodations and strategies used to include people with disabilities have much wider applicability that can help address thorny public health issues, such as universal design for learning, person-centered planning, and others. Finally, we believe that addressing ethical issues that touch the lives of people with disabilities within the framework of disability justice and the newly revised and adopted Code of Ethics of the American Public Health Association provides an opportunity for public health professionals to live out this impressive code as it becomes more inclusive of disability. Those more focused on disability and ethics now have the opportunity to learn from this revised Code's emphasis on understanding the ways that history impacts health care and the importance of seeking community input, especially that of communities that have often been disenfranchised at every stage of the assessment, program development, and evaluation of public health initiatives.

6.2   Evolving Conceptions of Healthcare Ethics and Disability

Conceptions of health and healthcare ethics have evolved since the birth of bioethics as a unique field in the 1960s and 1970s. As medical technology became more sophisticated and clear abuses of power by physicians and medical researchers were exposed, a group of theologians and philosophers rose to prominence with the goal of resolving new ethical challenges that had arisen as a result of scientific advancements. Initially, it appeared that bioethicists and disability rights advocates shared much in common. Both groups were concerned with protecting vulnerable patients, combating medical paternalism, and respecting patient autonomy. It soon became clear, however, that bioethicists generally favored a biomedical model of disability, which views disability as an individual problem to be prevented, cured, or mitigated through medicine. Although the number of bioethicists who draw from a disability rights perspective is on the rise, much of mainstream bioethics continues to endorse and reflect the biomedical model of disability. Upholding this understanding of disability has created heated debates between mainstream bioethicists and disability rights advocates concerning issues such as prenatal diagnosis, selective abortion, and physician-assisted suicide. Historically, public health has suffered the same fate, endorsing a biomedical model of disability and focusing efforts on the prevention and containment of disability, although we will highlight understandings of health and disability as well as the goals of public health that are changing.

As bioethics has increased its scope to include public policy, law, health disparities, and social determinants of health, the lines between bioethics and public health ethics have been blurred (Bickenbach, 2010). What often begins as an ethical decision on an individual case in tertiary care has implications for public policy, prevention programs, and even government spending priorities. It is therefore worth briefly revisiting content areas where mainstream bioethics and disability rights advocates continue to clash, and the implications these debates have for public health.

All bioethical issues affect persons with disabilities. Disability is experienced by people of all sexes and genders across the lifespan, and persons with disabilities require health care as much as, and in some cases more often than, the nondisabled. At the same time, there are issues in bioethics that remain particularly important for disability rights advocates, because they have direct implications for persons with disabilities and their families. The areas of concern have remained relatively unchanged over the past 30 years, even though new technologies require bioethicists to revisit old debates. There are seven recurring areas that scholars have focused on that have important implications for persons with disabilities. Bickenbach (2010) has names for five of these: autonomy, reproductive rights, prenatal screening and genetics, end-of-life issues, and resource allocation and health system performance. In what follows, we briefly point out new issues that have arisen in these areas over the last decade and add two areas that have become increasingly salient in recent years: children's best interests and research ethics.

In many ways, autonomy is the prevailing concern in bioethics. Bioethics helped to usher in a new era in medicine wherein the rights of patients to medical information and control over medical decision-making now supersede medical paternalism or the deference of healthcare professionals to direct healthcare treatment decisions for individuals. The right to self-determination, however, has historically been limited. Patients with mental illness and other developmental and intellectual disabilities, for example, are not always allowed to make their own treatment decisions. In some cases, court-appointed guardians were given the authority to make medical decisions on behalf of such patients. Clinical assessments for "decision-making capacity," however, have evolved to ensure that mental illness or disability do not prima facie restrict a person from his or her right to medical decisions. Ideally, decision-making capacity is individually assessed and is targeted toward a particular decision, rather than an overall judgment about a person's competency (Ganzini, Vocier, Nelson, Fox, & Derse, 2005). Increasingly, bioethicists are also arguing that the preferences of persons with diminished mental capacity should be taken into consideration when determining what is in their best interest (Navin, Wasserman, & Haiman, 2019). Disability advocates have also helped to push the need for supported decision-making, which enables people with disabilities to make and communicate their decisions *with* supportive partners, rather than allowing guardians make decisions *for* them. Supported decision-making has obviated the need for legal guardians to take over decision-making on behalf of their wards, and about one-fifth of state laws now recognize this ethically stronger policy approach.

Within the realm of reproductive rights, the right to parent and selective abortion based on predicted disability remain important topics. According to the National Council on Disability, parents with disabilities often face barriers to parenting, including lack of access to reproductive health care and adoption as well as increased risk of losing custody of their children (NCD, 2012). Persons with disabilities are often unfairly denied access to assisted reproductive technologies due to discriminatory practices against them by healthcare providers and insurance companies. Moreover, according to the US Department of Justice, reports of discrimination against parents with disabilities within State child welfare agencies are widespread (DOJ, 2015). The NCD also reports that "the child welfare system is ill-equipped to support parents with disabilities and their families" and that states must "eliminate disability from their statutes as grounds for termination of parental rights" (NCD, 2012). Appropriate parental assessments that take into account one's context and access to supportive services would go a long way toward remedying this situation. Some states are undergoing legal reform to reflect the need for reproductive justice for people with disabilities.

On the other end of the spectrum, prenatal screenings are increasingly sensitive and noninvasive, making it easier to detect embryonic and fetal differences. When disabilities are detected, abortion remains the preferred "therapeutic" option. Regardless of their stance on abortion in general, many disability rights advocates are concerned that selective abortion sends the message that persons with disabilities are unwelcome in our society. That is, abortion can be seen to "solve" the problem of disability by eliminating future persons living with disability, rather than working to improve the accessibility of our society (Asch, 2000). Our society's continued large investment in screenings signals that preventing the birth of children with disabilities is a social good and part of high-quality prenatal care (Parens and Asch, 2000). Moreover, disability rights advocates contend that the "choice" to abort is often influenced by misinformation and stigma surrounding disability (de Graaf, Buckley, & Skotko, 2015; Shakespeare, 2007). Until ableism ("Discrimination or prejudice against people with disabilities" Merriam-Webster, 2019) is dismantled and disability rights are achieved, the choice to abort will be constrained.

Genetic screenings and technologies raise similar questions concerning what kinds of lives are worth living and how public resources should be invested. Preimplantation genetic diagnosis (PGD) allows parents to choose to implant embryos that do not have single gene disorders and chromosomal differences. PGD and other genetic therapies have created renewed concerns over eugenics. Unlike the earlier practice of compulsory sterilization, contemporary genetic interventions remain optional, but once again, it is questionable how free the "choice" to use technologies to prevent or ameliorate disabilities is in a society that stigmatizes and fails to accommodate disability. New advancements in CRISPR-Cas9 technology, which promises to engineer human embryos, are once again raising questions about whether eliminating disability is a social good. Increasingly, disability bioethicists are claiming disability is worth conserving because it is essential to human diversity (Garland-Thomson, 2012).

The proper treatment of children with disabilities has raised new questions as well. Within bioethics, parents are generally seen as the appropriate medical decision makers for their children. Parental decision-making can be overruled however, when parent's decisions cause avoidable harm to their child. The Baby Doe regulations (1985),[1] for example, were passed after several widely publicized cases of parents denying their disabled newborns low-risk, lifesaving medical treatments. The regulations ensure access to lifesaving medical interventions, food, and fluids for newborns with disabilities.

More recently, the case of Ashley X has raised new concerns over parents' authority to direct their disabled child's medical care. In the case of Ashley X, physicians approved a parental request to administer growth attenuation therapy, including high-dose estrogen, prophylactic hysterectomy, appendectomy, and breast bud removal to their 6-year-old daughter with profound developmental disabilities. The parents' desire was to keep Ashley's stature small and prevent her maturation, so that they could continue to care for her at home (Gunther & Diekema, 2006). Many disability rights advocates were disturbed by the treatments, noting the treatments violated Ashley's rights, were not medically necessary (as they did not treat any underlying pathology), infantilized Ashley by disallowing her to be seen as a future adult, and sterilized her without her voluntary consent (as is required by law) (AAIDD, 2012). The authority of parents to alter their disabled children's bodies continues to be debated as more and more parents seek to permanently alter their children with disabilities without the child's consent.

End-of-life issues remain contentious in bioethics in part because of fears of the overreach of medicine. Physician-assisted suicide/Physician-assisted death (PAS/D) is now legal in eight US states as well as the District of Columbia, with many more states considering passing similar legislation. Whereas PAS/D was initially framed as an option for people in intractable pain, evidence shows pain is not the major driver for patients who choose PAS/D. The top motivations for seeking PAS/D include loss of autonomy, dignity, and becoming a burden on others, which is perhaps why the increased availability of palliative care has not decreased demand for assisted suicide as many had hoped (Oregon Health Authority, 2017). Many

---

[1] The Baby Doe regulations requires that states that receive federal aid under the Child Abuse and Protection and Treatment Act report instances of "medical neglect" wherein treatments are withheld from infants that are not irreversibly comatose or in which the treatment is virtually futile (USC 5101).

disability rights advocates note the reasons persons give for wanting PAS/D are often the very conditions under which people with disabilities live. Disability advocates argue that social circumstances and our collective failure to eradicate ableism—and not bodily impairments themselves—are driving these decisions to end one's life (Gill, 2004; Tuffrey-Wijne, Cerfs, Finlay, & Hollins, 2019). New controversies have also arisen in response to the detection of new states of disordered consciousness. Increasingly, many patients who were thought to be in vegetative states (or "non-responsive wakefulness syndrome") are now thought to be minimally conscious, raising new concerns about when it is appropriate to withdraw life sustaining treatments for persons who are not terminally ill and may have some chance of limited recovery (Stahl & Banja, 2018).

When it comes to resource allocation, worries remain that QALY (quality-adjusted life years) and DALY (disability-adjusted life years) assessments, which are used to measure the impact of various diseases and disabilities on the productivity and well-being of people, devalue and endanger the lives of persons with disabilities. QALYs and DALYs can be used to exclude new drugs, organ transplantation, and other healthcare treatments from health insurance programs because they are determined not be cost-effective (Ne'eman, 2018). Researchers have developed subjective, disability-friendly measures of quality of life (Renwick, Nourhaghighi, Manns, & Rudman, 2003), but such measures have not found much traction. There is now plenty of evidence that persons with disabilities rate their quality of life as high as the nondisabled, drawing into question the conceptual and measurement assumptions of these approaches (Albrecht & Devlieger, 1999; Hartoonian et al., 2013). Many bioethicists, however, dismiss such findings, claiming people with disabilities merely have "scaled down preferences" (Glover, 2006, p. 18). The idea that disability is a deficit that inevitably leads to a bad life remains well-entrenched in the medical field as well as in bioethics.

Finally, advancements in research ethics have had direct implications for persons with disabilities. Standards for responsible research conduct have existed since at least the Nuremburg trials. After the Willowbrook experiments (1956–1970) came to light, in which children who were considered "mentally retarded" were infected with live hepatitis with the hopes of developing a vaccine (Dubois, 2008), the protection of human subjects with developmental and intellectual disabilities has been given higher priority. Some researchers have suggested the pendulum has swung too far, however, and the effort to protect persons with disabilities from exploitation has resulted in a neglect of this population in research. In an effort to better understand important health disparities, health behaviors, and healthcare experiences in this population, public health researchers are working to improve the comprehensibility and accessibility of consent materials, avenues to communicate decisions, and ways to balance power dynamics (McDonald & Raymaker, 2013). Under its *Project INCLUDE* program, the National Institutes for Health (NIH, 2018) is increasing its efforts to include people with developmental disabilities in basic and clinical research to better understand what will improve their health and well-being. The goal of many researchers is now to work with persons with disabilities directly, rather than rely upon proxy reports.

Within each of these content areas, disability rights scholars and activists have pushed bioethics to reconsider whether so-called consensus opinions are sensitive to disability perspectives, including disability rights. This is especially important when inaccurate and unethical bioethical judgments influence health policy and other initiatives taken up within public health. The biomedical model of disability has dominated thinking about disability in health care, leading many to believe medicine's role is to prevent or "fix" disability. Public health, in turn, has sought to prevent and contain disability through various measures. When bioethics, including public health ethics, neglects the disability perspective or inclusive practices that make initiatives accessible, scarce resources can be directed to programs and projects that people with disabilities do not need nor want and the lives of persons with disabilities can be diminished and even put in danger. Moreover, when health is reduced to a biomedical lens, important services that could help improve the lives of persons with disabilities, including their health, might be overlooked.

6.3   A New Era of Flourishing and Disability Justice

Shifts in the goals of public health and its understanding of and approach to disability, however, may prove to be beneficial to people with disabilities. The 2019 American Public Health Association (APHA) Public Health Code of Ethics describes the role of public health as moving away from individual and population "health" to the notion of "flourishing" (p.3). The APHA recognizes that impairment and illness do not prohibit flourishing, so long as persons are given appropriate supports. Flourishing hinges not so much on individual health or biological functioning as it does on the social conditions and structures which enable people to live their lives well. The notion of flourishing then demands an account of human interdependence, which resonates with how many disability rights scholars have spoken about the structures and conditions of human life. Flourishing is a relational concept rather than an individualist one.

With the goal of flourishing in mind, health disparities take on a new importance in public health. There is strong evidence that persons with disabilities experience significant health disparities linked to avoidable social, economic, and environmental disadvantages rather than their individual impairments or the health conditions that led to one's disability. Enabling persons with disabilities to flourish requires eliminating such unjust disadvantages. The Centers for Disease Control and Prevention (CDC) have recognized that many of these disadvantages are linked to America's practices of institutionalization and eugenics as well as lack of educational, employment, and independent living opportunities (Krahn et al., 2015). Today, adults with disabilities are more likely to avoid receiving health care because of cost and accessibility (CDC, 2010), they are at higher risk for obesity, lack of physical activity and smoking (CDC, 2006), and they are at increased risk for cardiovascular disease (Reichard, Stolzle, & Fox, 2011). People with disabilities are also more likely to be injured and victims of violent crimes and sexual assault (Rand

& Harrell, 2007), and they are less likely to receive adequate social and emotional support (Kinne, Patrick, & Doyle, 2009). Enabling people with disabilities to flourish requires understanding the cause and remedy to these health disparities.

Additionally, flourishing requires increased attention to the social determinants of health for people with disabilities, and thus demands increasing responsibility to address these root causes of inequities in the work of public health. Researchers have long known that health outcomes are linked to non-physiological determinants, including behaviors, education, and income. People with disabilities fare poorly in all these categories (Kessler Foundation, 2010). Discrimination and lack of access ensure people with disabilities live in a cycle of poverty and poor health, which can be devastating for their overall flourishing. To combat these disparities, *Healthy People 2020* has outlined a number of objectives, including recommendations for disability-friendly systems and polices, ways to overcome barriers to health care and measures to improve the environment, and activities and participation of people with disabilities (DHHS, 2019). Although they do not use the language of flourishing, the US Department of Health and Human Services clearly recognizes people with disabilities face various avoidable obstacles that can be remedied through appropriate public health measures designed with inclusion and accessibility in mind.

There is no reason, however, to believe that disability is antithetical to health or that persons with disabilities cannot flourish. Public health services can work to improve the social and environmental conditions of persons with disabilities to ensure their well-being and flourishing within our society. Health remains important for persons with disabilities, which is why the health disparities of this population are worthy of systematic attention. According to the APHA (2019), human flourishing recognizes that all persons are interdependent and that their social and cultural environments contribute to their flourishing. Humans fail to flourish when they experience "domination, inequity, discrimination, exploitation, exclusion, suffering, and despair..." (p. 3). Disability justice, therefore, ought to be a goal of public health. As we consider the ethical challenges that arise in health care and public health more generally, we cannot neglect to attend to this vision of justice.

As public health embraces flourishing as its organizing goal and acknowledges the significant role structural factors play in fostering—and impeding—this outcome, the reach of public health into diverse social institutions, rises to the fore. Yet explicit and systematic attention to people with disabilities as an important health disparities population is glaringly absent from mainstream public health practice. Public health has an ethical imperative to fully and unquestionably understand disability as natural part of the human experience and embody disability rights as a guiding ethical principle informing all public health practice. That is, a disability justice perspective necessitates that we center disability rights—equal access and full inclusion—into efforts to articulate, interpret, and apply ethical principles into public health (Parens & Asch, 2003). This also means taking efforts to dismantle ableism—multi-faceted discrimination against people with disabilities and its insidious effects on health and well-being—as an important aspect of public health.

Commitment to public health ethical principles requires that we move public health from the damaging grip of past efforts to segregate, control, and eliminate people with disabilities to efforts that understand the distinctions between health and disability and see people with disabilities as a population demographic worthy of systemic attention. Such attention would involve full inclusion in all public health work as well as focused attention to the ways in which disability may need to be accommodated to promote flourishing. Centering disability justice, public health would encourage efforts to help the millions of people living with disabilities avoid preventable secondary conditions, experience equal access to their communities as they desire (e.g., accessible and welcoming community-based health promotion opportunities including play areas for children and community recreation areas, opportunities for the community living, education, and employment options that one desires) and health-promoting policies and institutions (e.g., health insurance that appropriately enables positive health outcomes including removing the institutional bias of Medicaid, SNAP benefits that allow food choice and are responsive to the food and nutrition needs of people with disabilities), and lead the full lives that are hallmarks of flourishing (Kaiser Family Foundation, 2018; Larson et al., 2018; National Council on Disability, 2012; Association of University Centers on Disabilities and the American Association on Intellectual and Developmental Disabilities, 2015). Centering disability justice requires that public health reflect the universality of disability, meaning disability is everywhere, among all populations and all issues that public health addresses—in children, in racial and ethnic minorities, in refugees, in sexual minorities, in people aging, etc. Centering disability justice would result in people with disabilities having a seat at the table in professional capacities and as community members in public health planning efforts to ready for and respond to emergencies and disasters so that they do not fare worse than others in these events or to help set public policy addressing structural conditions affecting health.

6.3.1 Disability Ethics and Justice as an Ally and Asset to Public Health Practice

As noted, the American Public Health Association's Public Health Code of Ethics (APHA, 2019) recognizes the imperative to hear and honor the voices of multiple communities who have been historically marginalized:

> A given action might have permissible consequences—such as gaining new knowledge that can be used beneficially in the future—but nonetheless be the type of action that is prohibited on the basis of social, cultural, and historical experience and consensus. One clear example of an impermissible actions is torture; another is discrimination based on race, gender, ethnicity, or functional impairment. Such actions violate values that today are recognized as central to the mission of public health. pp. 7–8

The Code encourages the practitioners of public health to both invite and seek out the voices and participation of diverse communities from the beginning of assessment and planning through design, implementation, and evaluation.

> 4.4.7 Be attuned to cultural, social, and historical contexts that influence community health and receptivity to public health partnerships. Attunement to cultural, social, and historical contexts is particularly important when addressing health disparities because communities burdened by excess illness and disease may also be socially disadvantaged by discrimination related to race, ethnicity, age, social class, geography, immigrant status, and sexual orientation and gender identity, among other differences reflected in social hierarchies. (p. 18)

The Code also recognizes that public health systems wield significant power (Section 3: Guidance for Ethical Analysis, pp. 7–10). Using that power in ways that build trust, mutual respect, and participation is an imperative for communities that have felt powerless, or experienced abuses of power in the past. If public health initiatives are to succeed, they need to *include* community members in ways that build a shared sense of responsibility and commitment rather than *impose* a plan of action. As the Code says, public health thus lives out its foundational values of professionalism and trust, health and safety, health justice and equity, interdependence and solidarity, human rights and civil rights, and inclusivity and engagement (Section 2: Public Health Core Values and Related Obligations).

Thus, from the perspective of disability justice, one could say that the newly revised Code of Ethics almost seems like it was written to address issues that disability rights advocates have raised with public health. Initial success in raising explicit and systematic attention to people with disabilities is also reflected in the inclusion of relevant goals in in the Healthy People 2010 and 2020. For example, inclusion in all forms of community life, including education, employment, civic life and health care, has been the major goal and vision for disability communities for the past 50 or more years. Self-determination has also guided multiple forms of public policy and practice. "Nothing about us without us" has been one of the rallying cries of disability advocates and their allies.

Although we recognize that *functional impairment* may reflect a less stigmatized label than disability and be a useful framework for creating some forms of access to public health functions, it fails to capture the structural aspects of disability and misses the opportunity to normalize the label of disability as a natural part of the human condition. The APHA Code of Ethics can be strengthened by using the word "disability" rather than "functional impairment" in the first quote from the Code above because it would be a more inclusive example of communities impacted by the "type of action that is prohibited on the basis of social, cultural, and historical experience and consensus" (Andrews et al., 2019). Moreover, its addition to the Section 4.4.7 listing (see above) of "communities burdened by excess illness and disease may also be socially disadvantaged by discrimination related to race, ethnicity, age, social class, geography, immigrant status, and sexual orientation and gender identity, among other differences reflected in social hierarchies" would go a long way toward a rational for enhancing the visibility of disability in public health initiatives (Krahn & Havercamp, 2019). That visibility is even more important because of what one might call "double marginalization," i.e., the frequent margin-alization of people with disabilities within other marginalized communities. This oversight of naming disability signals the need for explicit and systematic attention to disability justice in public health. Invisibility yields, at best, a failure of opportu-nity to benefit from public health initiatives and, at worst, direct harm from public health initiatives (Krahn & Havercamp, 2019).

Promoting equal rights and opportunity, hallmarks of justice, through education and public policy have been major avenues for enhancing inclusion and participa-tion for people with disabilities. Along the way, other creative policies, strategies, and tools have developed to build the ethical policies, accommodations, and rela-tionships needed to include people with disabilities and to strengthen their level of participation in multiple arenas of community life. A number of them have great potential for contributing to the ethical practice of public health as a whole. Stated another way, resources and strategies that have been developed to assist people with disabilities turn out to have universal application, i.e., to be good for all of us. We highlight six exemplars.

First, at a conceptual level, the WHO definition and functional construct of dis-ability is that of an impairment that is impacted by personal and environmental fac-tors (i.e., attitudes, beliefs, interpretations, coping mechanisms, etc.) which then together affect participation in all aspects of community life. As such, its biopsycho-social model integrates much of the social model of disability, whose central prem-ise is that those constructs and social barriers do more to disable people than the actual impairments, while also holding space for other forms of intervention to posi-tive impact the lives of people with disabilities. The WHO definition thus lines up with an understanding of public health that is becoming intensely aware of the social determinants of health, i.e., the impact of malleable environmental conditions such as poverty, poor housing, education, ableism, pollution, and other socioeco-nomic factors that both impact human flourishing and lead to major healthcare ineq-uities. The rationale is then obvious for seeking, *including*, and *engaging* the input of people with disabilities as one of the communities impacted by public health policies and programs and, further, *hiring* people from that community as one way of building trust and collaboration (APHA Code of Ethics, 2019, 4.8.2, p. 24 and 4.11.2, p. 28). Looking closely at the physical and geographical accessibility of public health programs and other social barriers that may hinder participation is another implication of both theoretical approaches.

Second, the theory and practice of Universal Design is one promising practice process to promote inclusion, although individual accommodations may still be needed. Universal Design for Learning (UDL) emerged as inclusive education learned that the accommodations necessary to enhance inclusion and learning for children with disabilities in typical educational settings led to recognition that chil-dren and adults learn in multiple ways. Then, learning environments should be designed in ways that seek to include everyone from the beginning, rather than fit-ting some children into what was considered "typical."

The three main principles of UDL are: (1) provide multiple means of engagement (the "why" of learning), (2) provide multiple means of representation (the "what" of learning), and (3) provide multiple means of action and expression (the "how" of learning). Therefore, one must stimulate interest and identify ways to maintain motivation and engagement, present information in different ways, and allow people to express their ideas in different ways (AUCD, SOI, CDC, and Golisano Foundation, 2018).

The principles of Universal Design for Learning are being expanded to envision universal design for programs and services. If they became a driving principle for public health education, training and service programs, people from very diverse backgrounds and with different levels of ability could be included from their beginning in both professional roles and as engaged community members.

Third, one of the tenets of UDL and inclusive practices with people with various forms of disabilities is that people communicate in a variety of ways. Besides the obvious example of the importance of signing for working with deaf individuals and communities, inclusion of people with intellectual and developmental disabilities, including people on the autism spectrum, has led to a much greater awareness of the importance of writing in plain English, the use of pictures and symbols, the use of video, and other accommodations that engage multiple senses. (See Sect. 6.5.) Many of those strategies and tools have obvious overlaps with public health initiatives that seek to engage diverse communities where English skills are limited. An example is the *Books Beyond Words* series that comes out of the UK picture books that tell a story, with a possible text, but primarily geared for a conversation between a person with limited reading skills and a counselor or assistant. The topics now cover multiple areas of social life, community living, and health care, including personal health care, coping with depression, abuse, dealing with diabetes, dental care, going to the hospitality, nutrition, and more. The point is not that those particular books might have a much larger audience, but that the principles involved, e.g., simplified English, pictures, scenes out of community life, and guided discussion all have potential for enhancing communication, enhancing learning, and engaging multiple audiences.

Fourth, one of the cautions taken in the new APHA Code of Ethics is recognizing that inclusion and participation by individuals and communities is often impacted by stigma and discrimination, by failing to hear the voices of everyone, and the need to recognize that everyone has a right to be involved in choices and decisions impacting their lives and communities, with a goal of enhancing everyone's agency (Code of Ethics, Introduction, p. 3, and Domain 4, pp. 17–21). Self-determination has been a core value and programmatic goal in disability services and supports for more than 20 years, leading to changes in program planning, the right to participate in planning bodies, and more control over individual use of public funds (National Center on Self Determination, n.d.). A relatively new process called supported decision-making also enables people with an array of disabilities to receive support in understanding, making, and guiding decisions impacting their lives (National Resource Center on Supported Decision Making). The process involves people who know an individual best, thus indicating a promising applicability not only to elicit the contributions and participation of people with disabilities but also people from cultures where no one would consider making a decision without consulting family members or others in their community. Public health could readily take advantage of this emerging model for supporting individuals in contributing to public health policy and planning decision-making processes.

Fifth, in the world of intellectual and developmental disabilities, the methods and practices of person-centered planning arose as a counterpoint to care planning in which professional voices held sway and individuals had little say. One form, *Essential Lifestyle Planning* (Smull & Sanderson, 2005), seeks the answers to two questions: "What is important *for* someone?" and "What is important *to* someone?" (Smull & Sanderson, 2005). Another form called the *PATH* (*Planning Alternative Tomorrows with Hope*) (Pearpoint, O'Brien & Forest, 1991) process starts with the dreams and hopes that someone has for their life rather than with the deficits that need to be addressed. The principles and practices of person-centered planning are easily applicable with almost anyone and become a way of helping to build the trust that professionals are truly listening. Like supported decision-making, person-centered planning processes recognize the embeddedness of individuals in communities by encouraging an individual to include people who are close to them. Person-centered planning also impacts public policy by affirming the right and importance for the voices of people to be included in public discourse on polices, issues, and resources. This approach resonates with public health's emphasis on community assessments, rather than needs assessments, so that community strengths and resources are identified and leveraged to further encourage positive community health. Integrating these approaches may yield unique insights into public health initiatives more inclusive of people with disabilities. With the new Code's emphasis on partnership and collaboration, an organizational approach would be to develop alliances with self-advocacy organizations, Centers for Independent Living, and other advocacy organizations run by people with disabilities and/or their families.

In a world where one trait or difference for individuals or populations often becomes the single or dominating identity, person-centered planning is a way of recognizing what Nigerian writer Chimamanda Ngozi Adichie calls "the danger of a single story":

> All of these stories make me who I am. But to insist on only these negative stories is to flatten my experience and to overlook the many other stories that formed me. The single story creates stereotypes, and the problem with stereotypes is not that they are untrue, but that they are incomplete. They make one story become the only story…Power is the ability not just to tell the story of another person, but to make it the definitive story of that person (Adichie, 2009).[2]

Thus, envision that people with disabilities are affected by all the public health issues as listed by the APHA on its website, as are other minorities (APHA, 2019). The importance of seeing the multiple stories in one's life, said another way, is another way of describing the intersectionality of disability with multiple issues of

---

[2] Chimamanda Ngozi Adichie, The danger of a single story, TED2009. To watch the full talk, visit TED.com.

concern in public health delivery. Disability is but one facet of one's identity and lived experience.

All of these inclusive processes from the world of disability -- definitions and models of disability (e.g., WHO) that include social determinants of health, universal design for learning and service delivery, utilizing multiple forms of communication, self-determination/supported decision-making and person-centered planning -- share a common belief that every person has worth, value, and dignity by explicitly noting that people with disabilities have strengths and gifts as well as weaknesses and deficits. These tools can be leveraged to infuse disability justice into public health while also providing ways for public health to address and include other minorities. Seeking individual and community capacity beyond a single story defined by a stereotype has multiple implications for working with diverse communities and populations too often defined by a single healthcare issue, or other stereotypes as noted in the Code of Ethics (4.1.5; 4.2.6; 4.5.5; 4.7.3). Adjectives become nouns, and we work with "the aging," "diabetics," alcoholics, the "obese," and multiple other groups. In the past decades, learning about how to build community inclusion and participation by and with people with disabilities has also utilized and allied with the theory and practice of asset-based community development (Kretzmann & McKnight, 1993) to go looking for the strengths of stereotyped communities and build from those assets in addressing issues of inclusion and participation. "Capacity vision," as it is sometimes called, can thus be a crucial foundational premise for seeking to include devalued populations in public health planning, programming, and evaluation with the premise that they have skills, gifts, and insights to bring to the table. *Community Conversations* (Swedeen, Cooney, Moss, & Carter, 2011) is one specific tool for getting input from groups of people as well as their buy-in to potential strategies for addressing community health issues.

6.4   Conclusion

Ethics is the very essence of an arena where voices from multiple disciplines and perspectives are needed to help define core values and principles that influence and guide policies and practice. Cultural, legal, moral, philosophical and religious traditions shape that context, bringing insights from centuries of human experience into a time when both old and new issues arise from new developments in arenas such as health care, technology, economics, and politics. For example, the perfect storm of the industrial age, mass immigration, and scientific hubris from the latter part of the nineteenth century to the middle of the twentieth shaped questions around people with disabilities into deep and wounding stereotypes, damaging policies and laws, and oppressive practices (Rose, 2017; Smith & Wehmeyer, 2012). It took the multiple voices of people with disabilities, their families, legal advocates, as well as changing philosophies in human services to change those policies and practices, all of them appealing to historical understandings of rights, freedoms, human values, and understandings of community, including the belief that the righteousness and justice of a society can best be measured by how it treats its most vulnerable citizens.

This chapter has reviewed the evolving history of healthcare ethics and disability, noting growing attention to the ethical questions in systems of care in addition to ethical questions in individual cases within hospital settings. Models, constructs, and definitions of disability have evolved in ways that have reflected and led those changes. Disability justice has always been concerned with individuals and society, as well as rights to equal opportunity, community inclusion, and participation. Lessons learned about effective strategies for accessibility, inclusion, and participation in the arena of disability turn out to have universal applicability and thus can support the growing understanding in public health ethics that all voices need to be heard and all parts of a community included in planning, service delivery, and evaluation processes.

In that history, as in the discussions in this chapter, there are four basic lessons to remember. First, the lived experience of disability, whatever its cause, raises fundamental questions for many about the essence of what it is to be human, what it means to be community, and the relationship between assumed suffering and flourishing in describing quality of life. Second, disability is a part of lived experience, a possibility for anyone's life that is not going to go away given life's vulnerabilities and limitations. People with disabilities as well as other conditions can indeed flourish, in their own eyes and in those of others. Third, just as the voices of people with disabilities and their allies led to multiple changes in the last eighty years, so should any discussion about ethics, health, and public policy involve people with disabilities and their families at all levels, their voices heard, and their agency honored. Fourth, we know that when people experience and know a sense of belonging in their communities, it helps their flourishing, including their level of health.

Ethics direct us from what is wrong toward what is right and are expressed in cultural narratives and laws. Commitments to what is morally right, therefore, have far-reaching tentacles and implications on people's lives. As we have reviewed, prior wrongs can re-emerge under new guises. APHA's Code of Ethics articulates professional standards and expectations for public health. While this newly adopted code resonates implicitly with a disability justice orientation, from a disability justice perspective, disability needs to be named as one of the populations that experiences health disparities so that public health initiatives can intentionally be designed to help people with disabilities flourish. Said another way, invisibility fosters a lack of explicit and systematic attention to disability justice, especially because people with disabilities often are marginalized within other marginalized populations. The disability rights movement and the institutions that seek to promote disability rights are a natural and beneficial resource to public health professionals. Public health and its initiatives also need to be seen as a natural ally for people with disabilities, their families, and professionals who work with them. Ethics, after all, is expressed in cultural narratives and laws, but it comes from, and goes back to, relationships; relationships between people, between people and organizations, and between organizations. We encourage all to take deliberate actions to weave together the knowledge, resources, and goals of each to help all people with disabilities, and everyone else, flourish..

6.5   Resources for Further Exploration

American Medical Association Journal of Ethics April 2016, Volume 18, Number 4. Focus issue on medicine, disability and ethics.

Foundational Principles and Guidelines for the Sustainable Inclusion of People with Intellectual Disability, AUCD and Special Olympics. See, in particular, the resources suggested for strategies to implement the principles and guidelines. There is significant correlation with, and applicability for, the new APHA Code of Ethics.

Intellectual and Developmental Disabilities, 2019, Vol. 57, No.5, 476-481. October, 2019. Focus issue on Population Health and People with Intellectual and Developmental Disabilities.

National Council on Disability: Bioethics and Disability Report Series. https://www.ncd.gov/publications/2019/bioethics-report-series.

Plain Language Resources: https://centerforplainlanguage.org/; https://www.sabe-usa.org/wp-ontent/uploads/2014/02/GuideToCreatingAccessibleLanguage.pdf; https://selfadvocacyinfo.org/resource/plain-language.

What Is Universal Design? http://universaldesign.ie/What-is-Universal-Design/

References

Adichie, C. N. (2009). *The danger of a single story. TED Talk*. Retrieved December 10, 2019, from https://www.ted.com/talks/chimamanda_adichie_the_danger_of_a_single_story?language=en

Albrecht, G., & Devlieger, P. (1999). The disability paradox: High quality of life against all odds. *Social Science & Medicine, 48*(8), 977–988. https://doi.org/10.1016/s0277-9536(98)00411-0

American Association on Intellectual and Developmental Disabilities. (2012). *Position statement: Growth attenuation*. Retrieved December 10, 2019, from https://www.aaidd.org/news-policy/policy/position-statements/growth-attenuation

American Public Health Association. (2019). *Public health code of ethics*. Washington: APHA Issue Brief.

Andrews, E. E., Forber-Pratt, A. J., Mona, L. R., Lund, E. M., Pilarski, C. R., & Balter, R. (2019). SaytheWord: A disability culture commentary on the erasure of disability. *Rehabilitation Psychology, 64*(2), 111–118. https://doi.org/10.1037/rep0000258

Asch, A. (2000). Why i haven't changed my mind about prenatal diagnosis: Reflections and refinements. In E. Parens & A. Asch (Eds.), *Prenatal testing and disability rights*. Washington, DC: Georgetown University Press.

Association of University Centers on Disabilities and the American Association on Intellectual and Developmental Disabilities. (2015). *Community living and participation*. Washington, DC: The Association of University Centers on Disabilities and the American Association on Intellectual and Developmental Disabilities.

Association of University Centers on Disabilities (AUCD), Special Olympics International (SOI), Centers for Disease Control and Prevention National Center for Birth Defects and Developmental Disabilities, and Golisano Foundation. (2018). *Foundational principles and guidelines for sustainable inclusion of people with intellectual disability.*

Baby Doe Amendment, §§ 5106a. (1985). in Kappel, B. (2009). Moral and ethical issues specific to developmental disabilities: Guardianship, involuntary servitude, sterilization, Baby Doe,

euthanasia. Retrieved from http://mn.gov/mnddc/honoring-choices/cnnReports/Moral_and_
Ethical_Issues-Kappel.pdf.

Buck vs. Bell, 274 US 200, paragraph 4. https://scholar.google.com/scholar_case?c
ase=1700304772805702914&q=Buck+v.+Bell,+274+U.S.+200.+(1927&hl=en
&as_sdt=6,44&as_vis=1

Bickenbach, J. E. (2010). Disability issues in health care ethics and law in the public health curriculum. In D. J. Lollar & E. M. Andresen (Eds.), Public Health Perspectives on Disability:
Epidemiology to Ethics and Beyond. New York, NY: Springer: 211–226.

Carey, A. C. (2009). *On the margins of citizenship: Intellectual disability and civil rights in
twentieth-century America*. Philadelphia, PA: Temple University Press.

Centers for Disease Control and Prevention. (2010). Quick-Stats: Delayed or forgone medical care
because of cost concerns among adults aged 18-64 years, by disability and health insurance
coverage status—National Health Interview Survey, United States, 2009. *MMWR Morbidity
and Mortal Weekly Report., 59*(44), 1456.

Centers for Disease Control and Prevention. (2006). *Disability and health state chartbook: Profiles
of health for adults with disabilities*. Atlanta, GA: Centers for Disease Control and Prevention.

Center for Self Determination. (n.d.). Retrieved from http://www.self-determination.com

Charlton, J. (1998). *Nothing about us without us: Disability oppression and empowerment*.
Berkeley, CA: University of California Press.

de Graaf, G., Buckley, F., & Skotko, B. G. (2015). Estimates of the live births, natural losses, and
elective terminations with Down syndrome in the United States. *American Journal of Medical
Genetics, 167a*(4), 756–767. https://doi.org/10.1002/ajmg.a.37001

Department of Justice. (2015, January 29). *Letter from the U.S. Department of Justice, Civil Rights
Division and U.S. Department of Health and Human Services, Office for Civil Rights to the
Massachusetts Department of Children and Families*. Retrieved December 10, 2019, from
www.ada.gov/ma_docf_lof.pdf,   www.hhs.gov/ocr/civilrights/activities/examples/Disability/
mass_lof.pdf

Dubois, J. M. (2008). Solving ethical problems: Analyzing ethics cases and justifying decisions. In J. M. Dubois (Ed.), *Ethics in mental health research* (pp. 46–57). Oxford: Oxford
University Press.

Ganzini, L., Vocier, L., Nelson, W. A., Fox, E., & Derse, A. R. (2005). Ten myths about decision
making capacity. *Journal of the American Medical Directors Association, 6*(5), S99. https://
doi.org/10.1016/j.jamda.2005.03.021

Garland-Thomson, R. (2012). The case for conserving disability. *Journal of Bioethical Inquiry,
9*(3), 339–355. https://doi.org/10.1007/s11673-012-9380-0

Gill, C. (2004). Depression in the context of disability and the 'right to die'. *Theoretical Medicine,
25*, 171–198. https://doi.org/10.1023/B:META.0000040058.24814.54

Glover, J. (2006). *Choosing children: Genes, disability, and design*. Oxford: Oxford University Press.

Gunther, D. F., & Diekema, D. S. (2006). Attenuating growth in children with profound developmental disability: A new approach to an old dilemma. *Archives of Pediatric and Adolescent
Medicine, 160*, 1013–1017. https://doi.org/10.1001/archpedi.160.10.1013

Hartoonian, N., Hoffman, J. M., Kalpakjian, C. Z., Taylor, H. B., Krause, J. K., & Bombardier,
C. H. (2013). Evaluating a SCI-specific model of depression and quality of life. *Archives
of Physical Rehabilitation and Medicine, 95*(3), 455–465. https://doi.org/10.1016/j.
apmr.2013.10.029

Kaiser Family Foundation. (2018). *Waiting list enrollment for Medicaid Section 1915(c) home and
community-based services waivers*. Retrieved December 10, 2019, from https://www.kff.org/
health-reform/state-indicator/waiting-lists-for-hcbs-waivers/?

Kessler Foundation. (2010). *NOD survey of Americans with disabilities*. Retrieved December 10,
2019, from http://www.adminitrustllc.com/wp-content/uploads/2013/12/Kessler-NOD-2010-
Survey.pdf

Kinne, S., Patrick, D. L., & Doyle, D. L. (2009). Prevalence of secondary conditions among people with disabilities. *American Journal of Public Health, 94*(3), 443–445. https://doi.org/10.2105/ajph.94.3.443

Krahn, G., Klein, D., & Correa-De-Araujo, R. (2015). Persons with disabilities as an unrecognized health disparity population. *American Journal of Public Health, 105*(S2), S198–S206. https://doi.org/10.2105/AJPH.2014.302182

Krahn, G., & Havercamp, S. (2019). From invisible to visible to valued: Improving population health of people with intellectual and developmental disabilities. *Intellectual and Developmental Disabilities., 57*(5), 476–481. https://doi.org/10.1352/1934-9556-57.5.476

Kretzmann, J., & McKnight, J. (1993). *Building communities from the inside out: A path toward finding and mobilizing a community's assets.* Chicago, IL: ACTA Publications. Also see: The ABCD Institute: https://resources.depaul.edu/abcd-institute/Pages/default.aspx

Larson, S. A., Eschenbacher, H. J., Anderson, L. L., Taylor, B., Pettingell, S., Hewitt, A., … Bourne, M. L. (2018). *In-home and residential long-term supports and services for persons with intellectual or developmental disabilities: Status and trends through 2016.* Retrieved December 10, 2019, from https://risp.umn.edu/archive

McDonald, K. E., & Raymaker, D. M. (2013). Paradigm shifts in disability and health: Toward more ethical public health research. *American Journal of Public Health, 103*(12), 2165–2173. https://doi.org/10.2105/AJPH.2013.301286

The Merriam-Webster.com Dictionary, Merriam-Webster Inc. (2019). *Ableism.* Retrieved December 12, 2019, from https://www.merriam-webster.com/dictionary/ableism

National Council on Disability. (2012). *Deinstitutionalization toolkit.* Retrieved December 12, 2019, from https://ncd.gov/publications/2012/DIToolkit

National Institutes of Health. (2018). *The INCLUDE Project Research Plan. 2018.* Retrieved December 12, 2019, from https://www.nih.gov/include-project/include-project-research-plan

Navin, M., Wasserman, J., & Haiman, M. H. (2019). Treatment over objection: Moral reasons for reluctance. *Mayo Clinical Proceedings, 94*(10), 1936–1938.

Ne'eman, A. (2018, October 29). Formulary restrictions devalue and endanger the lives of disabled people. *Health Affairs.* https://doi.org/10.1377/hblog20181025.42661/full/

Oregon Health Authority Public Health Division. (2017). *Oregon Death with Dignity Act 2017 data summary.* Retrieved from https://oregon.gov/oha/PH/ProviderPartnershipResources/EvaluationResearch/DeathwithDignityAct./Documents/year20:pdf.

Parens, E., & Asch, A. (2003). Disability rights critique of prenatal genetic testing: Reflections and recommendations. *Mental Retardation and Developmental Disabilities Research Review, 9*(1), 40–47. https://doi.org/10.1002/mrdd.10056

Pearpoint, J., O'Brien, J., & M. Forest. (1991). Planning positive possible futures, planning alternative tomorrows with hope (PATH). Toronto, Canada: Inclusion Press

Rand M. R., & Harrell E. (2007). *National crime victimization survey: Crime against people with disabilities, 2007.* Bureau of Justice Statistics Special Report. https://www.bjs.gov/content/pub/pdf/capd07.pdf.

Reichard, A., Stolzle, H., & Fox, M. H. (2011). Health disparities among adults with physical disabilities or cognitive limitations compared to individuals with no disabilities in the United States. *Disability and Health Journal, 4*(2), 59–67. https://doi.org/10.1016/j.dhjo.2010.05.003

Reinders, H., Stainton, T., & Parmenter, T. (2019). The quiet progress of the new eugenics: Ending the lives of persons with intellectual and developmental disabilities for reasons of presumed quality of life. *Journal of Policy and Practice in Intellectual Disabilities, 16*(2), 99–112. https://doi.org/10.1111/jppi.12298

Renwick, R., Nourhaghighi, N., Manns, P., & Rudman, D. (2003). Quality of life for people with physical disabilities: A new instrument. *International Journal of Rehabilitation Research, 26*(4), 279–287. https://doi.org/10.1097/00004356-200312000-00005

Rose, S. (2017). No right to be idle: the invention of disability 1840s – 1930s. Chapel Hill: University of North Carolina Press.

Shakespeare, T. (2007). Arguing about genetics and disability. In J. Swinton & B. Brock (Eds.), *Theology, disability and the new genetics: Why science needs the church*. New York, NY: T&T Clark.

Shapiro, J. (1994). *No pity: People with disabilities forging a new civil rights movement*. New York, NY: Three Rivers Press.

Smith, J. D., & Wehmeyer, M. L. (2012). *Good blood, bad blood: Science, nature, and the myth of the Kallikaks*. Washington, DC: American Association on Intellectual and Developmental Disabilities.

Smull, M., & Sanderson, H. (2005). *Essential lifestyle planning for everyone*. Stockport: HSA Press.

Stahl, D., & Banja, J. (2018). The persisting problem of precedent autonomy among persons in a minimally conscious state: The limitations of philosophical analysis and clinical assessment. *AJOB Neuroscience, 9*(2), 120–127. https://doi.org/10.1080/21507740.2018.1459932

Swedeen, B., Cooney, M., Moss, C., & Carter, E. W. (2011). *Launching inclusive efforts through community conversations: A practical guide for families, services providers, and communities*. (Downloadable) Also see https://www.erikwcarter.com/communityconversations, and Centers for Disease Control. *Community conversations tool kit: Instructions for conveners and facilitators*.

Tuffrey-Wijne, I., Cerfs, L., Finlay, I., & Hollins, S. (2019). Because of intellectual disability, he couldn't cope: Is euthanasia the answer? *Journal of Policy and Practice in Intellectual Disabilities, 16*(2), 113–116. https://doi.org/10.1111/jppi.12307

US Department of Health and Human Services. (2019). *The secretary's advisory committee on national health promotion and disease prevention objectives for 2020*. December 10, 2019, from https://www.healthypeople.gov/2020/About-Healthy-People/History-Development-Healthy-People-2020/Advisory-Committee

World Health Organization. (2001). *International classification of functioning, disability and health (ICF)*. December 10, 2019, from https://apps.who.int/iris/bitstream/handle/10665/42407/9241545429.pdf

Chapter 7
International Public Health and Global Disability

Donald J. Lollar and Mary Chamie

Disability and human functioning are global public health concerns. Unfortunately for those who live with disabling conditions and in environments not conducive to accommodate them, public health has traditionally focused on eliminating the conditions under which they occurred—communicable diseases, birth defects, injuries, chronic medical conditions, or aging. By virtue of its close traditional connection with medicine through prevention of communicable diseases, primary prevention is crucial. It is altogether fitting, even noble, for public health practitioners to work to reduce the conditions contributing to the etiology of a limitation—disease outbreaks, automobile crashes, falls, lead contamination, nutritional inadequacies, or lack of exercise, as examples. Public health's mission has been and still is the prevention or reduction of mortality, morbidity, and disability. Throughout the world, primary prevention activities to reduce these unfavorable outcomes are a principle public health direction.

Nonetheless, "More than one billion people in the world live with some form of disability, of whom nearly 200 million experience considerable difficulties in functioning" (Chan & Zoellich, 2011), representing an astounding number of individuals live with disabilities in spite of public health's best primary prevention efforts. By all accounts, the prevalence of disabling conditions is increasing as a result of a convergence of better life-saving medical interventions, an increase in chronic health conditions, and extended life spans in most countries. The health of people with disabilities has not been a focus traditionally for public health activities around the globe. Public health has assumed that medical and rehabilitation services are responsible and will manage any health needs. Public health has assumed any secondary condition associated with a primary disabling condition or health promotion activities a lesser priority. This public health bias and approach to the training of public health professionals is finally being challenged. Broadening public health

D. J. Lollar (✉)
School of Public Health, Oregon Health & Science University, Portland, OR, USA

M. Chamie
International Disability Statistics Consultant, Portland, OR, USA

United Nations Statistics Division (former), Demographic and Social Statistics, New York, NY, USA

© Springer Science+Business Media, LLC, part of Springer Nature 2021
D. J. Lollar et al. (eds.), *Public Health Perspectives on Disability*,
https://doi.org/10.1007/978-1-0716-0888-3_7

149

activities to include preventing secondary conditions and health promotion for people with disabilities represent an emerging global public health enterprise.

In the past 50 years, a confluence of activities around the globe has placed a greater emphasis on affording individuals with disabilities and their families equal footing with the general population—including health and well-being. Much of this emphasis began with a movement in several countries by people with disabilities themselves. Grassroots organizations began to advocate for greater autonomy and inclusion in their lives. International organizations began to take note of this movement and include people with disabilities in their planning and directions of their agencies. This chapter will outline the primary global entities that have lead public health and advocacy efforts alongside people with disabilities. The chapter will characterize global issues for people with disabilities beyond traditional medical or health concerns. The World Health Organization in its most cogent document thus far recognizes that there are three distinct but related issues for people with disabilities globally (WHO, 2014). First, disability is a **human rights issue** because people with disabilities live with stigma, isolation, discrimination, and inequality. These societal attitudes undermine access to opportunities for a full life to which all are entitled. Second, disability is a **development issue** in that many individuals with disabilities live in poverty whether in lower-income or higher-income countries. Poverty and disability interact and contribute to further disability through malnutrition, poor health care, lack of transportation, and overall toxic environments in which they must live, work, or go to school. Opportunities for education and employment are similarly lacking for this population. Disability, it would follow, is both an outcome of social determinants as well as a demographic factor affecting social and economic status. Finally, disability is a **global public health issue** because people with disabilities have poorer health outcomes than the general population, have difficulty with access to health care and rehabilitation, and can be healthy in the presence of a disabling condition. That is, people with disabilities can be healthy, and their disability status should not be equated with illness.

7.1 Stigma and Discrimination

International health programs confront a wide range of interpretations and understandings of population functioning and disability by communities. Social and cultural attitudes, for example, can sometimes stand in the way of delivering needed services to a person who has a disability. Family members or others in the community may believe disability is punishment for some past behavior on the part of a relative. As a result, a household which includes a person with a disability—or even a household associated with disability—may be so ashamed or fearful of discrimination that they prefer to keep the disability hidden.

In some settings, disability or association with it may mean facing cultural, political, religious, or even legal proscriptions. People with disabilities may be discouraged from appearing in public and may not be able to participate in common daily activities, vote, marry, or attend public schools. Because of the grave effects of these exclusionary practices, more and more rights advocates have come to see community inclusion of persons with disabilities as a human rights goal.

7.2 Disability as a Human Rights Issue

The most fundamental and powerful mandates for people with disabilities are found in the international covenants from the United Nations, including the Convention on the Rights of Persons with Disabilities (CRPD) (United Nations, 2019a) and the Convention on the Rights of the Child. In addition, the health-focused policies, programs, and classifications developed through the World Health Organization (WHO) and the World Bank, including the *International Classification of Functioning, Disability and Health* (ICF), the approved derived classification for children and youth (ICF-CY), the *World Report on Disability*, and *Global Disability Action Plan 2014–2021*, provide the impetus and mandate for member states to improve the living conditions and opportunities for people with disabilities.

7.2.1 Disability Policies and Programs and Global Health

Global health data, policy, and programs are affected by international agreements. These agreements over time have built on one another to strengthen the rights and health of people with disabilities. Three major United Nations agreements have shifted the orientation of public health programs worldwide.

1. The *World Programme of Action Concerning Disabled Persons* (WPA) (United Nations General Assembly, 1982) informed concepts used in the *Standard Rules on the Equalization of Opportunities for Persons with Disabilities* (United Nations General Assembly, 1993).
2. The *Standard Rules* were adopted by the United Nations General Assembly at its 48th session in 1993 and were used as a basis for drafting the now internationally agreed human rights treaty as of 2006.
3. The *International Convention on the Rights of Persons with Disabilities (United Nations, 2019a).*
   In addition, the *International Convention on the Rights of the Child* completes the emphasis on the rights of every citizen, including children.

7.2.2 The World Programme of Action Concerning Disabled Persons (WPA)

The World Programme of Action Concerning Disabled Persons (WPA) was adopted by the United Nations General Assembly at its 37th session on 3 December 1982 by its resolution 37/52 (United Nations General Assembly, 1982). The World Programme laid out the major concepts proposed for the study of the general situation of people with disabilities and for monitoring program action. The *World Programme* identifies three key goals in the field of disability: (a) equalization of opportunities, (b) rehabilitation, and (c) prevention.

These same three program goals are agreed and elaborated upon in the *Standard Rules on the Equalization of Opportunities for Persons with Disabilities* adopted by the United Nations General Assembly at its 48th session on 20 December 1993 (resolution 48/96) (United Nations, 1993).

The following program descriptions apply:

- *Equalization of opportunities*: the process through which the general system of society, such as the physical and cultural environment, housing and transportation, social and health services, educational and work opportunities, and cultural and social life, including sports and recreational facilities, are made accessible to all.
- *Rehabilitation*: a goal-oriented and time-limited process aimed at enabling an impaired person to reach an optimal mental, physical, and/or social functional level, thus providing people with the tools to change their own life. It can involve measures to compensate for a loss of function or a functional limitation (e.g., by technical aids) and other measures intended to facilitate social adjustment or readjustment.
- *Prevention*: measures generally aimed at two broad health areas: (1) preventing the onset of mental, physical, and sensory impairments (primary prevention) and (2) preventing impairment when it has occurred, from having negative physical, psychological, and social consequences.

7.2.3 Standard Rules on the Equalization of Opportunities for Persons with Disabilities

The purpose of the Standard Rules is to ensure that planning for girls, boys, women, and men with disabilities, as members of their societies, may exercise the same rights and obligations as others. The Standard Rules noted that in all societies of the world obstacles remain that prevent persons with disabilities from exercising their rights and freedoms, thus making it difficult for them to participate fully in the activities of their societies. The Rules state that it is the responsibility of States to take appropriate action to remove such obstacles and that persons with disabilities and their organizations should play an active role as partners in this process. The fundamental concepts in disability policy were set out through the Standard Rules, including prevention, rehabilitation, and equalization of opportunity. These three policy concepts are explained in more detail below.

States are encouraged to support the exchange of knowledge and experience among non-governmental organizations, research institutions, representatives of field programs and professional groups, organizations of persons with disabilities, and national coordinating committees (p. 38). Moreover, States are asked to ensure that the United Nations and the specialized agencies, as well as intergovernmental and inter-parliamentary bodies at the global and regional levels, include in their work the global and regional organizations of persons with disabilities.

7.2.4   Convention on the Rights of Persons with Disabilities (CRPD)

The Convention on the Rights of Persons with Disabilities was adopted by the United Nations in 2006 (United Nations General Assembly, 2006). It was opened for signature in 2007 and entered into force in May 2008 (United Nations, 2020). The Convention is built upon the *World Programme of Action* and the *Standard Rules* and raises the agreements to the level of an international treaty. According to Don MacKay, the Chairman of the committee that negotiated the Treaty, the Convention endeavors to "elaborate in detail the rights of persons with disabilities and set out a code of implementation" (United Nations, 2020). There are eight guiding principles that underlie the Convention and each one of its specific articles. They are shown in the Box below, and each of these principles has implications for work in the area of health (United Nations).

7.2.4.1   Guiding Principles of the Convention

1. Respect for inherent dignity, individual autonomy including the freedom to make one's own choices, and independence of persons;
2. Non-discrimination;
3. Full and effective participation and inclusion in society;
4. Respect for difference and acceptance of persons with disabilities as part of human diversity and humanity;
5. Equality of opportunity;
6. Accessibility;
7. Equality between men and women;
8. Respect for the evolving capacities of children with disabilities and respect for the right of children with disabilities to preserve their identities.

The Convention states that it "takes to a new height the movement from viewing persons with disabilities as 'objects' of charity, medical treatment and social protection towards viewing persons of disabilities as 'subjects' with rights who are capable of claiming those rights and making decisions for their lives based on their free and informed consent as well as being active members of society" (United Nations, 2020).

Article 4 of the Convention indicates that countries joining in the Convention sign on to work to develop and carry out national policies, laws, and administrative measures for securing the rights recognized in the Convention and abolish laws, regulations, and customs and practices that constitute discrimination. Disability is an important area where policies, laws, and administrative measures must be addressed.

7.2.5   Convention on the Rights of the Child (CRC)

The United Nations recognized the greater vulnerability of children and youth under the age of 18 years and therefore, even before the CRPD, approved basic rights for this group (United Nations, 1989). Article 23 of that Convention focused on those children and youth who live with mental or physical disabilities as well as their families. One section addresses the right to available resources for the eligible young person and his/her caregivers. Clearly outlined in the Article is the right of the young person to have access to education, training, health care, rehabilitation, and preparation for employment and recreation opportunities. The outcome of these services would be that the child or youth achieve "the fullest possible social integration and individual development, including cultural and spiritual development." To meet these objectives, UN member states are mandated to promote the exchange of information in the field of preventive health care and medical, psychological, and functional treatment for this group.

Article 24 of the CRC continues the focus on health by recommending appropriate measures be taken to decrease infant and child mortality, ensure provision of health care with particular attention to primary health care, and ensure prenatal and postnatal care for mothers. Family planning education and services to parents related to preventive health care for their children was included. It is clear that these Articles were included to address both the prevention of disabling conditions and the interventions to assist children and youth who have not been spared physical or mental disabilities.

7.3   Disability as a Development Issue: Sustainable Development Goals

The relationship between poverty and disability has been well-established (CICH, 2000; Fujiura & Kiyoshi, 2000; Yeo & Moore, 2003). The Millennium Development Goals (MDGs) were established by the United Nations from 2000 to 2015 focusing on ending poverty in its various spheres of influence, including health. The MDGs, however, focused on developing countries, and while successful to some extent, highlighted the gap between "developing" and "developed" countries—primarily centered on Northern vs Southern hemispheres. The Millennium Development Goals were created for developing countries primarily by developed countries. The vast majority of people living with disabilities globally are in less developed countries. The MSG goals include the eradication of extreme poverty and hunger, achieving universal primary education, reducing child mortality, and ensuring environmental sustainability. James D. Wolfensohn, then World Bank Group President, reported that the MDGs established by the UN and World Bank could not be achieved without the inclusion of people with disabilities, since the overlap between disability and poverty is so great (Wolfensohn, 2004). Wolfensohn suggested that unless people with disabilities are contributing economically to a country's economy, their development goals could not be reached. To move forward more equitably, a much broader alliance, including both developing and developed countries, was formed to develop Sustainable Development Goals for 2015–2030 (ICLEI, 2015). As with the MDGs, once again, disability issues were not directly mentioned in the SDGs. Ending poverty, achieving food security, ensuring healthy lives, promoting well-being, and reducing inequality within and among countries are examples of the 17 worthy goals, but none can be met without working specifically with and for the more than one billion individuals in the world living with disabilities and their families.

A second element of disability as a development issue is found in the World Report on Disability (WPD) (World Health Organization & World Bank, 2011). The WPD frames prevention of health conditions as a development issue, with the assumption that environmental factors, such as unsafe water and sanitation, poor roads, and unsafe workplaces, often contribute to the incidence of disabling conditions, most notably through lower levels of human functioning. This intersection of development and public health broadens the scope and importance of the inclusion of people with disabilities in all aspects of community life.

7.4   Disability as a Public Health Issue

7.4.1   Health Classifications in Global Public Health

The first classification for "health" was developed in 1893 by the International Statistical Institute and entitled the *International List of Causes of Death* (WHO, 2019), addressing the etiology or causes of people dying. This mortality classification was revised every 10 years over several decades until World War II. WHO was tasked with oversight of the evolving classification in 1948 and published for the first time the inclusion of morbidity codes—illness, not just death. The classification continued to change over the decades with the most recent effort completed in 2018—the *International Classification of Diseases 11th Revision: The Global Standard for Diagnostic Health Information (ICD)* (WHO, 2019). The ICD "defines the universe of diseases, disorders, injuries, and other related health conditions" (WHO, 2019). The ICD is used to assess prevalence of diseases, track reimbursements, and trends in resource allocations.

An initial effort to add a disability classification to complement the mortality and morbidity classification was found inadequate by members of the global disability community (*International Classification of Impairments, Disabilities, and Handicaps, 1980*) (WHO, 1980); therefore, member states of the WHO in 2001 approved a substantially stronger conceptual and coding framework called the *International Classification of Functioning, Disability and Health (ICF)* (WHO, 2001). In contrast to the ICD efforts focusing on etiology of death or morbidity, the ICF provides a system for classifying states of functioning, health, and well-being. The ICF transitioned from a medical model to a biopsychosocial model, identifying body impairments, and basic human activities, such as seeing, hearing, walking, and learning. Beyond these two dimensions, ICF included major areas of participation, such as play, school, work, social relationships, and voting, and, in addition, identifies environmental factors affecting the three preceding domains—impairments, activities, and participation. Environmental factors include physical, policy, and attitudinal elements and are a unique feature among health classifications.

Several conceptual notions are included in the ICF. First, the ICF describes functioning, but it does not categorize people. Second, the ICF is not about disability per se, but rather the ICF can describe anyone's functioning. Third, it is important to note that individuals with the diagnosis can have extreme differences in functioning that will affect medical and public health interventions. Conversely, individuals with different diagnoses and different impairments, for example, may have very similar functional levels for which similar interventions will be effective. The coding system of ICF allows for a description of the individual's functional issues (impairments, activities limitations, and participation restrictions) along with the environmental factors, whether barriers or facilitators.

7.4.2 The ICF Framework for the Study of Human Functioning and Disability

In virtually all societies, the concept of disability arises when people compare their physical and mental health states. In the newly agreed ICF, these comparisons are encompassed in the umbrella framework of human functioning, seen from a neutral perspective. Three key domains of functioning are described:

1. Individual *body structure and function*
2. Human *activities*
3. Community *participation*

Disability is also part of the umbrella framework of ICF, seen through a problematic lens (WHO, ICF, p. 3); i.e., it indicates a limitation in one of the three domains of functioning:

1. *Impairments* of *body structure and function*
2. *Limitations* of *human activities*
3. *Restrictions* in community *participation* (WHO, 2001, p. 3)

In the ICF framework, there are three important factors affecting human functioning: (a) contextual factors of the environment, having the capacity to both facilitate and debilitate human functioning; (b) characteristics of the person, such as age and sex; and (c) conditions of health (see Fig. 7.1).

Human functioning is a broad social, environmental, and biological concept. Figure 7.1 describes the way in which the three domains of environment, person, and health states are related in a broad framework of human functioning. The ICF framework recognizes that overall levels of human functioning and disability (problems of human functioning) are the result of interactions of persons with the environment, recognizing the general state of health conditions and while taking into

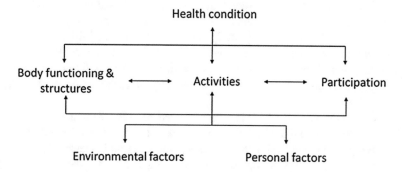

Fig. 7.1 Model of functioning and disability. (Reproduced with permission from International Classification of Functioning, Disability, and Health—Children & Youth Version, World Health Organization, Copyright 2007)

consideration demographic and social characteristics such as age, sex and residence, and other factors.

In the ICF, the concept of "person" in Fig. 7.1 is bracketed because personal characteristics, while recognized as influencing functioning, are not classified in ICF; they refer to sex, age, education, occupation, ethnicity, and other demographic, social, and economic characteristics classified elsewhere (WHO, 2001, p. 3).

ICF uses the term "disability" with specific meanings that may differ from its everyday usage. Both in the vernacular and the official health classification, disability as a concept largely refers to *restriction, loss, and limitation* of functioning, whether at the community, individual, or body level.

ICF classifies *environments* and communities according to products and technology designed and utilized; natural environmental characteristics and human-made changes to the environment; types of community and family support and relationships in place; attitudes and norms of society, family, and health professionals among others; and services, systems, and policies in place.

The *body functions and structures* of people are described and classified according to global and specific *mental functions* including consciousness, intellectual functions, temperament and personality functions, sleep functions, attention, memory, psychomotor functions, emotional, perceptual, and thought functions, and the like. *Sensory functions* such as seeing, hearing, taste, smell, touch, and pain among others are described and classified. Also described and classified are *voice and speech functions, functions of the cardiovascular, hematological, immunological, and respiratory systems; digestive metabolic and endocrine systems; genitourinary and reproductive functions, neuro-musculoskeletal and movement-related functions; and functions of the skin and related structures*. At the *body structure* levels, classifications of the nervous system, eye, ear, and related structures and structures involved in voice and speech and movement, for example, are also described.

Activities of people are described and classified with reference to learning and applying knowledge; general tasks and demands; communication activities; mobility; self-care; domestic life; interpersonal interactions and relationships; and according to *participation in major life areas* of education, work and employment, economic life and community, social and civic life. It should be noted that "at the time of the revision process of the ICIDH was in a final stage it seemed to be possible to distinguish activity and participation at the level of definitions. However, it was not possible to reach agreement about the related classifications. For this reason (in the ICF) there is one classification for activity and participation (domains) with four suggestions on how to use this in an activity or participation mode" (WHO 2001, p. 255).

ICF is a multipurpose classification designed to serve various disciplines. Its stated aims are threefold. First, it aims to provide a scientific basis for understanding and studying health and health-related states, outcomes, and determinants. Second, it aims to establish common language for describing health and health-related states in order to improve communication between healthcare workers, researchers, policy-makers, and the public, including people with disabilities. And third, the ICF provides a systematic coding scheme for health information systems (WHO, 2001, p. 5, item 2).

ICF has numerous applications. It may be used, for example, as:

- A *statistical* tool, in the collection and recording of data—for example, in population studies or management information systems.
- A *research* tool to study outcomes, quality of life, or environmental influences.
- A *policy* tool for risk adjustment related to reimbursement, social security planning, compensation systems, and policy design and implementation.
- An *educational* tool—for example, to design curriculum, raise awareness, or encourage action. (WHO, 2001, p. 5, item 2.1)

The ICF was a major triumph for the disability community who were intimately involved in its development and passage. Immediately, however, it was clear to many in the development process that functions related specifically to children and youth had not been well integrated into the original ICF. A working group was established by WHO and funded by the US Centers for Disease Control and Prevention's Disability and Health group to fill the gaps on behalf of children and youth (ICF-CY). Developmental issues and family emphases that were minimized in the original ICF were included, along with an emphasis on inclusion of terminology accessible to families around the globe. The ICF-CY was officially approved in 2005 (WHO, 2007) and became a derived ICF classification, currently being used in clinical, educational, and public health research and programs. Research using the ICF-CY has been particularly useful for children and youth in health and education settings (Hamlin et al., 2017; Lollar, Hartzell, & Evans, 2012; Rowland et al., 2016).

The ICF, when used for public health functions of assessment, policy development, or assurance, is a powerful framework. Collaborative work between ICD and ICF/ICF-CY has the potential for providing a substantially stronger description of the population involved in healthcare assessment and interventions.

7.5   Assessment

Public health assessment is defined as the regular, systematic collection and analysis of information on the health of a community or population. Data should include health status, health needs of the population, and epidemiological and other studies of health problems. The most basic tenet of assessment is a case definition, i.e., how does one identify what is to be assessed. Historically, definitions of disability and identification of individuals living with disabilities have varied greatly in public health. A traditional approach would merely equate a person in a diagnostic category (ICD code) with having a disability, such as cerebral palsy, or arthritis, or autism. This approach, however, as indicated earlier, assumes similar characteristics beyond just etiology. Functional equivalence is not revealed even if severity of diagnosis is included. Another definitional approach has been to focus on a person's impairment, for example, unable to hear in one or both ears or having lost an arm or leg.

Most countries have used one of these approaches to defining disability in surveys or censuses. The United Nations Statistics Division (UNSD) published the first compendium of disability statistics in 1990 (UN, 1990) that included data from 55 countries that provided prevalence estimates, but from differing case definitions. For example, countries trying to assess disability using a question, such as "Is anyone in the household deaf, blind, or mute?" will find a prevalence of disability in the 1–2% range. On the other hand, when an activity-oriented question or set of questions, asking, for example, "Does anyone in your household have difficulty seeing a friend across the street?" or "Does anyone in your household have difficulty taking care of themselves in eating, drinking, toileting, or dressing?", the prevalence rate of disability reaches double digits and, in some countries, might approach 20% (UN, 1990).

Since that initial effort, the UNSD has published the *Guidelines and Principles for the Development of Disability Statistics* (UN, 2001). This document was much clearer about how national statistical offices could improve the questions used, collection methods employed, and overall approach to dissemination of data. The UN guidelines used the ICF framework to assist countries as they work toward harmonization and comparability in disability data.

In 2001, the UNSD convened a group of disability experts from around the world to address the need for disability measures to be more standardized. From this conference emerged the Washington City Group on Disability Measurement (United Nations, 2019b). (City groups are a mechanism used by the UN to focus on specific topics and are named after the city in which they meet first.) This international group developed a short set of six functional questions, based on the ICF model, that are being used in several countries and recommended for use around the globe to encourage comparability of census data on disability. The domains are basic and universal, identifying a person's difficulty seeing, hearing, walking or climbing stairs, remembering or concentrating, washing oneself, and communicating (UN, 2019; United Nations, 2019b). An Extended Set of questions has been developed by the same group for use in surveys.

More recently UNICEF coordinated an effort to expand the use of the six functional questions to children and youth (Loeb, Cappa, Crialesi, & de Palma, 2017). The project focused on basic and universal functions of children and youth ages 2–17, with two divisions—2–4 years and 5–17 years of age. A proxy respondent using the mother or other primary caregiver is assumed. The base question, "Compared with children of the same age…," is followed by the identified functional domain. In addition, thresholds were added so that levels of difficulty can be collected, that is, no difficulty, some difficulty, a lot of difficulty, or can't do at all. To account for developmental differences inherent in assessing child and youth functioning, beyond the six basic domains, additional items were included according to the ages of the child or youth. For the preschool group, picking up small objects, playing, and aggressive behavior were added, while for the school-age group, accepting routines, making friends, anxiety, depression, and controlling behavior were added. This set of questions was used in the recent Multiple Indicator Cluster Surveys (MICS6) implemented by countries under the program developed by the UN Children's Fund to provide comparable, statistically rigorous data on the circumstances of women and children (UNICEF, 2019).

The US National Survey of Children with Special Health Care Needs used a similar activity-oriented approach more explicitly following the ICF-CY model: it included 13 questions and questions related to social and emotional limitations (Maternal and Child Health Bureau, 2010). An analysis by Lollar et al. (2012) found that children with special healthcare needs present clinically with various functional difficulties across an array of health conditions. The data demonstrate that functional difficulties contribute significantly to outcomes, such as emergency room visits, parental work patterns, and limitations in daily activities. Including functional difficulties alongside diagnostic/health conditions provides opportunities to provide richer characterization of children with disabilities for public health practice, training, policy, and research.

7.5.1 Disability: A Burden of Disease?

It is important that data collected to enhance the health and well-being of people with disabilities are, indeed, developed and used for this purpose. Over the years, international efforts to predict disability from disease conditions have drawn criticism both in terms of practical accuracy and for their human rights implications. The best-known of these predictive efforts is the Global Burden of Disease (GBD) schema (Murray & Lopez, 1996).

Those undecided about the merits of this conceptual and methodological approach to disability are encouraged to consider the period 1933–1945 in the life of US President Franklin Delano Roosevelt. According to the Global Burden of Disease, the quality of those years of life would have been adjusted for "years of life lost" from disability based on FDR's known status as a person with polio. As a professor and former federal disability program director living with a disability once concluded, "According to GBD, I would be better off dead!"

In essence, GBD purports to derive *lost years of productive life* from disability through estimates of disease. The weighting schemes used to calculate disability in the GBD are based upon the views and values of a jury of approximately 100 (mostly physicians and public health students, none of them disabled) claiming some knowledge of one or more of 63 known diseases. Jurors gave their opinion as to how much disability they thought would be associated with a specific disease and to what extent this specific disability would be a burden, by type of burden. Based on these opinions, weights were calculated that were widely criticized both conceptually and methodologically; for example, see Anand and Hanson (1997), Arnesen and Nord (1999), Groce, Chamie, and Me (1999). In light of the conceptual and measurement problems associated with this approach to estimate disability weights, it is proposed that one part of the calculation of the Global Burden of Disease what is called "disability-adjusted life years" be rejected as a measure of disability (Gross, Lollar, Campbell, & Chamie, 2009).

Mont (2007) suggested that DALYs were a poor indicator of how public health interventions affect or improve the lives of people with disabilities. He reported that the primary objective in the development of this indicator was to implement a metric that could help national policy makers in allocating resources to reduce poor health. Given the competing needs of people and the minimal resources available, governments have to make difficult decisions regarding public health improvement. Mont concluded that "an indicator that does not properly embody the intended goals can build in systematic bias against achieving them" (Mont, 2007). The use of DALYs to inform public health policy should be rejected, and methods incorporating increased levels of participation by people with disabilities compared to people without disabilities should be developed. Mont and Loeb (2008) have developed a protocol for addressing impact of activity limitations and impairments on participation using population-based data from Zambia. This approach provides a more scientific and generalizable approach to measuring the impact of disabling conditions on people with disabilities. In addition, it allows monitoring of changes in participation across the population and for comparisons across populations.

7.6   Policy Development

The World Program of Action (WPA), the Standard Rules for the Equalization of Opportunity for Persons with Disabilities, the Convention on the Rights of Persons with Disabilities (CRPD), and the Convention on the Rights of the Child (CRC) were described under the section on *Disability as a Human Rights Issue*. These documents are the foundation for public health policy development even though they often do not directly mention "health."

The Standard Rules are divided into three groups—preconditions for equal participation (Rules 1–4), target areas for equal participation (Rules 5–12), and implementation measures (Rules 13–22). The end product of these rules is that people with disabilities have an opportunity to participate in society equal to that of people without disabilities. It is a step beyond traditional public health and moves beyond the emphasis on preventing disease, injury, and disability to embrace the higher-order outcome of participation. However, this is the move made when the World Health Organization adopted as its mission "to improve health and well-being" around the globe. This broader interpretation is the result of an ongoing interaction between public health professionals and the disability community.

It is noteworthy that Rules 2 and 3—medical care and rehabilitation—are the traditional rules acknowledged by public health. Emphasis in Rule 2 medical care is on early detection, assessment, and treatment of *impairment* that can "prevent, reduce, or eliminate disabling effects." Also, states are encouraged to provide regular treatment and medication needed for people with disabilities to maintain or improve functioning. Rule 3 recommends that national rehabilitation programs for all people with disabilities should be developed. Programs should focus on the activities and access of needs of the individuals with the goal of full participation and equality. Recommendations are that individuals be involved in their own reha-bilitation, that services be available in the local community, and that advocacy groups be included in national program planning.

Implementation measures are, in fact, the processes that must be in place for the preconditions and target areas to be addressed. Most of the target areas are really the specific outcome areas in which opportunities should arise—e.g., education, employment, recreation and sports, culture, and religion. Throughout the document, the term "health" is rarely found. The notion of health promotion is also absent and can only be found by a generous reading of early detection, assessment, and treat-ment of impairment or the provision of healthcare and related services to all people to reduce or prevent the "disability effects of impairment" (UN, 1993). An emerging area for public health intervention focuses specifically on promoting health and preventing secondary conditions often associated with primary disabilities—such as decubitus ulcers or skin sores among persons with spinal injuries. Physical activ-ity and nutrition, smoking, and alcohol abuse, for example, are clear areas for public health policy and assurance in many countries. People with disabilities, however, are often not seen as a vulnerable population for public health messages. Formulation of policy addressing not only rehabilitation and medical services, but also health promotion and secondary condition prevention are important areas to be addressed among people with disabilities.

South Africa provided arguably the most complete national strategy interpreting the UN Standard Rules (Office of the Deputy President, 1997). The White Paper on an Integrated National Disability Strategy includes policy guidelines for the major areas of the Standard Rules, including prevention, health care, and rehabilitation. Secondary prevention is included and suggests that the results might be the preven-tion of complications, such as contractures for those with cerebral palsy. Inclusion of secondary prevention is a critical element in health policy relative to disability. A national data base is being developed to provide an array of medical- and disability-related services, as well as collect information on health-related needs and inci-dence of impairments. The policy objectives for data and research focus on the gaps between physical and/or mental conditions and their resources, including the envi-ronmental factors influencing their lives.

Since 2007, 137 countries have signed the first United Nations convention of the new century—a convention establishing the rights of people with disabilities—indi-cating their intent to ratify (UN, 2012). The United Nations Convention on the Rights of Persons with Disabilities (CRPD) continues to provide a roadmap to end discrimination and marginalization of people with physical or mental conditions and has as a goal to eliminate exploitation and abuse of this population. Its premise is that people with disabilities have an inherent right to life equal to that of people living without disabilities and will receive equal protection and rights, including controlling their own financial affairs and the right to privacy. A shift in perspective is explicit in the CRPD. People with disabilities are not objects of pity or charity but rather are citizens with rights and dignity, with the capacity to contribute to their society.

Health is addressed by establishing both a right to health and ensuring the access to health care for persons with disabilities (Article 25). Article 25 addresses equal opportunity to the same quality and range of services for people with disabilities as for the general population. Services to identify disabling conditions early followed by appropriate interventions are mandated. This includes the prevention of secondary conditions for this population across the lifespan. Ethical decisions such as preventing the withholding of food or fluids or basic health care and services are also addressed in Article 25. Training of health professionals to provide clinical or public health services equally across the population is another tenet of Article 25 of the CRPD. Consistent with CRPD is the move by countries to include disability as part of their national health agenda. Countries have begun to formulate public health policy by setting national health goals.

Healthy People 2020 (HP 2020) is the national public health agenda for the United States. The inclusion of a chapter in this volume focusing on improving the health and well-being of people with disabilities was a major step forward for public health policy in the United States. As a foundation for setting these objectives, DATA2010 was used to identify specific health disparities for this population. The disparities of greatest concern include not getting needed health care, participating less in activities to encourage physical fitness, using tobacco more, having a higher percentage of overweight or obesity, receiving less social-emotion support, and more emotional distress. In addition, annual dental visits are fewer and fewer women with disabilities have mammograms and pap tests when appropriate (Department of Health and Human Services, 2010).

Another international policy-focused project was mandated by the World Health Assembly of WHO. The directive was initiated to develop a world report on disability. The *World Report on Disability* (WPD) was published in 2011 and provides a comprehensive compendium of international disability information (WHO, 2001). A chapter is devoted to health among people with disabilities with the most important premise that people with disabilities are not, by definition, sick or ill. Rather, people with disabilities may live healthy lives. While certain conditions are associated with poor health, the common assumption of disability equaling illness undermines public health emphases to improve and maintain the health of this population. The WPD goes on to address secondary conditions, general health needs, as well as the need for specialty care. Specific emphasis is given to ensuring that people with disabilities benefit equally from public health programs as do the general population.

7.7 Assurance of Health and Health Care

Assurance focuses on the certitude that needed services will be provided to individuals and communities so that health goals can be reached. Assurance also suggests that services must not only be present but also maintained so that goals can be met. Implicit in these assertions is the notion that there are challenges or barriers to the provision and use of services which must be addressed. Assurance suggests, when needed, the use of authority may be required so that services will be provided and that they will not be too costly to access (IOM, 1990).

Assurance of services includes not only the presence of services but also the access to those services. Access includes physical proximity or transport to reasonably travel to the services, physical accessibility to the services, policies and systems that allow financial access, and attitudes that encourage participation in the services. The services include clinical preventive services usually set as a baseline for everyone in any particular country, health promotion activities, and prevention of secondary conditions, in addition to basic medical care and rehabilitation.

7.7.1 Poverty and Disability

A basic barrier to assurance of public health services and attention is poverty. Poverty not only contributes to acquiring a disability, but the presence of a disability contributes to poverty, particularly in low-income countries. Braithwaite and Mont (2008) surveyed poverty assessments and disability for the World Bank and concluded that the poor data on disability status keeps us from accurately estimating the relationship that "common sense and anecdotal evidence would suggest." Data that indirectly suggests this relationship, however, is available. For example, employment rates among people with disabilities are substantially lower (in the United States, 75% vs. 37% for individuals with and without disabilities, respectively) compared to people without disabilities (DOL, 2020). In lower-resource countries, we can assume the proportion of people with disabilities working is even lower.

Primary prevention programs are extremely important in public health across the life span. However, even with intense efforts to prevent birth defects, developmental disabilities, injuries, and chronic illnesses, for the foreseeable future, children and adults will continue to live with disabling conditions. Children and adults will be affected by poor nutrition, prenatal exposures and events, poorly controlled diseases, conflicts, and environmental factors. A Canadian report reflects that children with disabilities or children with parents who have disabilities experience some of the worst income equality (CICH, 2000). The relationship between poverty and disability, as noted, has long been established, alongside the general relationship between health status and poverty (Fujiura & Kiyoshi, 2000; Park, Turnbull, & Turnbull, 2002; UKPHA, 2012). Yeo and Moore (2003) in discussing the relationship between poverty and disability and health status, concluded that people with disabilities are among the poorest of the poor and are not represented in international development organizations and activities. It is often the case that people with disabilities, for reasons such as stigma, few resources, or transport, are unable to access appropriate health, medical, or rehabilitation services. It is clear that in many countries, public health activities are difficult to implement for any of the general population.

7.8   Public Health Services

Equal access to care and equal access to public health prevention is as important for people with disabilities as it is for the general public. Barriers to health care include high costs as well as transportation, particularly in low-income countries. For example, 33% non-disabled people are unable to afford health care compared to 53% of people with disabilities (WHO, 2019). Research in Indian states of Uttar Pradesh and Tamil Nadu conclude that lack of appropriate services is second only to cost of services (WHO, 2019). Inaccessible hospitals and health centers, along with inaccessible medical equipment, especially for women with mobility limitations are extremely common, undermining both preventive and interventional services. Disparities in access to preventive health care is documented in some countries, although, as we described above, data for monitoring disparities is not universal nor consistent. Violence against women and children with disabling conditions is a prime example of the need for equal access to prevention and care. Ortoleva and Lewis (2012) reported on the international problem of violence toward women with disabilities, addressing both the commonalities with women in general who experience violence while also highlighting the unique forms, causes, and results for this population of women. Services for women experiencing violence is seen as a public health issue, and women with disabilities must be included for screening, services, and programs addressing this major problem. Likewise, children with disabilities are at greater risk of being victims of violence according to a systematic review of international studies appearing in the *Lancet* (Jones, Bellis, et al., 2012). The analysis reported odds ratios of 3.68 for combined violence measures, 3.56 for physical violence, and 2.88 for sexual violence for children with disabilities using children without disabilities as the comparison. Any violence against children is unacceptable, but this disparity is appalling and contrary to the UN conventions focusing on the rights of children and people with disabilities. Public health programs and services should be a top priority for national efforts on behalf of this vulnerable population.

Primary prevention messages can be of equal importance for all segments of the population, including persons with disabilities. People with disabilities, for example, might be just as vulnerable, or more so, to heart problems than the general population. Public health messages often are not tailored so that those living with disabilities feel included. It is sometimes the case that people with disabilities are even included in messages as the outcome of inappropriate behavior, such as showing someone in a wheelchair in a message that promotes safe driving. It is important, therefore, that public health prevention messages are developed to acknowledge that people with disabilities can be affected by the same images as the general population. There are also times when public health messages should be tailored to reach individuals with disabilities. People who have limited mobility are at greater risk for weight gain than the general population because of reduced physical activity (DOL, 2020). It is, however, also the case that some in the disability community might interpret primary prevention activities related to injuries or screening for birth defects as inimical to their being alive and thus feel suspicious, if not angry, about public health prevention activities. Communication between public health professionals and the disability community is critical so that important public health education can occur with appropriate input from people living with disabilities, but without losing poignant public health messages.

Perhaps the most important public health message for individuals with disabilities is consistent with that for the general population. Encouraging children, youth, and adults to be responsible for their own health is a powerful message that is particularly cogent for people with disabilities. For anyone who experiences multiple medical interventions, there can develop a sense of losing control over one's body and equating that loss of control over medical procedures with a loss of control over one's health. At both the individual and population level, self-efficacy, a belief in one's ability to have control over one's life and health, is an important mediating variable for positive health outcomes.

Beyond public health education are the clinical services that all countries, whether well or less developed, attempt to provide their citizens (US Preventive Services Task Force, 1996). These services include immunizations, cancer screenings for both men and women, health guidance regarding nutrition and physical activity, sexuality and pregnancy education, as needed, drug use education including alcohol and smoking, and other important health information. In more developed countries, medical care and rehabilitation are emphasized, while clinical preventive services are not. Often, rehabilitation becomes equated with medical rehabilitation, and providers focus on the disabling condition and its medical complications. Primary care is not emphasized, with the assumption that medical care generalists will provide the immunizations, health screenings, education, and other primary care activities. Also, specialists might not be familiar with or sensitive to the need for these services in this population. Many individuals with disabilities, if they have specialized care, do not use primary care and, therefore, might not receive appropriate services. Jones and Kerr (1997) reported that individuals with cognitive impairments did not receive annual health screenings. Austin (2003) found that people with disabilities in the US state of Oregon using services funded through public mechanisms are at greater risk of developing smoking-related cancers, were more likely to be diagnosed at a later stage of cancer, and, therefore, do not receive timely screening for cancer. In addition, treatment was more often delayed among this population. A public health responsibility is to ensure that people with disabilities are not lost to the provision of clinical preventive services.

The World Health Organization begins with the notion that many countries whether developing or developed have medical care and rehabilitation consistent with their resources. These services subsequently are equated with public health. This translation of medicine and rehabilitation into public health is a necessary, but not sufficient, approach to improving the health and well-being of people with disabilities. Medical care is important, even critical, for all citizens regardless of disability status. Rehabilitation services, whether medical, educational, vocational, or social, are specific services focused on outcomes related to the designated area—e.g., work or school. The lived experience of individuals with disabilities is much broader than just medicine or rehabilitation, even defined broadly. Public health must encompass these services, as needed, but must also include health education, preventive services, prevention of secondary conditions, and environmental facilitators of health and well-being.

Toward this end, WHO community-based rehabilitation activities (CBR) have been developed in more than 90 countries and strive to provide comprehensive strategies to include people with disabilities in the life of their communities (WHO, 2007). This emphasis, sponsored by WHO, focuses on providing equal access to medical and rehabilitation services but also to education, employment, and numerous other community activities. Monitoring human resources for health-related rehabilitation services is also a function of CBR (Lollar and Andresen, 2015). Public health professionals, in conjunction with CBR staff, can collaborate to provide the expertise from both public health and the disability community that will improve the health of people with disabilities. The *WRD* provides a strong case for the utility of CBR throughout the world (WHO, 2011).

7.9   Directions for Global Public Health and Disability

WHO took a major step toward addressing improved health and well-being for people with disabilities in publishing the *WHO Global Disability Action Plan 2014–2021* (WHO, 2014). The plan enumerated three objectives:

1. To remove barriers and improve access to health services and programs.
2. To strengthen and extend rehabilitation, habilitation, assistive technology, assistance and support services, and community-based rehabilitation.
3. To strengthen collection of relevant and internationally comparable data on disability and support research on disability and related services.

Specific actions were outlined for each objective followed by proposed inputs for the member states, inputs for the secretariat, and proposed inputs for international and national partners.

To implement these activities successfully, as with all public health activities, there must be communication among the partners, leading to cooperation among the parties and states, and finally coordination of data collection, policy initiatives, and assurance activities. All activities should be undergirded by the conceptual framework of the *International Classification of Functioning, Disability and Health* (ICF), and training for public health professionals must be inclusive of the health and well-being of people with disabilities. It is hard to believe that this one billion subgroup is not the largest minority yet to be addressed by public health as a profession.

References

Anand, S., & Hanson, K. (1997). Disability-adjusted life years: A critical review. *Journal of Health Economics, 16*, 658–702.

Arnesen, T., & Nord, E. (1999). The value of DALY life: Problems with ethics and validity of disability-adjusted life years. *British Journal of Medicine, 319*, 1423–1425.

Austin D. (2003). *Disabilities are Risk Factors for Late Stage or Poor Prognosis Cancers.* Paper presented at Changing Concepts of Health and Disability: Science and Policy Conference, Oregon Health & Science University, Portland, OR.

Braithwaite, J., & Mont, D. (2008). *Disability and poverty: A survey of World Bank poverty assessment and implications.* Social Protection Discussion Paper, No. 0805. New York: World Bank.

Canadian Institute of Child Health (2000). *The Health of Canada's Children.* Ottawa: Canadian Institute of Child Health.

Chan, M., & Zoellich, R. B. (2011). Preface in World Bank and World Health Organization. In *World Report on Disability.* Retrieved July 30, 2019, from www.who.int

Department of Health and Human Services. (2010) *Healthy people 2020: Disability and health.* Retrieved August 1, 2019, from www.healthypeople.gov

Department of Labor (2020). *Disability Employment Statistics.* Washington DC: Office of Disability Employment Policy. Online dol.gov. Accessed January, 2020.

Fujiura, G. T., & Kiyoshi, Y. (2000). Trends in demography of childhood poverty and disability. *Exceptional Children, 66*(2), 187–199.

Groce, N., Chamie, M., & Me, A. (1999). Measuring the quality of life: Rethinking the World Bank's disability adjusted life years. *International Rehabilitation Review, 49*, 12–15.

Gross, S. D., Lollar, D., Campbell, V., & Chamie, M. (2009). Disability and disability-adjusted life years (DALYs): Not the same. *Public Health Reports PHRN, 124*, 197–202.

Hamlin, T., Foster, J., Lantz, J., Northrup, M., Villavicencio, T., Simeonsson, R., & Lollar, D. (2017). Measuring complexity for autism interventions: TCFS's inventory of neuroeducational complexity. *Journal of Childhood & Developmental Disorders, 3*(2), 1–7.

ICLEI. (2015). *From MDGs to SDGs: What are the sustainable development goals?* Retrieved July 29, 2019, from November 2015, ICLEI Briefing Sheet—Urban Issues, No 01.

Institute of Medicine (1990). *The Future of Public Health.* Washington DC: National Academy Press

Jones, R. G., & Kerr, M. P. (1997). A randomized control trial of an opportunistic health screening tool in primary care for people with intellectual disability. *Journal of Intellectual Disability Research, 41*, 409–415.

Jones, L., Bellis, M. S., & Wood, S. et al. (2012). Prevalence and risk of violence against children with disabilities: A systematic review and meta-analysis of observational studies. *The Lancet, 380*, 899–907.

Loeb, M., Cappa, C., Crialesi, R., & de Palma, E. (2017). Measuring child functioning: The UNICEF/Washington group module. *Salud publica de mexico, 50*(4), julio-agosto.

Lollar, D. J., & Andresen, E. M. (2015). People with disabilities. In Detels R, Gulliford M, Karim QA, & Tan CC. *Oxford Textbook of Global Public Health.* Oxford: Oxford University Press, 1392–1407.

Lollar, D. J., Hartzell, M. S., & Evans, M. A. (2012). Functional difficulties and health conditions among children with special health needs. *Pediatrics, 129*(3), 714–722.

Maternal and Child Health Bureau. (2010) *National survey—Children with special health care needs: Chartbook 2009–2010.* Retrieved August 1, 2019, from www.mchb.hrsa.gov

Mont, D. (2007). Measuring health and disability. *The Lancet, 369*, 1658–1663.

Mont, D., & Loeb, M. (2008). *Beyond DALYS: Developing indicators to assess the impact of public health interventions on the lives of people with disabilities.* Social Protection Discussion Paper, No 0815. New York: World Bank.

Murray, C., & Lopez, A. (Eds.). (1996). *Global burden of disease.* Cambridge: Harvard University Press.

Office of the Deputy President. (1997). *Integrated national disability strategy: A white paper.* Ndabeni, South Africa: Office of the Deputy President.

Ortoleva, S., & Lewis, H. (2012). *Forgotten Sisters: A Report on Violence against Women with Disability: An Overview of its Nature, Scope, Causes, and Consequences.* Northeastern University School of Law Research Report, No. 104. Boston MA: Northeastern University School of Law.

Park, J., Turnbull, A. P., & Turnbull, H. R. (2002). Impacts of poverty on quality of life in families of children with disabilities. *Exceptional Children, 68*(2), 151–170.

Rowland, C., Fried-Oken, M., Bowser, G., Granlund, M., Lollar, D. J., Phelps, R. J., … Steiner, S. M. (2016). The communication supports inventory—Children & youth (CSI-CY). *Disability and Rehabilitation, 38*(19), 1909–1917.

UNICEF. (2019). *Multiple indicator cluster survey (MICS).* Retrieved July 31, 2019, from www.mics.unicef.org

United Nations. (1989). *Convention on the rights of the child.* Retrieved July 28, 2019, from https://www.ohchr.org/en/professionalinterest/pages/crc/aspx

United Nations. (1993). *Standard rules on the equalization of opportunities for persons with disabilities.* Retrieved July 28, 2019, from https://www.un.org/esa/socdev/enable/dissre01.htm

United Nations. (2019a). *Convention on the rights of persons with disabilities.* Retrieved July 28, 2019, from https://www.un.org/development/desa/disabilities/convention-on-the-rights-of-persons-with-disabilities.html

United Nations. (2019b). *Washington group question sets.* Retrieved July 31, 2019, from www.washingtongroup-disability.com

United Nations (2001). Guidelines and Principles for the Development of Disability Statistics. Series Y, No. 10. New York: UN

United Nations. (2020). *Guiding principles of the convention.* Retrieved April 9, 2020, from https://www.un.org/development/desa/disabilities/convention-on-the-rights-of-persons-with-disabilities/guiding-principles-of-the-convention.html

United Nations General Assembly. (1982). *The World Programme of Action concerning disabled persons.* Retrieved from http://www.unorg/disabilities/default/asp?id=23

United Nations Statistical Office, Department of International Economic and Social Affairs. (1990). *Disability statistics compendium.* (ST/ESA/STAT/SER.Y/4).

United Nations Statistics Division, Department of Economic and Social Affairs. (2006). *Fundamental principles of official statistics.* Retrieved from http://unstats.un.org/unsd/methods/statorg/FP-English.htm

United Kingdom Public Health Association (2012). *The State of Britain's Health: Poverty and Inequality.* Online http://www.ukpha.org.uk. Accessed January, 2020.

US Preventive Services Task Force (1996). *Guide to Clinical Preventive Services* (2nd Edition). Alexandria VA: International Medical Publishing.

Wolfensohn, J. D. (2004). *Disability and inclusive development.* Keynote presentation. World Bank Conference, Washington DC, December 1.

World Health Organization. (1980). *International classification of impairments, disabilities, and handicap.* Geneva: WHO.

World Health Organization. (2001). *International classification of functioning, disability and health.* Geneva: WHO.

World Health Organization. (2007). *International classification of functioning, disability, and health—Children & youth version.* Geneva: WHO.

World Health Organization (2011). *World Report on Disability.* Geneva: WHO.

World Health Organization. (2014). *WHO global disability action plan 2014–2021.* Retrieved July 28, 2019, from https://www.who.int/disabilities/actionplan/en/

World Health Organization. (2019). *International classification of diseases 11th revision.* Retrieved July 30, 2019, from www.icd.who.int

World Health Organization, & World Bank. (2011). *World report on disability summary.* Retrieved July 30, 2019, from www.who.int

Yeo, R., & Moore, K. (2003, March). Including disabled people in poverty reduction work: "nothing about us, without us". *World Development, 31*(3), 571–590.

Part II
Public Health Applications

Chapter 8
Disability and Health Programs: Emerging Partners

Dot Nary and Lindsey Catherine Mullis

Because people with disabilities experience significant health disparities (Krahn, Walker, & Correa-De-Araujo, 2015; Reichard & Stotzle, 2011; Reichard, Stotzle, & Fox, 2011), programs aimed at surveilling and promoting the health of members of this population are critical to ensuring their ability to fully participate in society. However, transition from the public health community's emphasis on disability prevention to recognition that health can exist in the context of disability and to the development of programs to promote health for persons with disabilities occurred gradually and was influenced by numerous societal changes and events over the last 50 years. The increasing number of people living with disabilities and chronic conditions due to medical research and public health interventions prompted public health to go beyond disease prevention to "pay attention to outcomes beyond mortality" (Lollar, 2001, p. 756) for this growing population. Successful surveillance efforts and evidenced-based health promotion programs have been initiated and expanded to address the needs of the larger, diverse population of individuals living with disability (e.g., National Center on Health, Physical Activity and Disability [NCHPAD]) but also developed to serve those with specific conditions (e.g., Christopher and Dana Reeve Paralysis Foundation, Special Olympics). Still, significant barriers remain due to centuries of equating disability with ill-health and a belief that people with disabilities cannot be healthy. Efforts continue to raise awareness that individuals with disabilities of all ages with all types of limitations

D. Nary (✉)
Developmental and Child Psychology, Research and Training Center on Independent Living, Institute for Health and Disability Policy Studies, Kansas Disability and Health Program, Life Span Institute, University of Kansas, Lawrence, KS, USA
e-mail: dotn@ku.edu

L. C. Mullis (✉)
Kinesiology and Health Promotion, Human Development Institute, Kentucky Disability and Health Program, University of Kentucky, Lexington, KY, USA
e-mail: lindsey.c.mullis@uky.edu

© Springer Science+Business Media, LLC, part of Springer Nature 2021
D. J. Lollar et al. (eds.), *Public Health Perspectives on Disability*,
https://doi.org/10.1007/978-1-0716-0888-3_8

are capable of health and that they require access to programs that support their health promotion efforts. The following sections present a brief historical context of increased interest in disability and health; some developments that shaped public health programs; the growth of disability and health programs within Centers for Disease Control and Prevention (CDC); and a description of ongoing challenges and efforts to meet the health promotion needs of the growing population of individuals living with disabilities.

8.1 Increased Interest in Health for People with Disabilities

As the disability rights and independent living movements gained a foothold in the 1970s and developed momentum in subsequent years, a group of individuals regarded as having severe disabilities advocated for the right to live and work in their communities and to access support services for community living (DeJong, 1979; Shapiro, 1994). Their advocacy influenced passage of the Rehabilitation Act of 1973, which included regulations that prioritized vocational rehabilitation services for people with the most severe disabilities and mandated affirmative action programs for the employment of disabled persons within the federal government and with its contractors. These mandates presented some of the first widespread opportunities for well-paying jobs with benefits, economic security, and self-sufficiency for a population viewed as so disabled that they had typically been regarded as unemployable (DeJong, 1979; Longmore, 2003).

Similarly, an advocacy movement among parents of children with developmental and intellectual disabilities influenced the passage of groundbreaking legislation, the Education for all Handicapped Children Act of 1975 (later reauthorized as the Individuals with Disabilities Education Act [IDEA]), which mandated that children with disabilities receive a free and appropriate education in the least restrictive environment (Yell, Rogers, & Rogers, 1998). For the first time, children with disabilities had the legal right to be educated alongside their peers in their own communities, laying the ground for a life of raised expectations for inclusion. A subsequent, watershed civil rights law, the Americans with Disabilities Act of 1990 (ADA), was conceived of and promoted by a collaboration of multiple segments of the disability community. These groups had previously advocated for the needs of their individual constituencies but finally recognized and organized around a critical, common barrier of discrimination against persons with any type of disability (Shapiro, 1994). The ADA bars discrimination against people with disabilities in employment, public services, public accommodations, and telecommunications. The combined result of these three legislative acts (the Rehabilitation Act, the Education for All Handicapped Children Act, and the ADA) was increased opportunities in the mainstream of society for children and adults with disabilities, raising the importance of health in order to take advantage of these opportunities. At this time, people with disabilities largely rejected the public health model that focused on prevention of disability rather than health in the context of disability, viewing the former perspective as devaluing their lives (Lollar, 2001).

Concurrently, the public health community's view of health for people with disabilities was evolving. Internationally, culmination of the World Health Organization's 10-year effort to develop the International Classification of Functioning, Disability and Health (ICF) resulted in a fundamentally different foundation for understanding health and disability that eschewed a sole emphasis on the medical model for a more interactive one (WHO, 1991). The ICF includes an assessment of how the environment interacts with an individual's ability to participate in the community versus a sole focus on their limitations resulting from a physical, mental, or emotional condition (Lollar & Crews, 2003).

In the United States, the Centers for Disease Control and Prevention (CDC) was changing how it viewed disability within the field of public health, with the focus expanding from surveillance and preventing primary disabilities to also preventing secondary health conditions and promoting health for individuals with disabilities. This change represented a turnaround from regarding "disability as a negative outcome equated with illness and injury to viewing it as a health state experienced by the person and influenced by the environment, as well as accepting the premise that persons with disabilities can be healthy" (Lollar, 2001, p. 756). As a result of this shift in focus, disability was to be regarded as a demographic, similar to race or age, versus an inalterable state. The emphasis on secondary conditions as preventable health problems, as described below, highlighted the need for prevention-oriented systems and programs for this population.

In 1979, US Department of Health and Human Services initiated Healthy People, a program establishing national health improvement priorities for the population, to be updated every 10 years and including both policy and assurance objectives (USDHHS, 2019). In a subsequent iteration, the objectives for Healthy People 2010 represented a significant advancement for the health of people with disabilities with its chapter titled "Disability and Secondary Conditions." Reflecting the emphasis on preventing secondary conditions versus primary disability prevention, this chapter's objectives addressed both (a) the identification of people with disabilities in all Healthy People surveillance instruments and (b) issues related to the health and well-being of this population not addressed in other chapters (e.g., reducing the number of people with disabilities reporting environmental barriers to participation in home, school, work, or community activities) (https://www.healthypeople. gov/2010/Document/pdf/Volume1/06Disability.pdf). Subsequent iterations of Healthy People have continued to address health disparities experienced by people with disabilities. Healthy People 2020 also included a chapter of disability and health objectives, and it is likely that Healthy People 2030, currently in the planning stage, will do the same. These efforts help to keep disability-related health disparities on the public health agenda.

Thus, as people with disabilities asserted their civil rights and as legislation was passed to protect those rights; as a new way of measuring disability increased emphasis on the role of the environment in functioning and participation; and as the

U.S. public health system shifted its focus from prevention of disabilities to preventing secondary conditions and promoting health, and incorporated the health of people with disabilities into its planning, an unmet need for programs to promote health for individuals living with disabilities became increasingly evident.

8.2   Shaping Disability and Health Programs

As the need for programs to promote health for people with disabilities was recognized, other developments in theory shaped program development.

Originating in Great Britain, the social model of disability countered the prevailing medical model by asserting that disability results not from individual impairment that needs to be "fixed" by an expert but rather from society failing to accommodate impairment-related needs and excluding those with impairments from the mainstream (Shakespeare, 2017). This presentation of disability as a social construction versus a personal shortcoming fits well with the ICF's emphasis on the role of the environment on functioning and with the disability rights movement's view of people with disabilities as a minority oppressed by the barriers in society. This model encouraged efforts to alter environments through programs to remove barriers and promote health.

The World Health Organization echoes the social model of disability in its statement, "Disability is now understood to be a human rights issue. People are disabled by society, not just by their bodies" (https://www.who.int/features/factfiles/disability/en/). The ICF presents a biopsychosocial model, based on an integration of the social and medical models of disability (Ustun, Chatterji, Bickenbach, Kostanjsek, & Schneider, 2003). This integrated model is reflected in the ICF's conceptualization of a person's levels of functioning, activity, and participation as dynamic interactions between their health conditions, environmental factors, and personal factors. This interaction is portrayed in Fig. 8.1, in which all elements of disability (i.e., body functions, activity, and participation) are noted and depicted as being able to interact with each other. All three elements are affected by contextual factors (i.e., environmental and personal).

By recognizing the importance of both environmental and personal factors, this biopsychosocial model elevated the importance of disability and health programs, as these programs can alter environments (e.g., increase the availability of accessible exercise classes, provide sign language interpreters in prenatal classes), change personal factors (e.g., increase knowledge regarding pressure ulcer prevention, provide materials on healthy nutrition in simple language), or do both.

In 2005, the promotion of health in the context of disability was re-asserted when the US Surgeon General issued the *Call to Action to Improve the Health and Wellness of Persons with Disabilities* (USDHHS, 2005). This report asserted the potential for people with disabilities to lead long, healthy, and productive lives and

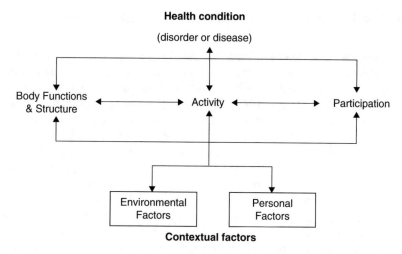

Fig. 8.1 Interactions between the components of the ICF. (Reprinted with permission from *Towards a Common Language for Functioning, Disability and Health: ICF*, World Health Organization, p. 9, Copyright 2002)

again highlighted the role of the environment in facilitating health for this population. The report emphasized the need for "health care providers who see and treat the whole person, educators willing to teach about disability, a public that sees beyond the person with a disability to see a whole person, and a community that provides accessible health and wellness services for persons with disabilities" (USDHHS, 2005). By presenting this vision in the form of four goals with accompanying strategies to achieve them, the Surgeon General affirmed the health of persons with disabilities as a public health concern and called on all segments of society to respond to the call.

As these developments progressed, the World Health Organization had begun to emphasize social determinants of health (SDOH) as a major factor in differences in health status (WHO, 1986). The WHO defines SDOH as the "conditions in which people are born, grow, live, work and age that are shaped by the distribution of money, power and resources at global, national and local levels" (https://www.who.int/social_determinants/sdh_definition/en/). Given the disadvantages that the population of people with disabilities has experienced historically, this emphasis on SDOH provided a framework to recognize and begin to address these disadvantages in a public health context.

Each of these developments set the stage for the growth of a comprehensive national program to promote the health of individuals with disabilities that involved multiple stakeholders, including the public health community and those living with disabilities and their advocates.

8.3 Evolution of CDC Disability and Health Programs

The Centers for Disease Control and Prevention (CDC) has been involved in health and disability since 1988 when it became the lead agency for establishment of the Disability Prevention Program, with a major emphasis on primary prevention of the causes of disabilities (Marge, 1988). This program awarded grant funds to 29 states to address prevention of injuries, birth defects, and chronic conditions under the leadership of the National Center for Environmental Health (NCEH).

In that same year, the introduction of the term "secondary disabilities" identified disabilities that occurred after the onset of the primary disability and were related to that disability (e.g., visual problems related to diabetes or pressure ulcers related to spinal cord injury) (Marge, 1988). This term later evolved into "secondary conditions." This concept, with accompanying emphasis on health promotion and wellness for persons with disabilities, quickly gained traction as it was used to "describe a broader understanding of problems to which persons with disabilities are vulnerable" (Lollar, 1999, p. 42). Several CDC-sponsored conferences from 1990 to 1994 explored the role of secondary conditions in the health of persons with disabilities and, notably, brought together public health professionals, clinicians, individuals with disabilities, and other stakeholders to recognize the need of addressing conditions that developed after the primary diagnosis and rehabilitation. These efforts prompted establishment of the Office of Disability and Health at the CDC.

As the field continued to evolve, the focus of the Office of Disability and Health changed in the 1996 announcement for state grants from disability prevention to a broader focus on disabilities and health. These programs spanned diagnostic categories primarily addressing issues of individuals who experienced limitations in mobility or cognition, with funding evenly split between science and programming. The science component included recommendations for criteria of disability surveillance systems, including a Behavioral Risk Factor Surveillance System (BRFSS) disability module, and states were asked to develop research projects around the programs being initiated. The recommended criteria reflected progress that had been made in the field and included focusing disability surveillance from specific diagnoses to activity limitations and, also, disseminating information to stakeholders. Importantly, it also involved including individuals with disabilities in the planning and delivery of activities (Hough, 1999).

In 2002, passage of the Children's Health Act stimulated creation of the National Center on Birth Defects and Developmental Disabilities (NCBDDD) at CDC, whose fourfold mission addresses issues specifically related to birth defects, developmental disabilities, blood disorders, and, also, improving the health of people living with disabilities. Within the NCBDDD is the Disability and Health Promotion Branch, with a major program emphasis to "promote the health and full participation in society by people with disabilities across the lifespan" (CDC, 2019; https://www.cdc.gov/ncbddd/disabilityandhealth/aboutus.html).

CDC Disability and Health works to improve the health of people with disabilities by (a) monitoring health disparities; (b) identifying risk factors for disease and secondary conditions; (c) supporting the inclusion of people with disabilities in public health programs; and (d) improving overall health and quality of life. This work focuses on identifying and addressing barriers to equitable health for persons with disabilities; developing and implementing disability-inclusive health policy; providing support and research for intervention strategies; and supporting programs that educate families, professionals, and the public on disability and health.

To address the need for ongoing surveillance and accomplish the activities listed above, in May of 2014, the CDC Disability and Health Promotion Branch launched the Disability and Health Data System (DHDS) to provide quick and easy access to state and national level data on health topics for adults with disabilities analyzed from the Behavioral Risk Factor Surveillance System (BRFSS). The goal of this system is to provide crucial information necessary to address the health needs of adults with disabilities. Data collected works to promote inclusive communities that foster health programs and services to address the need for improvement of health for this population. With customizable searches, data can be sorted by geographic location or by more than 30 health indicators and converted to maps, charts, or tables. Health factors include smoking, obesity, heart disease, diabetes, cancer screenings, and more. In addition to comparing state data to other states or national rates, disability status and type can also be further aggregated by age, sex, race/ethnicity, or veteran status, as well as demographics such as income, education, marital status, or employment. As demonstrated below in Fig. 8.2, the DHDS shows that adults with disabilities in the United States are more likely to experience health disparities than adults without disabilities.

The Disability and Health Data System [DHDS] can help to identify specific health disparities between adults with and without disabilities that can be used in presentations, reports, or fact sheets that inform and advocate the inclusion of disability in health efforts. These data can be easily customized and used for advocacy in presentations, reports, grant applications, and to inform stakeholders. Users can access DHDS information on six functional disability types in accordance with the

According to DHDS*, compared to adults without disabilities, adults with disabilities in the U.S are more likely to		
	With Disabilities	Without Disabilities
Have obesity	39.5%	26.3%
Smoke	27.8%	13.4%
Have heart disease	10.7%	3.6%
Have diabetes	16.2%	7.1%

*2017

Fig. 8.2 Disability-related health disparities revealed by the Disability and Health Data System. (Reprinted from Disability and Health Data System (DHDS) Fact Sheet, CDC, Disability and Health Branch, 2017)

data collection standards from the US Department of Health and Human Services (2011). These disability types are identified by using six questions which are answered with a Yes or No and are used as a set for the most accurate and encompassing results. These disability types and questions address:

1. Hearing ("Are you deaf or do you have serious difficulty hearing?")
2. Vision ("Are you blind or do you have serious difficulty seeing, even when wearing glasses?")
3. Cognition ("Because of a physical, mental, or emotional condition, do you have serious difficulty concentrating, remembering, or making decisions?" (5 years old or older)).
4. Mobility ("Do you have serious difficulty walking or climbing stairs?" (5 years old or older)).
5. Self-Care ("Do you have difficulty dressing or bathing?" (5 years old or older)).
6. Independent Living ("Because of a physical, mental, or emotional condition, do you have difficulty doing errands alone such as visiting a doctor's office or shopping?" (15 years old or older)) (US Department of Health & Human Services, 2011).

An individual is considered to have a disability if they answer Yes to any one of the six questions. Changes to the questions in this set are not permitted although additional questions may be included. For example, in 2004 the state of Montana added a visitability question to define a visitable home. Respondents were asked "If a person who uses special equipment, such as a wheelchair, came to visit you, could they get into your house without being carried up steps or over other obstacles?" Respondents with a disability who reported living in a visitable home were less likely than those who did not to report days of poor mental health in the past month and prompted discussion on independence of living at home and association of living in a visitable home and health outcomes (Seekins, Traci, Cummings, Oreskovich, & Ravesloot, 2008).

The six disability demographic questions define disability from a functional perspective and collectively provide a meaningful measure of disability for data collection and reporting. The inclusion of this question set in the BRFSS provides an important level of detail that supports more targeted interventions and programs that can provide direction for current health programs and services to make the necessary adaptations for inclusion of adults living with the specific disabilities captured (Stevens, Courtney-Long, Okoro, & Carroll, 2016).

Additionally, these questions comply with the most recent uniform data collection standards set forth by the US Department of Health and Human Services in accordance with the 2010 Affordable Care Act (ACA), Section 4302 as outlined by Secretary of the Department of Health and Human Services, Sylvia Burwell (2014):

> Section 4302(a) of the Affordable Care Act amended the Public Health Service Act (PHS Act) to add new section 3101, and requires the Secretary of HHS to develop data-collection standards for five demographic categories: race, ethnicity, sex, primary language, and disability status. Federally conducted or supported health care or public health programs, activities, and surveys are required, under section 3101 of the PHS Act, to collect and report data on these categories, to the extent practicable. (p. 2)

This inclusion of disability status as a demographic variable in the ACA was a major achievement in addressing the needs of people with disabilities in the field of public health and fulfilled a goal set by the Office of Disability and Health in 1996.

8.4   CDC Disability and Health Programs

The CDC has national reach with its Disability and Health Program efforts by funding 15 or more state and local programs or affiliates across the United States through varied state organizations such as University Centers for Excellence in Disabilities to state departments for public health or behavioral health. Local efforts include the adaptation and implementation of evidence-based strategies in their local communities. These programs develop, implement, evaluate, and report on services and activities that aim to address the health disparities for people with disabilities compared to those without disabilities while working to improve the health of individuals with cognitive or mobility disabilities across the lifespan.

CDC's Disability and Health Promotion Branch also currently funds two National Centers on Disability with the intent to support the development, implementation, evaluation, and reporting on activities focused at decreasing health disparities for individuals with disabilities as compared to those without disabilities that will ultimately improve the quality of life for this population across the lifespan. Descriptions of these Centers follow.

National Center on Health, Physical Activity and Disability (NCHPAD) The Center, founded in 1999, operates as a public health practice and resource center on health promotion with a mission to improve the health, wellness, and quality of life for those with disabilities through supporting local, state, and national public health organizations in incorporating NCHPAD's developed guidelines, recommendations, and suggested adaptations that promote inclusion in public health practices. This effort to achieve health equity for individuals with disabilities is accomplished through four main objectives:

1. Identify successful models, programs, practices, and policies and incorporate inclusion adaptations for youth and adults with mobility limitations.
2. Develop unique training materials on inclusion and accommodation strategies for individuals with mobility limitations.
3. Assist local providers to implement inclusion adaptations and strategies into existing programs, practices, and services.
4. Expand and advocate for the best practices on inclusive physical activity, nutrition, and obesity reduction strategies in community settings.

NCHPAD's primary goal is to develop the infrastructure to support accessibility and inclusion of people with disability in existing and future public health promotion programs focused on improving physical activity, nutrition, and healthy weight management. NCHPAD is the premier resource for information on physical activity, health promotion, and disability, serving persons with physical, sensory, and cognitive disability across the lifespan and features a variety of resources or services that can benefit all ages and populations. More information can be found at www. nchpad.org.

Special Olympics. The CDC Disability and Health Branch partners with the Special Olympics to address barriers to inclusive health services and programs challenge misperceptions and eliminate stigma in order to improve the health of individuals with intellectual disabilities. Together the CDC and Special Olympics are working toward equal health care and inclusion in programs that promote long-term good health. The efforts to accomplish this are through Special Olympics Healthy Athletes® and Healthy Communities programs that provide Special Olympic athletes access to free health screenings, education, and medical referrals for follow-up care, in addition to year-around health promotion and disease prevention programming. Core components of this partnership include (a) healthcare professional training to direct Healthy Athletes® screening events across the nation and (b) increased availability of data during and after screening events to improve the capacity to evaluate the effectiveness of health interventions and provide disability awareness training to healthcare professionals, community partners, educational settings, and other collaborative partnering organizations with limited to no experience working with individuals who have intellectual disabilities. These initiatives not only benefit the health of Special Olympic athletes, but also by training healthcare professionals worldwide to take inclusive strategies back to their home base practices, the activity increases knowledge and compassion for individuals with intellectual disabilities and improves their experience in obtaining health care. From 2002 to 2019, this partnership has allowed for approximately one million Healthy Athlete screenings in the United States alone at over 5000 events and supported specialized training for more than 100,000 US healthcare professionals on inclusion of individuals with intellectual disabilities in health practices.

CDC Disability and Health offers additional support to Special Olympics through the Center for Inclusive Health which is a virtual clearinghouse for healthcare providers, fitness and wellness professionals, business, and professional associations like the American Public Health Association. This center provides online resources, training, and technical assistance for mainstream inclusion to help ensure that individuals with intellectual disabilities are intentionally and successfully included in health policies, laws, programs, services, research, and funding opportunities in order to address health disparities experienced by individuals with intellectual disabilities. For more information, go to: https://inclusivehealth.specialolympics.org.

The CDC also currently funds several other organizations that support the health of persons with disabilities through targeted efforts to address health disparities in a variety of ways.

National Association of County and City Health Officials (NACCHO). The mission of NACCHO is "to improve the health of communities by strengthening and advocating for local health departments." Through support from the CDC and the National Center on Birth Defects and Developmental Disabilities, NACCHO's Health and Disability Program promotes the inclusion and engagement of people with disabilities in all local health department programs, products, and services.

Key activities of the program include a fellowship program for emerging leaders in the health and disability field; a technical assistance program to assist local health departments with inclusion efforts; maintenance of a Health and Disability Workgroup; and communication activities to educate local health departments on inclusion best practices. Additionally, NACCHO's Health and Disability Program provides an online Health and Disability 101 training resource for health department employees that includes foundational knowledge about individuals with disabilities, disability-related health disparities, and how local health department staff can promote inclusion in programs and services. Efforts of NACCHO's Health and Disability Program have aided local health departments to build capacity in developing and growing inclusive focused partnerships, implementing inclusive practices, and bringing awareness of inclusion to staff and local communities. For more information, go to: https://www.naccho.org/programs/community-health/disability.

Association of University Centers on Disabilities (AUCD). The AUCD works in every state and territory to advance policies and practices that improve the health, education, social, and economic well-being of all people with disabilities, their families, and their communities. AUCD connects public health partners for systems change efforts as a multidisciplinary network of university-based training and service centers and programs. Through research, training, service, and advocacy, the AUCD network helps people with disabilities to overcome barriers to inclusion and wellness. AUCD works on public health efforts with the mantra that "public health is for everyone." This effort aims to build the capacity of the public health workforce by encouraging collaboration between public health partners and AUCD university network centers to collectively address health disparities for individuals with disabilities. The AUCD supports the National Center on Disability in Public Health which uses evidenced-based strategies to develop and increase the ability of public health professionals to include people living with disabilities. Among the plethora of resources available, AUCD has created three "getting started" resources for disability inclusion in public health:

1. *Public Health is For Everyone Toolkit*: www.phetoolkit.org

   (a) Online toolkit with capacity building fact sheets, resources, and training for public health professionals.

2. Including People with Disabilities—Public Health Workforce Competencies: https://disabilityinpublichealth.org

   (a) Provides foundational knowledge around the relationship between disability and public health programs and outcomes.

3. *Foundational Principles for Sustainable Inclusion of People with Intellectual Disability*: https://nationalcenterdph.org

   (a) With support from Special Olympics, this document provides organizations with principles and guidelines to ensure full and sustainable inclusion of people with intellectual disabilities in health policies, programs, services, trainings, and funding streams.

For more information on AUCD, go to: www.aucd.org/.

Christopher & Dana Reeve Foundation. The Christopher & Dana Reeve Foundation is a nonprofit dedicated to improving the quality of life for people and families living with paralysis. It works to cure spinal cord injury by funding innovative research and to improve the quality of life for people living with paralysis through grants, information, and advocacy. Since 2002, its Paralysis Resource Center (PRC) has served as the support side of the Reeve Foundation's twin missions to provide "Today's Care" and to strive for "Tomorrow's Cure." This center provides a free comprehensive national source of information for people living with paralysis and their caregivers with the goal of promoting community inclusion, health promotion, and improved quality of life. The PRC focuses on the daily challenges of independent living by offering a variety of services, support communities, and programs. In partnership with the Administration for Community Living under the US Department of Health and Human Services, the PRC strives to address the environmental, social, and systemic barriers to health and community living for individuals with all forms of paralysis by offering trained Information Specialists, a Peer and Family Support Program, a Military and Veterans Program, and a Multicultural Outreach Program. Data collected from 100,000 individuals with paralysis and families help to inform the creation of new programs and materials so that the PRC continues to provide the most comprehensive and up-to-date resources. These insights are also used to educate the public and policymakers on the realities and needs of the greater paralysis community. For more information: www.christopherreeve.org.

The CDC is committed to protecting the health and well-being of individuals with disabilities throughout the lifespan. Through efforts of the CDC Disability and Health Branch and its State Disability and Health Programs and national collaborations, work will continue toward decreasing health disparities experienced by people with disabilities. To advance this goal, CDC resources are dedicated to providing information and resources for health professionals and caregivers or support networks of people with disabilities as well as individuals with disabilities themselves. Several CDC Disability and Health Program expected outcomes for future directions include improved monitoring of health and healthcare utilization and increased availability and access to inclusive health promotion resources that include evidence-based and innovative health programs.

8.5   Challenges and Future Directions

While substantial advances have been made in promoting the health and wellness of persons with disabilities, much remains to be done as members of this population continue to experience significant disadvantages regarding health and barriers to health care (Peacock, Iezzoni, & Harkin, 2015).

Rimmer and Rowland (2008) echoed the Surgeon General's Call to Action in noting that health promotion interventions aimed at assisting people with disabilities to manage their health could significantly impact their health, functioning, community participation, and quality of life. Still, almost 10 years later, Wingo and Rimmer (2018) acknowledged deep-rooted socioeconomic disadvantages as well as community structural, programmatic, and attitudinal barriers within communities as major contributors to health disparities confronting people with disabilities. Examples of these barriers include obstacles in the built environment, such as inaccessible diagnostic equipment; absence of accommodations, such as sign language interpreters or large print materials, in health promotion programs; and lack of awareness about the needs and abilities of patients with disabilities exhibited by healthcare providers.

For those with disabilities who also experience racial and ethnic health disparities, disability-related barriers and disparities are even more significant. A 2017 report, titled *Compounded Disparities: Health Equity at the Intersection of Disability, Race and Ethnicity* (Yee et al., 2017), found embedded systemic structural and attitudinal discrimination that diminishes the health of this population. As Yee et al. (2017) noted:

> Many false assumptions about disability, race and ethnicity underlie the way we deliver health care, the historical development of our public health care systems, and the disregard for the health disparities experienced by some groups as a natural consequence of being in the group, rather than an inequity that needs to be addressed through multiple approaches. (p. 7)

Thus, addressing the complex problem of disability-related barriers added to those experienced by a growing population of persons belonging to ethnic and racial minorities will require systemic change well beyond our health-related institutions.

Still, there is reason for hope. CDC programs focused on improving the health of persons with disabilities continue to reach key populations across the nation. These programs employ five strategies to achieve this goal: (a) promoting the use of standardized disability identifiers in surveillance instruments; (b) advancing research that increases understanding of health disparities experienced by persons with disabilities; (c) discovering and developing evidence-based interventions to address the needs of persons with disabilities; (d) training healthcare and public health professionals regarding the needs of persons with disabilities; and (e) promoting accessible health care and other community environments for persons with disabilities. Additionally, implementation of the Affordable Care Act (ACA) has resulted in increased access to both healthcare coverage and care for persons with disabilities (Rudowitz & Antonisse, 2018). This access to coverage may help to reduce long-standing health disparities for this population. Researchers have also found that increased access to coverage through Medicaid expansion under the ACA is associated with higher employment rates for people with disabilities (Hall, Shartzer, Kurth, & Thomas, 2018). The importance of this increase cannot be underestimated as improved health and greater access to employment has the potential to substantially improve the lives of persons with disabilities and help to mitigate the pervasive socioeconomic disadvantages that this population experiences. A progress report of the National Council on Disability (2017) reported that only 32 percent of working-age people with disabilities are employed compared with 73% of those without disabilities. Thus, the impact of the ACA on both health and employment of persons with disabilities on a seemingly intractable problems is promising.

Public health leaders have noted that a key component of success in this work is to build strong collaborations with diverse stakeholders and partners, identifying common goals and integrating persons with disabilities into all facets of public health activities, including planning, surveillance, programming, education, and evaluation (CDC, 2013). Lollar (2001) went further to express a hope that "Over time it may be possible to integrate the best of public health services and practice into the advocacy and networks of people with disabilities to unite a powerful force for improving the health of this segment of the public" (p. 756).

Much progress has been made in health promotion programming aimed at addressing the health disparities experienced by individuals with disabilities; however there is still much more work that needs to be done. Future efforts should continue to emphasize the broad inclusion of individuals with disabilities across all programming efforts and policies and leverage partnerships between public health and disability and health programs.

References

Burwell, S. M. (2014, November). *Report to congress: Improving the identification of health care disparities in Medicaid and CHIP*. Department of Health and Human Services. Retrieved from https://www.medicaid.gov/medicaid/quality-of-care/downloads/4302b-rtc-2014.pdf

Centers for Disease Control and Prevention (CDC). (2013). CDC grand rounds: Public health practices to include persons with disabilities. *Morbidity and Mortality Weekly Report, 62*(34), 697–701.

Centers for Disease Control and Prevention (CDC), Disability and Health Branch. (2017). *Disability and Health Data System (DHDS)*. Retrieved from https://www.cdc.gov/ncbddd/disabilityandhealth/documents/DHDS_FactSheet-508.pdf

Centers for Disease Control and Prevention. (2019). Disability and Health Promotion. Retrieved from https://www.cdc.gov/ncbddd/disabilityandhealth/aboutus.html

DeJong, G. (1979). Independent living: From social movement to analytic paradigm. *Archives of Physical Medicine and Rehabilitation, 60*, 435–446.

Hall, J. P., Shartzer, A., Kurth, N. K., & Thomas, K. C. (2018). Medicaid expansion as an employment incentive program for people with disabilities. *American Journal of Public Health, 9*, 1234–1237.

Hough, J. (1999). Surveillance and outcome measurement systems for monitoring disabilities. In R. Simeonsson & L. N. McDevitt (Eds.), *Issues in disability and health: The role of secondary conditions and quality of life* (pp. 95–128). Chapel Hill: University of North Carolina, FPG Child Development Center.

Krahn, G., Walker, D. K., & Correa-De-Araujo, R. (2015). People with disabilities as an unrecognized health disparity population. *American Journal of Public Health, 105*(52), S198–S206.

Lollar, D. (1999). Clinical dimensions of secondary conditions. In R. Simeonsson & L. N. McDevitt (Eds.), *Issues in disability and health: The role of secondary conditions and quality of life* (pp. 41–50). Chapel Hill: University of North Carolina, FPG Child Development Center.

Lollar, D. (2001). Public health trends in disability: Past, present and future. In G. L. Albrecht, K. D. Seelman, & M. Bury (Eds.), *Handbook of disability studies* (pp. 754–771). Thousand Oaks: Sage.

Lollar, D., & Crews, J. E. (2003). Redefining the role of public health in disability. *Annual Review of Public Health, 24,* 195–208.

Longmore, P. K. (2003). *Why I burned my book and other essays on disability.* Philadelphia: Temple.

Marge, M. (1988). Health promotion for persons with disabilities: Moving beyond rehabilitation. *Journal of Health Promotion, 2,* 2944.

National Council on Disability. (2017). *National disability policy: A progress report.* Washington, DC: Author. Retrieved from https://www.ncd.gov/sites/default/files/NCD_A%20Progress%20 Report_508.pdf

Peacock, G., Iezzoni, L. I., & Harkin, T. R. (2015). Health care for Americans with disabilities-25 years after the ADA. *New England Journal of Medicine, 373*(10), 892–893.

Reichard, A., & Stotzle, H. (2011). Diabetes among adults with cognitive limitations compared to individuals with no cognitive disabilities. *Intellectual and Developmental Disabilities, 49*(3), 141–154.

Reichard, A., Stotzle, H., & Fox, M. H. (2011). Health disparities among adults with physical disabilities or cognitive limitations compared to individuals with no disabilities in the United States. *Disability and Health Journal, 4*(2), 59–67.

Rimmer, J., & Rowland, J. (2008). Physical activity for youth with disabilities: A critical need in an underserved population. *Developmental Neurorehabilitation, 11*(2), 141–148.

Rudowitz, R., & Antonisse, L. (2018). *Implications of the ACA Medicaid expansion: A look at the data and evidence.* San Francisco, CA: Kaiser Family Foundation. Retrieved from https://www.kff.org/medicaid/issue-brief/ implications-of-the-aca-medicaid-expansion-alook-at-the-data-and-evidence/

Seekins, T., Traci, M. A., Cummings, S., Oreskovich, J., & Ravesloot, C. (2008). Assessing environmental factors that affect disability: Establishing a baseline of visitability in a rural state. *Rehabilitation Psychology, 53*(1), 80–84.

Shakespeare, T. (2017). The social model of disability. In L. J. Davis (Ed.), *The disability studies reader* (5th ed., pp. 195–203). New York: Routledge.

Shapiro, J. P. (1994). *No pity: People with disabilities forging a new civil rights movement.* New York: Random House.

Stevens, A. C., Courtney-Long, E. A., Okoro, C. A., & Carroll, D. D. (2016). Peer of 2 Disability Measures, Behavioral Risk Factor Surveillance System, 2013. Preventing chronic disease, 13, E106. https://doi.org/10.5888/pcd13.160080.

U.S. Department of Health and Human Services. (2005). *The surgeon general's call to action to improve the health and wellness of persons with disabilities.* U.S. Department of Health and Human Services, Office of the Surgeon General.

U.S. Department of Health and Human Services. (2011). *Implementation guidance on data collection standards for race, ethnicity, sex, primary language, and disability status.* Retrieved from https://aspe.hhs.gov/basic-report/hhs-implementation-guidance-data-collection-standards-race-ethnicity-sex-primary-language-and-disability-status

U.S. Department of Health and Human Services, Office of Disease Prevention and Health Promotion. (2019). *Healthy people.* Retrieved from https://health.gov/our-work/healthy-people/

Ustun, T. B., Chatterji, S., Bickenbach, J., Kostanjsek, N., & Schneider, M. (2003). The International Classification of Functioning, Disability and Health: A new tool for understanding disability and health. *Disability and Rehabilitation, 25*(11–12), 565–571.

Wingo, B. C., & Rimmer, J. H. (2018). Emerging trends in health promotion for people with disabilities. *Journal of Environmental Research in Public Health, 15*(4), 742.

World Health Organization (WHO). (1986). *Ottawa charter for health promotion.* Geneva: World Health Organization. Retrieved from http://who.int/hpr/archive/docs/ottawa.html

World Health Organization (WHO). (1991). *International Classification of Functioning, Disability, and Health: ICF.* Geneva: Author.

World Health Organization. (2002). *Towards a common language for functioning, disability and health: ICF.* Geneva: World Health Organization. Retrieved April 7, 2020, from https://www. who.int/classifications/icf/icfbeginnersguide.pdf

Yee, S., Breslin, M. L., Goode, T. D., Havercamp, S. M., Horner-Johnson, W., Iezzoni, L. I., & Krahn, G. (2017). *Compounded disparities: Health equity at the intersection of disability, race, and ethnicity*. Berkeley, CA: Disability Rights Education and Fund.

Yell, M. L., Rogers, D., & Rogers, E. L. (1998). The legal history of special education: What a long, strange trip it's been! *Remedial and Special Education, 19*(4), 219–228.

Chapter 9
Children with Special Healthcare Needs

Rune J. Simeonsson and Kristina L. Simeonsson

Of the population of children from birth through age 17 in the USA accessing pediatric health care, about one-fifth are identified as children with special healthcare needs, CSHCN (Bethell, Read, Blumberg, & Newacheck, 2008). The standard definition of this group of children was established in 1998 by the US Maternal and Child Health Bureau (MCHB) as children "who have or are at increased risk for a chronic physical, developmental, behavioral or emotional condition and who also require health and related services of a type or amount beyond that required of children generally" (McPherson et al., 1998). This chapter describes the characteristics of this population, the screening and epidemiological basis for their identification, the nature and scope of care coordination to meet their complex needs, and consideration of policy and research issues related to serving CSHCN.

The definition of CSHCN within a public health perspective contributed to the systematic documentation of this population beginning in 2001 with the administration of the National Survey of Children with Special Health Care Needs. That survey included a screener, operationalizing the above MCHB definition, which became the basis for subsequent surveys in 2005/2006 and 2009/2010 and later in combination with the administration of the National Survey of Children's Health in 2016, 2017, and 2018. Whereas up to 20% of the population of children in the USA are identified as CSHCN (Bethell et al., 2008), a smaller subgroup is recognized as children with medical complexity (CMC). This subgroup of children accounts for 6.57% of the total group of CSHCN and represents children with chronic and/or severe medical conditions requiring comprehensive and intensive healthcare

R. J. Simeonsson (✉)
School of Education, University of North Carolina at Chapel Hill, Chapel Hill, NC, USA
e-mail: rjsimeon@email.unc.edu

K. L. Simeonsson (✉)
Department of Pediatrics, Brody School of Medicine, East Carolina University,
Greenville, NC, USA
e-mail: simeonssonk@ecu.edu

© Springer Science+Business Media, LLC, part of Springer Nature 2021
D. J. Lollar et al. (eds.), *Public Health Perspectives on Disability*,
https://doi.org/10.1007/978-1-0716-0888-3_9

services (Hofacer et al., 2019). In a paper describing this subgroup of children as a population with pervasive medical problems and intense service needs, Cohen et al. (2011) refer to descriptions of the children with a range of terms including complex, chronic, fragile, congenital, and multi-system conditions. Integrating the existing descriptions, they summarized the chronic and complex nature of children with CMC within a definitional framework of (a) elevated child service needs; (b) existence of one or more chronic conditions; (c) significant limitations of functioning; and (d) elevated utilization of health and health-related resources (Cohen et al., 2011). Given the complexity of their condition, children with CMC are likely to experience unmet needs, that is, the need for a specific health service but not receiving it. A secondary analysis of data from two administrations of the National Survey of Children with Special Health Care Needs (2005–2006 and 2009–2010) confirmed an overall twofold increase of an unmet healthcare need for children with CMC compared to children without CMC (Kuo et al., 2014). Reported unmet needs ranged from 0 to 14, with 44.2% of families of children with CMC reporting at least one unmet need and 11.5% reporting three or more unmet needs, compared to 19.1% and 2.6%, respectively, by families of children without CMC.

These findings and that of disproportionately higher unmet needs of families of children with CMC across race and ethnicity compared to those without CMC led the authors to conclude that "medical complexity itself can be a primary determinant of unmet needs" (Kuo et al., 2014, p. 2190). As such, the response of healthcare systems to children with CMC needs to encompass a clinical agenda that builds on a model of chronic care that includes a family-centered approach to care, knowledgeable providers at different levels of care, provision of supports for child and family functioning, and accessible, coordinated, and efficient care services (Cohen et al., 2011).

9.1 Identification of CSHCN

Screening and surveillance of CSHCN is based on the administration of a national, random digital dialing telephone survey of households in 50 states and the District of Columbia. The National Survey of Children with Special Health Care Needs (NS-CSHCN) was administered in 2001 and 2005/2006 and in 2009/2010 (Yu et al., 2015). The 2009-2010 administration yielded a sample of 40242 family interviews for children with special healthcare needs (Ross et al., 2018). Beginning in 2016, the NS-CSHCN was combined with the National Survey of Children's Health (NSCH) to obtain a representative sampling of the US population yielding weighted estimates of children with special healthcare needs between 0 and 17 years of age (Ghandour et al., 2018).

In the administration of the NS-CSHCN, the caregiver is interviewed using a screener to establish if there is a child with special healthcare needs in the household. The identification of CSHCN is based on a positive response to one of five screener items by the respondent. If more than one child with special healthcare needs was identified in the house hold, the respondent was asked to randomly select one child for whom additional data was gathered. The five screener items are "(1) need or use of prescription medications, (2) above-routine use of medical, mental health, or educational services compared with other children, (3) daily activity limitations, (4) need or use of specialized therapies; and (5) need or use of treatment or counseling for emotional, developmental or behavioral conditions" (Akobirshoev, Parish, Mitra, & Dembo, 2019). In the 2009/2010 administration of the NS-CSHCN the survey was administered to 196,159 households, involving a total of 372,698 children with the result of 40,242 children being identified as having special healthcare needs (Hofacer et al., 2019). The repeated administrations of the NS-CSHN and the NSCH using the five items of the CSHCN screener have yielded estimates of the prevalence of CSHCN within a consistent range for the USA and District of Columbia. Variability in estimates of the prevalence of CSHCN was examined in a study of earlier administrations of the NSCH (2003) and the NS-CSHCN (2001) and the Medical Expenditures Panel Surveys (2001–2004) all using the CSHCN screener items (Bethell et al., 2008). Prevalence estimates for CSHCN among children 0–17 years of age were found to differ as a function the survey, with the NS-CSHCN yielding a prevalence of 12.8% compared to 17.6% for NSCH and a range of 18.8% to 19.3% across the four administrations of the MEP. Variability in estimates was attributable to methodological differences in the surveys, leading to the conclusion that the prevalence of CSHCN should be viewed as a range rather than a point estimate.

A one-time administration of the NSCH in 2011/2012 in the territory of Virgin Islands yielded data indicating a lower prevalence of CSHCN than the surveys conducted in the USA. Specifically, whereas almost one-fifth (19.8%) of children in the US population had a SHCN, the prevalence for children in the Virgin Islands was about 10%, half the prevalence in the 50 states of the USA (Vladutiu, Lebrun-Harris, Carlos, & Petersen, 2019). This lower prevalence existed in spite of the fact that almost a third (31.3%) of children in the Virgin Islands were from households below 100% of the federal poverty level.

In addition to documenting the prevalence of CSHCN with repeated administrations of the NS-CSHCN and the NSCH, the surveys have also been used to examine characteristics of CSHCN and their associations with other child and environmental factors. The relationship of special healthcare needs and general health status with school functioning of 6- to 17-year-old children was examined in a study of data based on the administration of the 2007 NSCH. General health status was measured on a five-point scale from excellent to poor, and school functioning was assessed with five indicators related to special education, missed school days, number of problem reports, grade repetition, and lack of school involvement. On the basis of responses to the screener, 13% of the sample was identified on the basis of meeting one or more of the screener criteria as C-CSHCN, and 9% identified as CSHCN-RX based only on the screener criteria of medication use. Analyses indicated higher rates of problematic school outcomes of children with CSHCN ranging from 14.5 to 46.6% across the five indicators compared to 1.2–16.0% for children without SHCN. Although not of the same magnitude, the rates of problematic outcomes were similarly higher for CSHCN-RX, ranging from 1.6 to 18.4% compared to the rates for children without SHCN.

Analysis of CSHCN in relation to environmental factors has also taken the form of complementary use of the National Survey of Children's Health and other databases. A recent study combining the use of the NSCH and National Land Cover Database was designed to test the possible association of a nature variable, green space, and manifestation of anxiety in different groups of children (Larson et al., 2018). Drawing on data from the 2012 administration of the NSCH, three groups of children aged 6–17 years of age were identified, children without SHCN, children with CSHCN but not autism, and children with autism. The hypothesis of elevated anxiety with more exposure to impervious surfaces (gray space) and lower anxiety with more exposure to surfaces with tree canopy (green space) was not confirmed for children either with or without CHCN. Ironically, for children with autism, a low level of support was found for associations of both environmental settings with increased levels of anxiety. Although the authors recognize that inferences that can be drawn from the study are limited, they emphasize the value of national data sets in examining the impact of the environment on children with various developmental conditions.

9.2   Social Determinants of CSHCN

The items for screening CSHCN reflect the fact that family factors constitute significant determinants of this population of children. Central among social determinants of CSHN are demographic factors related to poverty including education, ethnicity, and incomes below the federal poverty level. In keeping with the screener items, greater health problems of CSHCN contribute to three times greater healthcare-related expenditures for their families (Newacheck & Kim, 2005).

A significant manifestation of social determinants of CSHCN are financial challenges faced by families of CSHCN in the form of inadequate or lack of stable housing. A cross-sectional study of families served in five major medical centers examined the relationship of housing instability and caregiving for a young child with special healthcare needs (Rose-Jacobs et al., 2019). An interview was developed using the CSHCN screener items of need for prescription medication, increased use of health and related services, functional limitations, use of specialized therapies and treatment for mental health problems to identify children under 4 years of age with special needs. In the interview, caregivers were asked about demographic, household, and financial characteristics of their family. In addition, caregivers reported whether or not their child was a recipient of Supplemental Security Income (SSI).

Drawing on data for the period of 2013–2017, the results of the interview yielded three groups of children, 11,408 without CSHCN, 2193 with CSHCN but without SSI, and 587 with CSHCN and SSI. In multiple comparisons, families of children with CSHCN were significantly more likely to report being behind on paying mortgage or rent (24.1% vs 19.7%) moving two or more times in the previous year (6.2% vs. 4.3%) and reporting lifetime homelessness (9.9% vs. 7.5%). Further analyses revealed that CSHCN but without SSI had greater adjusted odds ratios of being behind on payments for housing, moving more than twice a year and experiencing homelessness than the comparison group of children without CSHCN and the group with CSHCN and with SSI. The results of the study indicate that families of CSHCN who face higher numbers of challenges in family life are at increased risk for not having adequate or stable housing.

A social determinant of increasing significance related to CSHCN is household language with the changing demography of immigration. Limited proficiency in English is likely not only to be associated with lower socioeconomic status but also therefore with difficulties in accessing health care and related services by families of children with special healthcare needs. The relationship of limited English proficiency (LEP) of parents as a social determinant and health outcomes of CSHCN has been substantial focus of research. In a systematic review of literature, Eneriz-Weimer, Sanders, Barr, and Mendoza (2014) identified 31 studies that examined outcomes related to child health and access, utilization, costs, and quality of care. Parents with LEP were more likely to report that their CSHCN to be uninsured, lack a medical home, and less likely to report that they received, or satisfied, with family-centered care than parents who were proficient in English.

Addressing the same issue, Yu, Lin, and Strickland (2015) compared the problems experienced by Non-English Primary Language (NEPL) and English Primary Language (EPL) households in healthcare utilization using data from the 2009–2010 NS-CSHCN. Although there was no difference between NEPL and EPL children by gender, children from NEPL were among other factors more likely to be from poor households, to have parents that did not complete high school, and less likely to have private insurance. The focus of the study was to document the extent of disparities of healthcare quality indicators of CSHCN as a function NELP. The six healthcare quality indicators were: "(1) family partnership in decision-making and satisfaction with care, (2) receipt of care through a medical home, (3) adequate health insurance, (4) early and continuous screening and surveillance, (5) services that are organized for ease of use, and (6) effective transition planning for adult health care" (Yu et al., 2015, p. 5). Analyses of the data indicated significant disparities for all healthcare quality indicators for families with NELP in the form of discrepancies in percentage of indicators met ranging from 11.7 to 19.4% compared to ELP families. These findings were confirmed by regression analyses indicating significantly higher odds of NELP families not feeling partnership in decision-making, lacking access to a medical home, lacking adequate health insurance, and lacking continuous screening and necessary transition services.

Other determinants of health, compounding demographic factors are adverse childhood experiences (ACEs) such as exposure to abuse and violence. Focusing on psychosocial factors in children and youth with special healthcare needs (CYSHCN), Mattson, Kuo, Committee on Psychosocial Aspects of Child and Family Health, and Council on Children with Disabilities (2019) reviewed NSCH research indicating that exposure to two or more ACEs was twice as high (37%) for CYSHCN than for children without special healthcare needs (18%). These ACEs are not only another dimension of the complexity of CYSHCN but can compound the effects of other manifestations and contribute to the development of secondary conditions and elevation of risk for social and educational problems. Given the complexity of CYSHCN and the diversity of factors associated with their identification and care, implications of the findings are for more effective public health surveillance approaches and programs for outreach and support of this population underserved on the basis of social determinants.

9.3   Health and Health-Related Services for CSHCN

Consistent with the definition of CSHCN, access to, and heavy use of, a range of health services is a characteristic of this group of children and their families. The coordination of this range of health services is a central concept in providing services for CSHCN with care coordination defined by the American Academy of Pediatrics as "a process that links CSHCN and their families with appropriate services and resources in a coordinated effort to achieve good health" (American Academy of Pediatrics Council on Children with Disability, 2005). A comprehensive analysis of care coordination for children with medical complexity (CMC) was made by Hofacer et al. (2019) drawing on caregiver responses to the 2009–2010 National Survey of Children with Special Health Care Needs (NS-CSHCN). For this analysis, the identification of CMC was based on multiple positive responses to the five screener questions resulting in a subgroup of children with the most complex medical conditions, representing 6.57% of the total unweighted CSHCN population (38,506). Analysis of the four categories of care coordination support reported by families of CSHCN indicated that 11.39% received clinical support, 5.32% received family/social network support, and 4.02% received both clinical and family support with 79.09% receiving no support. In comparison, care coordination in the form of clinic support was higher (25.73%) for families of CMC and the proportion not receiving any support was lower (66.47%). The data confirm that a very large proportion of the population of CSHCN lack care coordination.

Given the fragmentation of services and lack of coordination of services for families with children with complex medical needs, the concept of the "medical home" was developed by the American Academy of Pediatrics (AAP, 2002). The medical home was defined as a medical setting that was accessible for the family and that could provide and coordinate services that were comprehensive, continuous, and sensitive to the culture and needs of the family. The significance of the medical home as a mechanism for insuring access to needed health services by families with and without children with special healthcare needs is evident by the fact that it is a national health objective in Healthy People 2020. Further, progress of the implementation of the medical home is tracked in the two national surveys (NS-CSHCN & NSCH) sponsored by the Maternal and Child Health Bureau (Akobirshoev et al., 2019).

Drawing on data from the 2016 NSCH, Akobirshoev et al. (2019) examined the health experiences of CSHCN and non-CSHCN families as a function of having and not having a medical home. Assessment of the medical home experience of 11,392 CSHCN and 38,820 non-CSHCN families in the 2016 NSCH involved caregiver responses to a composite measure involving five components of having (a) a personal healthcare provider, (b) a regular source of care that was (c) family-centered, as well as (d) experiencing responsiveness to referrals and provision of care coordination as needed. An analysis of demographic characteristics of families of CSHCN and non-CSHCN that did not have a medical home included a greater likelihood of minority status, a language other than English spoken in the home and low or no insurance coverage compared to families who had a medical home. The impact of not having a medical home for CSHCN was evident by the fact they were more likely to lack preventive dental care visits, have at least two emergency room visits, have unmet medical and dental care unmet needs, and are more likely to be perceived as having fair or poor overall health or oral health status compared to CSHCN with a medical home.

The impact of not having a medical home was very similar for non-CSHCN, in that they were more likely to lack preventive medical and dental care visits, have more emergency room visits, have more unmet medical and dental care needs, and are more likely to be perceived as having fair or poor oral health compared to non-CSHCN with a medical home.

Disparities in unmet healthcare needs as a function of differences in access to a medical home by minority families were examined in data from the 2007 NSCH (Bennett, Rankin & Rosenberg, 2012). The proportion of white CSHCN without a medical home was 43.0% compared to 60.4% of black CSHCN with a corresponding rate of 8.8% versus 15.3% unmet needs, respectively. Application of a mediation framework to examine the role of the medical home indicated that it could account for some disparity in accounting for unmet medical needs, but not all. This and the above findings highlight the contribution of a medical home to improve health outcomes of CSHCN and non-CSHCN with implications for insuring access to a medical home for any child in need of coordinated health services.

The importance of care coordination reflected by the medical home in serving CSHCN is also reflected in efforts to coordinate access of the children to other services in the community related to their special developmental and educational needs. For younger CSHCN, early intervention authorized under Part C of the Individuals with Disabilities Education Act (IDEA) requires states to offer a range of services to children under 3 years of age identified with developmental delay or assigned a mental or physical diagnosis. Given the substantial overlap of eligibility criteria for services for children as CSHCN and under Part C, utilization of early intervention by CSHCN should be substantial. Although all states are required to provide services under the IDEA legislation, there is significant state variability in the eligibility criteria and the nature and extent of early intervention (EI) services provided. Drawing on the 2009/2010 National Survey of Children with Special Health Care Needs, McManus, Magnusson, and Rosenberg (2014) grouped children in the survey on the basis of restrictiveness of eligibility criteria in terms of percent delay or standard deviation units from the mean on developmental measures. Of the 2208 CSHCN in the survey under 3 years of age, 923 met the criteria for EI eligibility and of that number, just over half (52.4%) reported utilization of EI services. There was however, a very large spread in utilization of EI services across states ranging from 6% in Washington to 87% in New Mexico. The substantial spread in utilization of services was attributed to variability of eligibility policy across states documented by a negative correlation of $r = -0.41$ ($p < 0.05$) between utilization of EI services and the restrictiveness of state eligibility policy. On the basis of modeling the data, the authors suggested that differences in eligibility policy across states explained more of the variability in utilization of EI services than the underlying health and developmental conditions of the children.

The above findings speak to the importance of coordination of policies as a key element for care coordination to insure access to comprehensive services by CSHCN. This point is reinforced by Adams, Tapia, and The Council on Children with Disabilities (2013) in their call for best practice related to collaboration of the medical home and EI services under Part C of IDEA. Central to their call is the shared focus of EI and the medical home on the provision of family-centered support that is comprehensive, coordinated, and culturally sensitive. To this end, Adams and Tapia advocate the concepts of working in the natural relationship environments of families and the approach of "coaching" support of families as best practice for EI and the medical home. They identified four groups served in the medical home for whom collaborative EI services would be particularly indicated, infants and toddlers experiencing abuse or neglect, experiencing mental health problems, coming from culturally diverse backgrounds, and/or experiencing economic deprivation. Advancing collaboration between the medical home and EI programs, Adams and Tapia's call for best practice include improved surveillance and identification of children with developmental needs, individualized and coordinated resources for families, and monitoring and evaluation of services.

What constitutes recommendations for best practice in terms of intervention programs supporting for families with CSHCN? Jackson, Liang, Frydenburg, Higgins, and Murphy (2016) conducted a systematic review to identify characteristics of education programs found effective for parents with CSHCN. Their review was international in scope, including seven studies from the USA, two from Australia, and four from the UK. The studies included children with disabilities as well as specific chronic conditions and met the criteria of methodological rigor and being based on theory. Characteristics that were common across the parent education programs were a narrative approach for families to tell their stories, an emphasis on strengthening family protective factors and strengthening parental understanding of the nature and developmental challenges of their child's condition. On the basis of a detailed review of the 13 studies ranging in sample size from 6 to 301, including children with disabilities and specific-health conditions, Jackson et al. (2016) reported positive outcomes of intervention in terms of improved family functioning, parenting skills, communication, problem-solving, and mental health.

In that care coordination is a key element of the medical home, coordination with schools becomes an important focus for CSHCN of school age. Drawing on previous research indicating that CSHCN were more likely to have a higher rate of school absences than peers without special needs, Willits et al. (2013) conducted a cross-sectional study of the 2005 NS-CSHCN to examine the role of the medical home on school functioning of CSHCN. Caregiver responses to the question of how many days the child missed school because of illness or injury in the previous 12 months were assigned to three categories, 0–3 days, 4–7 days, and 8–14 days. The results indicated that the category of most missed days of school was associated with CSHCN with a medical home. Further, even accounting for demographic and socioeconomic factors the presence of a medical home remained a significant factor in the prediction of missed days. Further, the odds of missing more school days were associated with increasing severity of functional limitations. Willits et al. (2013) conclude that the findings call for more effective interdisciplinary efforts in care coordination including consideration of a school-based medical home model.

9.4 Continuing Issues

As the formal identification of CSHCN as a group of children with complex medical and developmental needs has been relatively recent, issues related to practice, policy, and research related to coordination of their care continue to emerge. A central concern pertaining to care coordination is the issue of providing support for families of children with CSHCN that is comprehensive and family-centered. Given the complexity of a child's health condition, families of CSHCN may face a number of challenges related to understanding and coping with the nature of the child's health problems as well as to become advocates for their child and participants in their care. On the basis a scoping review of literature, DeHoff, Staten, Rodgers, and Denne (2016) have advocated for online social support as a key mechanism to empower families with CSHCN and to provide them with information they can apply in supporting their child. Parent-to-parent support has been recognized as perhaps the major factor facilitating how families cope with the demands of caring for children with chronic health conditions and disabilities. In this regard, DeHoff et al. (2016) advocate for investment in efforts to expand the use of digital technology, moving from mobile phones and texting to the increasing use of phone apps and social media, particularly given that such use is nearly universal among women under 30 for information and communication. A priority for healthcare providers is thus to advance online support of families of CSHCN including the development of online provider-to-parent support.

The provision of central aspects of healthcare policy for CSHCN with medical complexity (CMC), including care coordination and the medical home, should be evident in health outcomes of the children. A recent systematic review by Barnert et al. (2019) sought to identify the nature of health outcomes for this population of children. A review of the literature for the period from 1964 for Medline and 1985 for PsyINFO databases yielded 517 articles for data extraction. Using a systematic content analysis, a total of 5 domains and 24 sub-domains of health outcomes were found. In order of frequency, 50% of the articles pertained to the first domain of access and utilization of health care, 43% to the second domain of family well-being, 39% to the third domain of child health and well-being, 38% to the fourth domain of healthcare quality and for the fifth domain, and 25% to child adaptive functioning. Barnert et al. (2019) noted the lack of health outcomes measuring promotion of child health, child mental health, and family functioning, outcomes that should be the focus of a population health approach in the provision of services for children with medical complexity.

Although the formal designation of the CSHCN population was only made about 20 years ago, it is likely that pediatricians and other providers have in fact encountered the complex characteristics of at least some children with, as well as without, the designation of CSHCN in the context of providing healthcare services. Systematic training for pediatricians in providing comprehensive health care to CSHCN as well as to children with medical complexity has been limited (Huth, Long-Gagne, Mader, & Sbrocchi, 2018). In a study of five training programs in Massachusetts, Nazarian, Glader, Choueiri, Shipman, and Sadof (2010) reported that pediatric residents felt more comfortable caring for CSHCN in the hospital setting than addressing their needs in the community and at home and concluded that "Residents and faculty believe that residents would benefit from more formal training opportunities to learn directly from families and community representatives about caring for CYSHCN" (Nazarian et al., 2010, p. s183). Residents can learn from families and community partners caring for CSHCN; curricula can be enhanced by including a home visit with a family of a CSHCN as well as using parents and community partners as guest speakers/teachers in the program (Bogetz, Bogetz, Rassbach, Gabhart, & Blankenburg, 2015; Nazarian et al., 2010).

Limitation of resident training may not only limit the pediatrician's recognition of the complex nature and scope of the special healthcare needs but may also be a factor defining their confidence in the provision of care coordination and the medical home. In a focus group of 16 pediatric residents and recent graduates from a residency training program at a tertiary care center, four main challenges emerged in discussing the pediatrician's role in caring for CSHCN: (1) lack of care coordination, (2) complex technology management, (3) psychosocial needs, and (4) lack of effective healthcare provider training (Bogetz et al., 2015). These focus groups generated ideas to address these challenges during residency training including greater integration of primary care providers, attention to psychosocial needs through shared decision-making with families, and integration of longitudinal patient relationships into provider training.

In addressing training issues, Huth et al. (2018) developed a brief training module to inform pediatricians about the unique characteristics of children with medical complexity (CMC) including fragility of health, elevated service needs, limitations of functioning and dependence on technology, and their potential role in development of a medical home. The module was piloted with 15 residents in a pediatric residency program, most of whom (87%) had not had a rotation in complex care but had some prior exposure on the topic through informal teaching. Although the module was brief with a limited purpose, Huth et al. (2018) felt that it provided a valuable learning experience for providers with reference to the medical home and understanding of the challenges faced by families of children with CMC. Further, the module was seen as offering an important approach for providing care in collaboration with families and the interdisciplinary team, an approach equally useful for other members of interdisciplinary care teams. A similar training model to enhance integration of care for CSHCN was developed in the context of a resident continuity clinic (Linton et al., 2018). Implementation of the pilot curriculum involved a range of individual and group learning experiences resulted in improved perceptions of residents and nurses on the team-based care concept of the medical home in the continuity clinic.

A related issue in provider care was addressed by Braganza et al. (2020) focusing on confidence of providers in serving CSHCN. Building on prior literature describing factors limiting the work of pediatricians with CSHCN, a study was made of the confidence of resident and attending pediatricians in encounters with CSHCN. Of 381 encounters between resident patient, 49% were with CSHCN, and of 137 encounters between attending patient, 39% were with CSHCN. The percentage of children with complex needs for the respective encounters were 17 and 10%. Overall, providers expressed lower confidence in caring for CSHCN. Further, the odds of expressing confidence was lower with higher CSHCN score and was lower for resident vs attending pediatrician. Braganza et al. (2020) conclude that the results call for further emphasis on all aspects of health care for CSHCN.

The continuing emergence of CSHCN as a population of children presenting with multiple, chronic, and complex health conditions will be paralleled with the need for frameworks for defining coordination of services and measures to effectively document the outcomes of providing support. Addressing these issues, Cohen et al. (2011) have identified the importance of defining outcomes for reliable and valid evaluation of the dimensional framework (needs, chronic conditions, functional limitations, healthcare use) defining children with medical complexity (MCM). An important consideration in this regard is to distinguish between documentation of outcomes that define specific disease conditions including congenital anomalies and outcomes that are independent of specific conditions such as health-related quality of life, mental health, and functioning of families and caregivers.

Cohen et al. (2011) have proposed the International Classification of Functioning, Disability and Health-ICF (WHO, 2001) as a holistic approach that may be particularly useful to encompass the development of outcome measures. A complementary recommendation has been made for the use of the ICF as an overall framework for defining a dimensional approach, focusing on technology, family system, and team management in comprehensive care of children with medical complexity (Glader, Plews-Ogan, & Agrawal, 2016). The ICF version for Children and Youth- ICF-CY (WHO, 2007) encompasses domains of Body Functions and Structures, Activities and Participation, and Environmental Factors for documenting condition-specific and condition-independent outcomes for CSHCN and their families. Applications of the ICF-CY for health and health-related settings could take the form of documenting child characteristics interventions, drawing on ICF-CY codes for condition-specific and condition-independent outcomes as well as deriving content for evaluation measures (Lollar & Simeonsson, 2005; Simeonsson, 2009).

Adopting the ICF-CY can add value to enhance the provision of health care for CSHCN and children with medical complexity in clinical practice and public health in a number of ways. In addition to their multiple medical conditions, the psychosocial problems of children and youth with special healthcare needs (CYSHCN) can be viewed as both internal (e.g., emotional) and external (e.g., life experiences) in nature (Mattson et al., 2019). To address the complexity of medical and functional problems and associated internal and external factors of CYSHCN, a comprehensive approach is needed that can be used to document that complexity in assessment and care coordination. The dimensional framework and codes of Body Functions and Structures, Activities and Participation, and Environmental Factors and an associated qualifier designating severity provide a comprehensive language uniquely suited to document the diversity and complexity of child and family needs. Application of such taxonomic documentation has been widely implemented for children and adults with disabilities in other health and health-related settings.

A useful application of the ICF-CY in CSHCN care settings would be to more fully describe the complexity and severity of CSHCN with codes differentiating dimensions of the environment and functioning of the child. Such application could extend descriptive studies by Roman, Dworkin, Dickinson, and Rogers (2019), for example, in which the nature and frequency of use across 11 resource sectors was cross-linked to 13 diagnostic groups, 2 related to the diagnoses of Asthma and ASD, and the remaining 11 to broad groupings based on etiological, developmental or system-level factors. Specifically, ICF-CY codes and qualifiers could expand descriptions of individual differences of children and characteristics of resources in greater detail.

In a broader context, the ICF-CY can advance care integration by offering a universal language for interdisciplinary communication in the design and delivery of integrated care and evaluation of interventions. Further, as the commitment to identify and provide care for CYSHCN expands in other countries (Flores et al., 2016), the universal language of ICF-CY domains and codes may be of particular value in enhancing public health screening and surveillance as initiatives to identify and provide care for CYSHCN.

9.5   Questions for Discussion

1. Identify the social determinants that are associated with greater unmet needs by some parents of CSHCN and propose ways in which their utilization of services could be enhanced.
2. Describe the basis for differentiating the subgroup of Children with Medical Complexity from CSHCN and describe the nature and scope of the additional services they need.

3. Why are CSHCN more likely to experience adverse childhood experiences (ACEs) and what are implications for prevention?
4. Training programs for medical professionals have largely focused on issues related to provision of clinical care for CSHCN, what should be the focus of training for professionals in public health?
5. What are challenges in documenting the complexity and severity of conditions of CSHCN for identification and for care coordination?
6. How could application of the framework and taxonomy of the ICF-CY enhance documentation of CSHSN in clinical practice and in public health?

References

Adams, R. C., Tapia, C., & The Council on Children with Disabilities. (2013). Early intervention, IDEA Part C services and the medical home: Collaboration for best practice and best outcomes. *Pediatrics, 132*(4), e1073–e1088. https://doi.org/10.1542/peds.2013-2305

Akobirshoev, I., Parish, S., Mitra, M., & Dembo, R. (2019). Impact of medical home on health care of children with and without special health care needs: Update from the 2016 National Survey of Children's Health. *Maternal and Child Health Journal, 23*(11), 1500–1507. https://doi.org/10.1007/s10995-019-02774-9

American Academy of Pediatrics (AAP). (2002). The medical home. *Pediatrics, 110*(1), 184–186. https://doi.org/10.1542/peds.110.1.184

American Academy of Pediatrics Council on Children with Disability. (2005). Care coordination in the medical home: Integrating health and related systems of care for children with special health care needs. *Pediatrics, 116*, 1238–1244. https://doi.org/10.1542/peds.2007-2070

Barnert, E. S., Coller, R. J., Nelson, B. B., Thompson, L. R., Tran, J., Chan, V., ... Chung, P. J. (2019). Key population health outcomes for children with medical complexity: As systematic review. *Maternal and Child Health Journal, 23*, 1167–1176. https://doi.org/10.1007/s10995-019-02752-1

Bethell, C. D., Read, D., Blumberg, S. J., & Newacheck, P. W. (2008). What is the prevalence of children with special health care needs? Toward an understanding of variations in findings and methods across three national surveys. *Maternal Child Health Journal, 12*, 1–14. https://doi.org/10.1007/s10995-007-0220-5

Bennett, A. C., Rankin, K. M., & Rosenberg, D. (2012). Does a medical home mediate racial disparities in unmet healthcare needs among children with special healthcare needs? Maternal and Child Health Journal, 16 Suppl 2, 330–338. https://doi.org/10.1007/s10995-012-1131-7

Bogetz, J. F., Bogetz, A. L., Rassbach, C. E., Gabhart, J. M., & Blankenburg, R. L. (2015). Caring for children with medical complexity: Challenges and educational opportunities identified by pediatric residents. *Academic Pediatrics, 15*(6), 621–625.

Braganza, S. F., Tyrell, H., Rosen, C., Mogilner, L., Phillips, A., Slovin, S., & Sharif, I. (2020). Cornet Card Study # 1: Do You See What I See? Provider confidence in caring for children with special health care needs. *Academic Pediatrics, 20*(2), 250–257. https://doi.org/10.1016/j.acap.2019.10.005

Cohen, E., Kuo, D. Z., Agrawal, R., Berry, J. G., Bhagat, S. K. M., Simon, T. D., & Srivastava, R. (2011). Children with medical complexity: An emerging population for clinical and research initiatives. *Pediatrics, 127*(3), 529–538.

DeHoff, B. A., Staten, L. K., Rodgers, R. C., & Denne, S. C. (2016). The role of online support in supporting and educating parents of young children with special health care needs in the United States: A scoping review. *Journal of Medical Internet Research, 18*(12), e333. https://doi.org/10.2196/jmir.6722

Eneriz-Weimer, M., Sanders, L., Barr, D. A., & Mendoza, F. S. (2014). Parental limited English proficiency and health outcomes for children with special health care needs: A systematic review. *Academic Pediatrics, 14*(2), 128–136.

Flores, C. J. C., Lizama, C. M., Rodriguez, Z. N., Avalos, A. M. E., Galanti, D. L. P. M., Barja, Y. S., … Comite NANEAS Sociedad Chilena de Pediatria. (2016). Models of care and classification of "Children with special health care needs-CSHCN": Recommendations for the CSHCN Committee, Chilean Paediatric Society. *Revista Chilena de Pediatría, 87*(3), 224–232.

Ghandour, R. M., Jones, J . R., Lebrun-Harris, L. A., Jessica Minnaert, J., Blumberg, S. J., Fields J, Bethell C, & Kogan, M. D. (2018). The design and implementation of the 2016 National Survey of Children's Health. Maternal and Child Health Journal, 22(8), 1093–1102. https://doi.org/10.1007/s10995-018-2526-x

Glader, L., Plews-Ogan, J., & Agrawal, R. (2016). Children with medical complexity: Creating a framework for care based on the International Classification of Functioning, Disability and Health. *Developmental Medicine & Child Neurology, 58*, 1116–1123. https://doi.org/10.1111/dcmn.13201

Hofacer, R. C., Panatopoulos, A., Vineyard. J., Tivis, R., Nguyen, E., Jingjing, N., Lindsay, R. P. (2019). Clinical Care Coordination in Medically Complex Pediatric Cases: Results From the National Survey of Children With Special Health Care Needs. Glob Pediatr Health 7(6), 2333794X19847911. https://doi.org/10.1177/2333794X19847911

Huth, K., Long-Gagne, S., Mader, J., & Sbrocchi, A. M. (2018). Understanding the needs of children with medical complexity. *MedEdPortal, 14*, 10709.

Jackson, A. C., Liang, R. P. T., Frydenburg, E., Higgins, R. O., & Murphy, B. M. (2016). Parent education programmes for special health care needs children: A systematic review. *Journal of Clinical Nursing, 25*, 1528–1547. https://doi.org/10.1111/jocn.13178

Kuo, D., Goudie, A., Cohen, E., Houtrow, A., Agrawal, R., Carle, A. C., & Wells, N. (2014). Inequities in health care needs for children with medical complexity. *Health Affairs, 33*(12), 2190–2198. https://doi.org/10.1377/hlthaff.2014.0273

Larson, L. R., Barger, B., Ogletree, S., Torquati, J., Rosenberg, S., Gaither, C. J., … Schutte, A. (2018). Gray space and green space proximity associated with higher anxiety in youth with autism. *Health and Place, 53*, 94–102. https://doi.org/10.1016/j.healthplace.2018.07.006

Linton, J. M., Reichard, E., Peters, A., Albertini, L. W., Miller-Fitzwater, A., & Poehling, K. (2018). Enhancing resident education and optimizing care for children with special health care needs in resident continuity clinics. *Academic Pediatrics, 18*(4), 366–369.

Lollar, D. L., & Simeonsson, R. J. (2005). Diagnosis to function: Classification for children and youth. *Journal of Developmental and Behavioral Pediatrics, 26*(4), 323–330.

Mattson, G., Kuo, D. Z., Committee on Psychosocial Aspects of Child and Family Health, & Council on Children with Disabilities. (2019). Psychosocial factors in children and youth with special health care needs and their families. *Pediatrics, 143*(1), e20183171. https://doi.org/10.1542/peds.2018-3171

McManus, B. M., Magnusson, D., & Rosenberg, S. (2014). Restricting state Part C eligibility policy is associated with lower early intervention utilization. *Maternal and Child Health Journal, 18*, 1031–1037. https://doi.org/10.1007/s10995-013-1332-8

McPherson, M., Arango, P., Fox, H., Lauver, C., McManus, M., Newacheck, P. W., … Strickland, B. (1998). A new definition of children with special health care needs. *Pediatrics, 102*(1 pt1), 137–140.

Nazarian, B., Glader, L., Choueiri, R., Shipman, D., & Sadof, M. (2010). Identifying what pediatric residents are taught about children and youth with special health care needs and the medical home. *Pediatrics, 126*(3), S183–S189.

Newacheck, P. W., & Kim, S. E. (2005). A national profile of health care utilization and expenditures for children with special health care needs. *Archives of Pediatric Adolescent Medicine, 159*(1), 10–17.

Roman, S. B., Dworkin, P. H., Dickinson, P., & Rogers, S. C. (2019). Analysis of care coordination needs for families of children with special health care needs. *Journal of Developmental Behavioral Pediatrics, 41*(1), 58–64.

Rose-Jacobs, R., de Cuba, S. E., Bovell-Ammon, A., Black, M. M., Coleman, S. M., Cutts, D., … Sandel, M. (2019). Housing instability among families with young children with special health care needs. *Pediatrics, 144*, e20181704. https://doi.org/10.1542/peds.2018-1704

Simeonsson, R. J. (2009). ICF-CY: A universal tool for documentation of disability. *Journal of Policy and Practice in Intellectual Disabilities, 6*(2), 70–72.

Vladutiu, C. J., Lebrun-Harris, L. A., Carlos, M. P., & Petersen, D. N. (2019). Assessing child health and health care in the U.S. Virgin Islands using the National Survey of Children's Health. *Maternal and Child Health Journal, 23*, 1271–1280.

Willits, K. A., Troutman-Jordan, M. L., Nies, M. A., Racine, E. F., Platonova, E., & Harris, H. L. (2013). Presence of medical home and school attendance: An analysis of the 2005-2006 national survey of children with special health care needs. *Journal of School Health, 83*(2), 93–98.

World Health Organization (2001) International Classification of Functioning, Disability & Health. Geneva: WHO

World Health Organization (2007) International Classification of Functioning, Disability & Health- Children and Youth. Geneva: WHO

Yu, S., Lin, S., & Strickland, B. (2015). Disparities in health care quality indicators among US children with special health care needs according to household language use. *International Journal of MCH and AIDS, 4*(1), 3–12.

Chapter 10
Achieving Equity: Including Women with Disabilities in Maternal and Child Health Policies and Programs

Linda Long-Bellil, Anne Valentine, and Monika Mitra

10.1 Introduction and Historical Background

Enacted in 1935, one of the most far-reaching efforts to improve the health and well-being of women and children in the United States has been Title V of the Social Security Act. Title V is administered by the Maternal and Child Health Bureau (MCHB) within the Health Resources and Services Administration and is "the only federal legislation that focuses solely on improving the health of mothers and children" (Long-Bellil, 2012; Maternal and Child Health Bureau, 2002). The majority of Title V funds are administered through MHCB's Maternal and Child Health Services Block Grant program, a federal-state partnership designed to provide a wide array of health care and public health services to pregnant women, mothers, and children at risk of disability and their families. Since its enactment, programs funded through Title V have made significant improvements in the survival and well-being of generations of mothers and their children (Long-Bellil, 2012; Lu & Halfon, 2003; Maternal and Child Health Bureau, 2002).

Although women with disabilities may by chance be among the women it serves, the Maternal and Child Health Bureau does not specifically target any programs designed to support women with disabilities, including prospective mothers and mothers with disabilities. The MCHB primarily serves individuals with disabilities through its programs for children and youth with special health care needs (CYSHCN) and their families. These CYSHCN programs are generally focused on needs that are directly related to the child's disability and do not typically include

L. Long-Bellil (✉)
University of Massachusetts Medical School/Commonwealth Medicine,
Shrewsbury, MA, USA
e-mail: linda.long@umassmed.edu

A. Valentine · M. Mitra
Lurie Institute for Disability Policy, Brandeis University, Waltham, MA, USA
e-mail: anvalent@brandeis.edu; mmitra@brandeis.edu

© Springer Science+Business Media, LLC, part of Springer Nature 2021
D. J. Lollar et al. (eds.), *Public Health Perspectives on Disability*,
https://doi.org/10.1007/978-1-0716-0888-3_10

services related to sexual and reproductive health (Allen, 2011; Long-Bellil, 2012). In this respect, the MHCB's program neglects to fill a critical gap in the supports available to prospective mothers and mothers with disabilities and their families. This dichotomy is reflective of erroneous societal attitudes and assumptions toward the sexual needs and desires of people with disabilities.

While there has been substantial progress in federal and state policies toward people with disabilities over the past 40 years, there has been little focus on the sexual and reproductive health needs of people with disabilities. A concerted and coordinated approach to public policy, including maternal and child health policy, is needed to better address the sexual and reproductive health needs of people with disabilities and their families (Allen, 2011; Long-Bellil, 2012). The remainder of this chapter will explore this issue and propose ways in which maternal and child health programs can better support women with disabilities and their families. First, we present an overview of the needs and disparities in access and outcomes related to sexual and reproductive health of women with disabilities, followed by a discussion of the potential ways to achieve equity through inclusion.

10.2 Need and Disparities

Despite passage of the Americans with Disabilities Act more than 30 years ago, women with disabilities continue to experience significant health and social inequities including disparities in access and outcomes related to sexual and reproductive health, ranging from preventative health, preconception health, and family planning to pregnancy and postpartum health (Nosek, 2016; Wisdom et al., 2010). It is estimated that nearly 12% of reproductive-age women report a disability, and a significant proportion of these women report mobility or self-care limitations (Signore, 2012). Despite recognition that women with disabilities are owed access to comprehensive sexual and reproductive health services, including family planning and maternal and postpartum care, historically, their sexual and reproductive rights have been overlooked or disregarded (Iezzoni & Mitra, 2017; Meekosha, 1998). Data suggest that after controlling for sociodemographic characteristics, adults with disabilities, and women in particular, receive less access to appropriate and necessary health care services (Mahmoudi & Meade, 2015; Wisdom et al., 2010; Waldman & Perlman, 2016). In this section, we present the literature on disparities in sexual, reproductive, and perinatal health of women with disabilities.

A substantial body of research documents the exclusion of people with disabilities from public health programming and services; women with disabilities tend to experience unique barriers in accessing health care and health promotion services (Chevarley, Thierry, Gill, Ryerson, & Nosek, 2006; Silvers, Francis, & Badesch, 2016). Inaccessible examination rooms and/or medical equipment persist (Pendo, 2008), as do erroneous assumptions about the ability of women with disabilities to need or use comprehensive healthcare services (Horner-Johnson, Dobbertin, Andresen, & Iezzoni, 2014; Iezzoni, Wint, Smeltzer, & Ecker, 2015; McColl et al.,

2008; Silvers et al., 2016). Further, providers may lack familiarity with how disability type may affect salient aspects of the clinical encounter including the communication between a woman and her provider (McColl et al., 2008). These factors reduce access to evidence-based sexual, reproductive, and perinatal healthcare services for women with disabilities.

While there is no uniform definition of access to health care services, this term generally refers to the equitable opportunity to receive quality services; the availability, acceptability, and affordability of such services are integral to this construct and its application to women with disabilities (Levesque, Harris, & Russell, 2013). Extant literature suggests that a better understanding of the barriers and facilitators to comprehensive reproductive and maternal health care services (antenatal, perinatal, and postpartum) for women with disabilities is needed (Lawler, Lalor, & Begley, 2013; Mitra, Long-Bellil, Smeltzer, & Iezzoni, 2015). Research examining the experiences of women with disabilities accessing sexual and reproductive health services may improve care, facilitate choice, and enhance outcomes (Lawler et al., 2013; Mheta & Mashamba-Thompson, 2017).

10.2.1 Preconception Health

Preconception health refers to the health and well-being of women *prior* to pregnancy. For women desirous of pregnancy, preconception health care affords the opportunity to address modifiable risk factors and to discuss concerns related to conception, pregnancy, birth, and the postpartum period with a provider(s). Studies that have looked at risk factors for adverse pregnancy outcomes among women with disabilities report that women with physical disabilities have a higher body mass index (BMI) and are more likely to experience depression and to smoke during pregnancy as compared to women without physical disabilities (Iezzoni, Yu, Wint, Smeltzer, & Ecker, 2014; Iezzoni, Yu, Wint, Smeltzer, & Ecker, 2015). In specifically examining preconception health, Mitra and colleagues similarly found that women with disabilities are generally more likely to be obese and to smoke and are less likely to exercise compared to their counterparts without disabilities (Mitra, Clements, Zhang, & Smith, 2016).

There is a limited understanding of how preconception health status of women with disabilities is expressed *within* and across type of disability or disabilities. Overall, women with disabilities are more likely to report social isolation, to live in poverty, and have limited access to primary care (Chevarley et al., 2006; Emmett & Alant, 2006). These social and economic circumstances have an enormous influence on the health status and sense of well-being of women and are persistent drivers of health disparities among these women (Krahn, Walker, & Correa-De-Araujo, 2015). Similarly, disparities in maternal and child health indicators across race and ethnicity among women with disabilities are poorly understood. Despite an extensive body of research documenting significant disparities in healthcare access and outcomes among racial and ethnic minority groups in the United States (Nelson, 2002), research examining the intersection of race/ethnicity and disability in relation to perinatal care, complications, and outcomes is lacking. It is theorized, however, that systemic structural and economic barriers, stigma, racism, gender, and disability intersect in ways that exacerbate health care disparities in racial and ethnic minority women with disabilities (Correa-de-Araujo, 2016).

10.2.2 Family Planning and Contraception

Women with disabilities are often inaccurately stereotyped as having limited sexual desire, being asexual, or sexually inactive (O'Toole & Bregante, 1992; Silvers et al., 2016). As such, their desire for intimate relationships and family may be unexamined or underestimated as may be their need for contraception (Greenwood & Wilkinson, 2013; Nosek et al., 1995). A meta-analysis of 62 articles describing the results of 54 studies of contraceptive knowledge and use among women with intellectual, physical, and sensory disabilities described several barriers to contraceptive care ranging from negative attitudes among physicians to physical and communication barriers and lack of access to written materials. It also described the results of studies that reported that women who were deaf or hard of hearing and those with intellectual disabilities had lower knowledge of contraceptive methods than women without disabilities (Horner-Johnson et al., 2019).

One of the first investigations of sexually active women with physical disabilities observed that they were significantly less likely to use contraception than nondisabled women (42% vs. 33%) (Nosek, Wuermser, & Walter, 1998). A recent study using data from the 2013 Behavioral Risk Factor Surveillance System (BRFSS) found that despite similar rates of reported sexual activity and contraceptive use among respondents with and without disabilities, there were significant differences in the effectiveness of the contraceptive method endorsed across disability type (Haynes et al., 2018). Among all women reporting contraceptive use, those with disabilities were more likely to report use of a male or female permanent contraception method compared to women without disabilities (Haynes et al., 2018).

Studies examining contraceptive use among women with intellectual and developmental disabilities (IDD) find that rates of reported use are significantly lower compared to women without disabilities (Servais, 2006), with one study reporting next to no contraceptive use by this population (van Schrojenstein Lantman-de Valk, Rook, & Maaskant, 2011). Using the US National Survey of Family Growth, Wu and colleagues found that 27% of women with either physical or sensory disabilities at risk for unintended pregnancy did not report use of a contraceptive method at last intercourse (Wu et al., 2017). Further, disability was significantly associated with decreased odds of using a highly effective contraceptive method by this population of women (Wu et al., 2017). Research examining the reasons for discrepancies in contraceptive method and use are needed, but persistent barriers to appropriate reproductive care, including contraceptive services, are implicated (Mosher et al., 2017).

10.2.3   Pregnancy Care and Outcomes

Women with disabilities are nearly as likely to be pregnant as nondisabled women (Horner-Johnson, Darney, Kulkarni-Rajasekhara, Quigley, & Caughey, 2016). However, women with disabilities are more likely to avoid or forego prenatal care than women without disabilities (Mitra, Clements, et al., 2015; Mitra, Parish, Clements, Zhang, & Simas, 2018; Horner-Johnson, Biel, Caughey, & Darney, 2019). Concerns about accessibility, provider knowledge of disability, and the very real potential for negative reactions by clinicians—including erroneous assumptions that women with disabilities necessarily wish to terminate their pregnancies or are somehow aberrant for wanting children—are potential drivers of foregone care (Powell et al., 2017; Walsh-Gallagher, Sinclair, & Mc Conkey, 2012) and lower quality of prenatal care among women with disabilities. An emerging body of literature on pregnancy among women with disabilities suggests that they experience greater risk of morbidity and mortality resulting from pregnancy compared to women without disabilities (Akobirshoev, Parish, Mitra, & Rosenthal, 2017; Brown, Lunsky, Wilton, Cobigo, & Vigod, 2016; Mitra, Akobirshoev, McKee, & Iezzoni, 2016; Mitra, Long-Bellil, Iezzoni, Smeltzer, & Smith, 2016; Parish et al., 2015). Significant differences in maternal outcomes have been observed in studies that have examined outcomes by disability type, but relatively scant data exists for some populations, including deaf and hard of hearing women (Mitra, Akobirshoev, et al., 2016). A systematic review and meta-analysis of existing research found that women with *any* disability experience a significant increased risk for hypertensive disorders during pregnancy and are more likely to have caesarean sections compared to women without disabilities (Tarasoff, Ravindran, Malik, Salaeva, & Brown, 2020). It is unknown whether disparities in receipt of maternal care and pregnancy outcomes may be magnified in racial and ethnic minority women with disabilities because a dearth of clinical outcome studies exist to inform perinatal care for this population. Overall, it should be noted that studies examining the pregnancy experiences of women with disabilities, including factors that contribute to adverse maternal and neonatal outcomes in women with disabilities, are lacking (Long-Bellil, Mitra, Iezzoni, Smeltzer, & Smith, 2017). Accurate methods of capturing and categorizing disability in national survey data are limited and hinder the development of a more robust evidence base to inform clinical practice and policy (Iezzoni, 2002; Signore, 2012).

Pregnant women with disabilities may be subject to misdirected concerns about the relative riskiness of pregnancy and often report that their clinicians are ill-equipped to manage their care (Brown, Kirkham, Cobigo, Lunsky, & Vigod, 2016; Mitra, Clements, et al., 2015; Silvers et al., 2016). Labor induction and caesarean sections occur more frequently in women with disabilities, often in the absence of standard medical indicators (Brown, Kirkham, et al., 2016; Horner-Johnson, Biel, Darney, & Caughey, 2017; Biel, Darney, Caughey, Horner-Johnson, 2020). As noted, women with disabilities may have fewer prenatal care appointments than nondisabled women, receive inadequate prenatal care overall due to inaccessible equipment or clinical offices, and may not have access to pregnancy and childbirth classes that meet their physical and/or cultural needs (Mitra et al., 2017; Mitra, Parish, Clements, Cui, & Diop, 2015). Scant information exists to guide practitioners (Mitra et al., 2017). While the American College of Obstetricians and Gynecologists (ACOG) has taken steps to address existing knowledge gaps, there are no practice guidelines or recommendations to address the specific needs of women with disabilities by disability type. Lack of provider familiarity may result in diminished access to evidence-based reproductive and maternal health care for women with disabilities (McColl et al., 2008; Silvers et al., 2016; Smeltzer, Mitra, Long-Bellil, Iezzoni, & Smith, 2018).

10.2.4 Postpartum Health

Examination of the postpartum period and its potential threats to the physical and psychological well-being of women with disabilities is an emerging area of inquiry (Mitra, 2017). Population-based cohort studies of postpartum women with intellectual and developmental disabilities observe that women with IDD are significantly more likely to have emergency department visits and utilization of psychiatric services up to 42 days following childbirth compared to women without disabilities (Brown, Cobigo, Lunsky, & Vigod, 2017; Mitra, Parish, Akobirshoev, Rosenthal, & Simas, 2018). Results from these studies suggest the need for postpartum guidelines and comprehensive, coordinated postpartum care for women with IDD.

The year following childbirth is a critical touchpoint in the lives of women and their infants. The physical and emotional demands of pregnancy and childbirth, caring for a newborn, and adjusting to the enormous changes associated with parenthood may increase the potential for health problems and postpartum depression (Stewart, Robertson, Dennis, & Grace, 2003). Nationally, estimates suggest that postpartum depression affects approximately 10–20% of US mothers annually. Less is known about the incidence and prevalence of postpartum depression in women with disabilities (Mitra, Iezzoni, et al., 2015). Robust data on the prevalence, course, and treatment of depression specifically among individuals with disabilities is limited as individuals with disabilities, apart from older adults, have historically been excluded from traditional mental health research (Rotarou & Sakellariou, 2018). Postpartum depression may predispose women to subsequent behavioral health problems, including future episodes of depression, which negatively impact the maternal-infant bond and put strain in a woman's partner and family. Further, maternal depression increases the risk for disruptions in employment, material hardship, and poverty (Neckerman, Garfinkel, Teitler, Waldfogel, & Wimer, 2016). Given the increasing numbers of US women with disabilities who elect to become pregnant each year, examining the risks and prevalence of postpartum depression among this population is an important area of inquiry. A recent study by Mitra and colleagues (Mitra, Iezzoni, et al., 2015) found that compared to women without disabilities, women with disabilities experienced an increased likelihood of postpartum depression (RR 1.6, 9% CI 1.1–2.2), controlling for a number of sociodemographic and maternal characteristics related to perinatal depression and PPD (Mitra, Iezzoni, et al., 2015).

10.2.5 Considering the Social Determinants of Health

The social determinants of health refer to the social and economic circumstances in which individuals are born, live, work, and play. Social determinants are integral to an individual's quality of life, functioning, and health status (Braveman, Egerter, & Williams, 2011). As such, the emphasis placed on the social determinants of health forms the basis of many public health initiatives that seek to positively impact population health via the direct or indirect provision of resources, including adequate housing, food, transportation, and community-based opportunities for leisure and exercise.

The social determinants of health focus on discrete aspects of economic stability as opposed to the broader association between poverty and health (Silverstein, Hsu, & Bell, 2019). While a nuanced discussion of the social determinants of health as they relate to women with disabilities is beyond the scope to this chapter, any effort to address the reproductive health care needs of women with disabilities must consider the persistent and significant association between poverty and disability. Across race, ethnicity, and age, US adults with disabilities are twice as likely to live in poverty than those without disabilities. While *all* women are more likely to be poor than their male counterparts, women with disabilities experience markedly higher rates of poverty (30.7%) than women without disabilities (12.0%) (Tucker & Lowell, 2016). Of note, disparities in the poverty rate between women with and without disabilities are most pronounced in reproductive-aged women aged 18–44 years, a significant period in the life course when many women—irrespective of disability—opt to become parents, develop their skills and talents, and lay the groundwork for financial stability as they age.

Disability often results in poverty, and poverty may result in disability. Disability may make poverty particularly difficult to avoid or escape for women, given entrenched discrimination they experience in educational and labor market opportunities. Barriers to gainful employment, a lack of appropriate educational opportunities, a lack of transportation, a dearth of accessible and quality housing, increased medical care expenses, and high rates of interpersonal violence and other social risks are drivers of poverty among women with disabilities (Tucker & Lowell, 2016). While these drivers do not necessarily only pertain to women, women with disabilities often experience multiple intersecting forms of discrimination that increase the likelihood of poverty. Indeed, the poverty gap between women and men with disabilities is large and increasing (Tucker & Lowell, 2016). Persistent *within*-group disparities in the poverty rate also exist among women of color with disabilities. Racial and ethnic minority women with disabilities are more likely to live in poverty than white women with disabilities and constitute the most economically disadvantaged population in the USA (Tucker & Lowell, 2016). Poverty and material hardship are formidable threats to the health and well-being of women with disabilities, their children, and their family stability.

10.3 Achieving Equity Through Inclusion

10.3.1 Integrated Life Course Approach

An emerging body of evidence suggests that an ever-increasing number of women with disabilities are becoming mothers (Horner-Johnson et al., 2017; Iezzoni, Yu, Wint, Smeltzer, & Ecker, 2013; Shepard, Yan, Hollingsworth, & Kraft, 2018). Given the growth of this population, it is imperative to have an understanding of how the field of public health can address the sexual and reproductive health needs of these women. To identify the points at which public health can have an impact that promotes optimal outcomes for women with disabilities and their infants, it is necessary to apply an integrated life course approach.

An integrated life course approach describing the experiences of women with disabilities first requires an understanding and acceptance of the fact that women with disabilities are sexual beings. It is well-documented that women with disabilities of all kinds are commonly viewed as asexual (Esmail, Darry, Walter, & Knupp, 2010; Murphy & Elias, 2006; Sinclair, Unruh, Lindstrom, & Scanlon, 2015; Streur et al., 2019; Wendell, 2013). This perception not only constrains the life choices of women with disabilities and their ability to be fully integrated into the community, but since they are, in fact, sexual beings, it also puts them at risk of unplanned pregnancy, sexually transmitted infections, and sexual abuse (Esmail et al., 2010; Murphy & Elias, 2006; Sinclair et al., 2015; Streur et al., 2019). Secondly, an integrated life course approach requires improved access to sexual health education and reproductive health care over the life span. The evidence shows that women with disabilities have limited access to sex education, and that even when such education is available, it often does not address specific disability-related concerns (East & Orchard, 2014; Gougeon, 2009; Sinclair et al., 2015; Streur et al., 2019). The literature is also replete with evidence about lack of access to reproductive health care (Chernomas, Clarke, & Chisholm, 2000; Greenwood & Wilkinson, 2013; Holland-Hall & Quint, 2017; Iezzoni, Wint, et al., 2015; Lagu et al., 2013; Mitra, Clements, et al., 2016; Nosek et al., 1995; Silvers et al., 2016) as noted above.

To assist public health professionals and others in conceptualizing the many factors that affect women with disabilities throughout their lives and which may influence their experiences and the outcomes of perinatal care, it is useful to have a structure that explicates the many interdependent variables at play. In 2015, Mitra and her colleagues articulated a perinatal health framework for women with physical disabilities that outlined a life-span approach (Mitra, Long-Bellil, et al., 2015). This framework reflects the short- and long-term outcomes of pregnancy for women with physical disabilities as a result of the interaction of specific individual and mediating factors. This framework was guided by the World Health Organization's International Classification of Functioning, Disability, and Health (ICF) and drew upon the work of Misra, Evans, and Stoddart, Lu and Halfon, Aday and Anderson, and Nosek (Aday & Andersen, 1974; Evans & Stoddart, 2017; Lu & Halfon, 2003; Misra, Guyer, & Allston, 2003; Nosek et al., 1995; World Health Organization, 2001). The framework incorporates factors related to the social determinants of health and other influences present at various points throughout a woman's lifetime as well as around the time of pregnancy. These same factors are relevant, not only to women with physical disabilities but also to women with disabilities more broadly. Figure 10.1 shows a revised version of the framework which illustrates how it may apply to women with disabilities generally with a more expanded array of the individual and mediating factors that can lead to maternal and infant outcomes within the broader environmental context in which women with disabilities lead their lives (Mitra, Long-Bellil, et al., 2015).

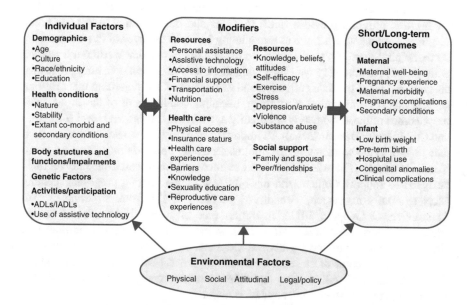

Fig. 10.1 Perinatal health framework for women with disabilities: individual, mediating, maternal, and infant outcomes and environmental context. (Reprinted from Disability and Health Journal, 8(4); Mitra, M., Long-Bellil, L. M., Smeltzer, S. C., & Iezzoni, L. I.; A perinatal health framework for women with physical disabilities, pp. 499–506, Copyright 2015, with permission from Elsevier (Mitra, Long-Bellil, et al., 2015))

10.3.2 Inclusion in Public Health Programs/Interventions

10.3.2.1 Existing Programs

Programs that provide support to families of children and youth with special health care needs (CYSHCN) operate to influence both the individual and mediating factors described in our framework as they relate to the health and well-being of women with disabilities beginning early in their lives. By providing information and referral along with other supports to families of CYSHCN, they enhance the health of these children and increase the ability of families to provide them with the care and support they need (Allen, 2011). Some of these programs have an emphasis on the transition to adulthood. For example, GOT Transition is a cooperative agreement between the Maternal and Child Health Bureau and The National Alliance to Advance Adolescent Health that aims to expand the use of Six Core Elements of Health Care Transition™ in pediatric, family medicine, and internal medicine practices to improve the transition from pediatric to adult health care; however, none of these six core elements addresses sexual and reproductive health. This program could be revised to include an explicit focus on this topic (National Alliance to Advance Adolescent Health, 2019).

The Maternal, Infant, and Early Childhood Home Visiting (MIECHV) program is among the most well-known maternal and child health programs. Funded by Title V and administered by the MCHB and the Administration for Children and Families (ACF), this program provides funds to states and other entities to operate home visiting programs which serve as a mediating factor in the lives of the women they serve, helping to promote positive maternal and infant outcomes. Although women with disabilities may very well be among those served by home visiting programs, an examination of the data collection and evaluation efforts regarding this program suggest that documentation of mothers' disabling conditions or of the experiences or outcomes of these women is not readily available at the national level (Maternal and Child Health Bureau, 2016). An important step forward would be to make such data regarding the women with disabilities served by home visiting programs more readily available. There is also a need to increase the research on interventions designed to support women with disabilities in home visiting programs (Garcia, McNaughton, Radosevich, Brandt, & Monsen, 2013; Monsen, Sanders, Yu, Radosevich, & Geppert, 2011). In the absence of such evidence, it not known whether the nurses and other staff visiting women in their homes are familiar with strategies to support mothers with disabilities and know how to adapt their methods to accommodate some of these mothers' unique needs. Such research could lead to the development of staff training and other strategies to support women with disabilities and require their implementation nationally.

Another separately funded MCHB program, Healthy Start, seeks to reduce disparities in maternal and infant health. As with MIECHV, it is possible that Healthy Start may also include mothers with disabilities and their infants among those it serves, but it has no specific strategies to address the needs of this population. As with home visiting programs, it would be beneficial to document to include a focus on the needs of mothers with disparate disabilities and also document the representation of mothers with disabilities among the families it serves. The data could then be used to understand the experiences and outcomes of mothers with disabilities and their infants and devise strategies to enhance the program's ability to serve this population.

One potential model for serving parents with disabilities is the Early Intervention Parenting Partnership, a home visiting program which includes a maternal and child health nurse, a mental health clinician, and a community health worker who work with families through pregnancy and up through a baby's first year. Provided by the Massachusetts Department of Public Health through its early intervention program and funded by a combination of Individuals with Disabilities Education Act (IDEA) Part C and state public health funding, it has served mothers with disabilities, and many of its practices could be incorporated into the Home Visiting, Healthy Start, or similar programs (Massachusetts Department of Public Health, 2019, K. Downs, personal communication, December 11, 2019).

10.3.2.2   New Initiatives

There are additional, targeted efforts that maternal and child health programs could undertake to educate transition-age and adult women with disabilities and their parents about sexual and reproductive health. One strategy would be for maternal and child health programs to leverage existing relationships with state agencies that serve people with disabilities and collaborate with them to identify opportunities to incorporate information about reproductive health into programs operated and funded by those agencies. Another approach would be to provide grants to or otherwise collaborate with community organizations which are organized around specific diagnoses, e.g., the ARC, the Spina Bifida Association, the National Down Syndrome Congress, and United Cerebral Palsy Association, among others. Families frequently turn to these organizations when their children are very young for information, along with professional and peer support. Many of these organizations have both national offices and state or local affiliates or chapters, and funding and collaboration could take place at either the national, state, or local level. Similar relationships could be forged with other community organizations that serve cross-disability populations, such as Family Voices, which is a national organization and grassroots network of families of children with disabilities, and independent living centers. In some states, independent living centers offer programming specific to transition-age youth, and this would be a reasonable place to incorporate education regarding sexual and reproductive health. Maternal and child health programs could also collaborate with community-based organizations such as these to provide support to adult women with disabilities who are either considering motherhood or who have already become mothers. Support groups or play groups would a be logical and relatively low-cost way to provide disabled women with relevant support, information, and resources (Long-Bellil, 2012).

State public health programs could also collaborate with local assistive technology programs to provide adaptive equipment to mothers with disabilities.
Given the documented need for adaptive parenting strategies and technology,
public health programs that provide baby boxes to mothers to promote safe
sleeping practices can also help to make mothers with disabilities aware of the
availability of adaptive equipment and perhaps provide funding for this purpose
in collaboration with other funding sources (Long-Bellil, 2012; Powell
et al., 2019).

10.3.3   Sexual and Reproductive Health (and Reproductive Justice)

A critical aspect of improving the sexual and reproductive health of women with
disabilities is to improve clinical care. The Maternal and Child Health Bureau
(MCHB) funds a program on Leadership Education in Neurodevelopmental and
Related Disabilities (LEND) which "provides interdisciplinary training to improve
the clinical expertise and leadership skills of professionals dedicated to caring for
children with neurodevelopmental and other related disabilities" (Maternal and
Child Health Bureau, 2002). Sexual and reproductive health are currently absent
from the list of competencies that LEND programs seek to develop in the clinicians
and other trainees that they serve (Humphreys et al., 2015). The MCHB could incorporate this competency into its requirements for its next round of funding, thereby
providing LEND programs with an incentive to prepare their trainees to address
sexual and reproductive health issues.

There are also some specialty clinics that serve youth and, in some instances,
adults with disabilities, and these settings are also potential sites where the
sexual and reproductive health needs of women with disabilities could be
addressed. There is evidence that clinics such as these do not routinely address
the sexual and reproductive health needs of women and transition-age girls with
disabilities (Streur, Schafer, Garcia, & Wittmann, 2018). Depending upon the
diagnosis, there may be disability-related issues that need to be addressed to
provide for these women's sexual and reproductive health needs effectively.
Therefore, incorporating sexual and reproductive health care into the work of
these clinics has the potential to address these needs in the most comprehensive manner.

To reach a broader cross section of clinicians beyond those with disability-related
expertise, the MCHB could support efforts to educate physicians and other
health care professionals at the earliest stages of their professional educations, starting in medical, nursing, and similar programs and throughout residency or other
advanced training. The MCHB, along with state maternal and child health programs, could also partner with professional societies, such as the American Academy
of Family Physicians, the American College of Obstetricians and Gynecology, and

similar provider organizations to provide educational sessions to their members on the importance of addressing sexual and reproductive health issues as part of routine primary care for women with disabilities, just as they should with nondisabled women (Long-Bellil, 2012). Many women with disabilities receive their primary or sexual and reproductive health care from clinicians who have no particular expertise in disability, so reaching these clinicians is critical.

10.3.4 Health Promotion

A multifaceted approach is required to eliminate the disability-related disparities in sexual and reproductive health outcomes, reduce the social risks and socioeconomic disadvantages, and the structural barriers to health care to optimal sexual and reproductive health of people with disabilities. This approach should include integrating persons with disabilities into all facets of MCHB initiatives, including programming, data and surveillance, and funding. Sustained support, including a mandate to develop programs to eliminate disparities in the sexual and reproductive health of people with disabilities, is a necessary next step.

10.4 Conclusion

Maternal and child health programs are uniquely qualified to address the sexual and reproductive health needs of all women, including women with disabilities. In some instances, such as the home visiting programs, they may already be doing so. Improving the documentation of their existing efforts to support these women and developing programs to enhance their ability to do so, perhaps in collaboration with agencies and organizations with a disability focus and expertise, would be an important step forward in meeting the needs of this growing population.

10.5 Discussion Questions

1. What challenges do women with disabilities face with respect to sexual and reproductive health?
2. How can public health programs targeted to youth with disabilities or special needs support teenage girls with disabilities in obtaining appropriate support for sexual and reproductive health?
3. How can public health programs support women with disabilities in obtaining appropriate support for sexual and reproductive health and parenting?

References

Aday, L. A., & Andersen, R. (1974). A framework for the study of access to medical care. *Health Services Research, 9*(3), 208.

Akobirshoev, I., Parish, S. L., Mitra, M., & Rosenthal, E. (2017). Birth outcomes among US women with intellectual and developmental disabilities. *Disability and Health Journal, 10*(3), 406–412.

Allen, D. (2011). Disability and maternal and child health. In *Public health perspectives on disability* (pp. 151–161). New York: Springer.

Biel, F.M., Darney, B.G., Caughey, A.B., & Horner-Johnson, W. (2020). Medical indications for primary cesarean delivery in women with and without disabilities. *Journal of Maternal-Fetal & Neonatal Medicine, 33*(20), 3391–3398. https://doi.org/10.1080/14767058.2019.1572740

Braveman, P., Egerter, S., & Williams, D. R. (2011). The social determinants of health: Coming of age. *Annual Review of Public Health, 32*, 381–398.

Brown, H. K., Cobigo, V., Lunsky, Y., & Vigod, S. (2017). Postpartum acute care utilization among women with intellectual and developmental disabilities. *Journal of Women's Health, 26*(4), 329–337.

Brown, H. K., Kirkham, Y. A., Cobigo, V., Lunsky, Y., & Vigod, S. N. (2016). Labour and delivery interventions in women with intellectual and developmental disabilities: A population-based cohort study. *Journal of Epidemiology and Community Health, 70*(3), 238–244. https://doi.org/10.1136/jech-2015-206426

Brown, H. K., Lunsky, Y., Wilton, A. S., Cobigo, V., & Vigod, S. N. (2016). Pregnancy in women with intellectual and developmental disabilities. *Journal of Obstetrics and Gynaecology Canada, 38*(1), 9–16.

Chernomas, W. M., Clarke, D. E., & Chisholm, F. A. (2000). Perspectives of women living with schizophrenia. *Psychiatric Services, 51*(12), 1517–1521.

Chevarley, F. M., Thierry, J. M., Gill, C. J., Ryerson, A. B., & Nosek, M. A. (2006). Health, preventive health care, and health care access among women with disabilities in the 1994–1995 National Health Interview Survey, Supplement on Disability. *Women's Health Issues, 16*(6), 297–312.

Correa-de-Araujo, R. (2016). *Integrated health care for women of color with disabilities.* In S. E. Miles-Cohen & C. Signore (Eds.), Eliminating inequities for women with disabilities: An agenda for health and wellness (p. 159–177)

East, L. J., & Orchard, T. R. (2014). Somebody else's job: Experiences of sex education among health professionals, parents and adolescents with physical disabilities in Southwestern Ontario. *Sexuality and Disability, 32*(3), 335–350.

Emmett, T., & Alant, E. (2006). Women and disability: Exploring the interface of multiple disadvantage. *Development Southern Africa, 23*(4), 445–460.

Esmail, S., Darry, K., Walter, A., & Knupp, H. (2010). Attitudes and perceptions towards disability and sexuality. *Disability and Rehabilitation, 32*(14), 1148–1155.

Evans, R. G., & Stoddart, G. L. (2017). Producing health, consuming health care. In *Why are some people healthy and others not?* (pp. 27–64). New York: Routledge.

Garcia, C., McNaughton, D., Radosevich, D. M., Brandt, J., & Monsen, K. (2013). Family home visiting outcomes for Latina mothers with and without mental health problems. *Public Health Nursing, 30*(5), 429–438.

Gougeon, N. A. (2009). Sexuality education for students with intellectual disabilities, a critical pedagogical approach: Outing the ignored curriculum. *Sex Education, 9*(3), 277–291.

Greenwood, N. W., & Wilkinson, J. (2013). Sexual and reproductive health care for women with intellectual disabilities: A primary care perspective. *International Journal of Family Medicine, 2013*, 642472.

Haynes, R. M., Boulet, S. L., Fox, M. H., Carroll, D. D., Courtney-Long, E., & Warner, L. (2018). Contraceptive use at last intercourse among reproductive-aged women with disabilities: An analysis of population-based data from seven states. *Contraception, 97*(6), 538–545.

Holland-Hall, C., & Quint, E. H. (2017). Sexuality and disability in adolescents. *Pediatric Clinics, 64*(2), 435–449.

Horner-Johnson, W., Biel, F. M., Darney, B. G., & Caughey, A. B. (2017). Time trends in births and cesarean deliveries among women with disabilities. *Disability and Health Journal, 10*(3), 376–381.

Horner-Johnson, W., Darney, B. G., Kulkarni-Rajasekhara, S., Quigley, B., & Caughey, A. B. (2016). Pregnancy among US women: Differences by presence, type, and complexity of disability. *American Journal of Obstetrics and Gynecology, 214*(4), 529–5e1.

Horner-Johnson, W., Dobbertin, K., Andresen, E. M., & Iezzoni, L. I. (2014). Breast and cervical cancer screening disparities associated with disability severity. *Women's Health Issues, 24*(1), e147–e153.

Horner-Johnson, W., Moe, E. L., Stoner, R. C., Klein, K. A., Edelman, A. B., Eden, K. B., … Guise, J.-M. (2019). Contraceptive knowledge and use among women with intellectual, physical, or sensory disabilities: A systematic review. *Disability and Health Journal, 12*(2), 139–154.

Horner-Johnson, W., Biel, F.M., Caughey, A.B., Darney, B.G. (2019). Differences in prenatal care by presence and type of maternal disability. *Am J Prev Med., 56*(3), 376–382.

Humphreys, B. P., Couse, L. J., Sonnenmeier, R. M., Kurtz, A., Russell, S. M., & Antal, P. (2015). Transforming LEND leadership training curriculum through the maternal and child health leadership competencies. *Maternal and Child Health Journal, 19*(2), 300–307.

Iezzoni, L. I. (2002). 4. Using administrative data to study persons with disabilities. *The Milbank Quarterly, 80*(2), 347–379.

Iezzoni, L. I., & Mitra, M. (2017). Transcending the counter-normative: Sexual and reproductive health and persons with disability. *Disability and Health Journal, 10*(3), 369–370.

Iezzoni, L. I., Wint, A. J., Smeltzer, S. C., & Ecker, J. L. (2015). Physical accessibility of routine prenatal care for women with mobility disability. *Journal of Women's Health, 24*(12), 1006–1012.

Iezzoni, L. I., Yu, J., Wint, A. J., Smeltzer, S. C., & Ecker, J. L. (2013). Prevalence of current pregnancy among US women with and without chronic physical disabilities. *Medical Care, 51*(6), 555.

Iezzoni, L. I., Yu, J., Wint, A. J., Smeltzer, S. C., & Ecker, J. L. (2014). General health, health conditions, and current pregnancy among US women with and without chronic physical disabilities. *Disability and Health Journal, 7*(2), 181–188.

Iezzoni, L. I., Yu, J., Wint, A. J., Smeltzer, S. C., & Ecker, J. L. (2015). Health risk factors and mental health among US women with and without chronic physical disabilities by whether women are currently pregnant. *Maternal and Child Health Journal, 19*(6), 1364–1375. https://doi.org/10.1007/s10995-014-1641-6

Krahn, G. L., Walker, D. K., & Correa-De-Araujo, R. (2015). Persons with disabilities as an unrecognized health disparity population. *American Journal of Public Health, 105*(S2), S198–S206. https://doi.org/10.2105/AJPH.2014.302182

Lagu, T., Hannon, N. S., Rothberg, M. B., Wells, A. S., Green, K. L., Windom, M. O., … Chen, A. (2013). Access to subspecialty care for patients with mobility impairment: A survey. *Annals of Internal Medicine, 158*(6), 441–446.

Lawler, D., Lalor, J., & Begley, C. (2013). Access to maternity services for women with a physical disability: A systematic review of the literature. *International Journal of Childbirth, 3*(4), 203–217. https://doi.org/10.1891/2156-5287.3.4.203

Levesque, J.-F., Harris, M. F., & Russell, G. (2013). Patient-centred access to health care: Conceptualising access at the interface of health systems and populations. *International Journal for Equity in Health, 12*(1), 18. https://doi.org/10.1186/1475-9276-12-18

Long-Bellil, L. M. (2012). Public policy and mothers with disabilities. In *Taking care: Lessons from mothers with disabilities.* Lanham: University Press of America.

Long-Bellil, L., Mitra, M., Iezzoni, L. I., Smeltzer, S. C., & Smith, L. D. (2017). Experiences and unmet needs of women with physical disabilities for pain relief during labor and delivery. *Disability and Health Journal, 10*(3), 440–444.

Lu, M. C., & Halfon, N. (2003). Racial and ethnic disparities in birth outcomes: A life-course perspective. *Maternal and Child Health Journal, 7*(1), 13–30.

Mahmoudi, E., & Meade, M. A. (2015). Disparities in access to health care among adults with physical disabilities: Analysis of a representative national sample for a ten-year period. *Disability and Health Journal, 8*(2), 182–190.

Maternal and Child Health Bureau. (2002). *Leadership education in neurodevelopmental and related disabilities (LEND) fact sheet*. Retrieved from https://mchb.hrsa.gov/training/documents/fs/factsheet-LEND.pdf

Maternal and Child Health Bureau. (2016). *Data, evaluation, & continuous quality improvement*. Retrieved from https://mchb.hrsa.gov/maternal-child-health-initiatives/home-visiting/home-visiting-program-technical-assistance/performance-reporting-and-evaluation-resources

McColl, M. A., Forster, D., Shortt, S. E., Hunter, D., Dorland, J., Godwin, M., & Rosser, W. (2008). Physician experiences providing primary care to people with disabilities. *Healthcare Policy, 4*(1), e129.

Meekosha, H. (1998). Body battles: Bodies, gender and disability. In *The disability reader: Social science perspectives* (pp. 163–180). London: Cassell.

Mheta, D., & Mashamba-Thompson, T. P. (2017). Barriers and facilitators of access to maternal services for women with disabilities: Scoping review protocol. *Systematic Reviews, 6*(1), 99. https://doi.org/10.1186/s13643-017-0494-7

Misra, D. P., Guyer, B., & Allston, A. (2003). Integrated perinatal health framework: A multiple determinants model with a life span approach. *American Journal of Preventive Medicine, 25*(1), 65–75.

Mitra, M. (2017). Postpartum health of women with intellectual and developmental disabilities: A call to action. *Journal of Women's Health, 26*(4), 303–304. https://doi.org/10.1089/jwh.2017.6382

Mitra, M., Akobirshoev, I., McKee, M. M., & Iezzoni, L. I. (2016). Birth outcomes among US women with hearing loss. *American Journal of Preventive Medicine, 51*(6), 865–873.

Mitra, M., Akobirshoev, I., Moring, N. S., Long-Bellil, L., Smeltzer, S. C., Smith, L. D., & Iezzoni, L. I. (2017). Access to and satisfaction with prenatal care among pregnant women with physical disabilities: Findings from a national survey. *Journal of Women's Health, 26*(12), 1356–1363.

Mitra, M., Clements, K. M., Zhang, J., Iezzoni, L. I., Smeltzer, S. C., & Long-Bellil, L. M. (2015). Maternal characteristics, pregnancy complications and adverse birth outcomes among women with disabilities. *Medical Care, 53*(12), 1027.

Mitra, M., Clements, K. M., Zhang, J., & Smith, L. D. (2016). Disparities in adverse preconception risk factors between women with and without disabilities. *Maternal and Child Health Journal, 20*(3), 507–515.

Mitra, M., Iezzoni, L. I., Zhang, J., Long-Bellil, L. M., Smeltzer, S. C., & Barton, B. A. (2015). Prevalence and risk factors for postpartum depression symptoms among women with disabilities. *Maternal and Child Health Journal, 19*(2), 362–372.

Mitra, M., Long-Bellil, L. M., Iezzoni, L. I., Smeltzer, S. C., & Smith, L. D. (2016). Pregnancy among women with physical disabilities: Unmet needs and recommendations on navigating pregnancy. *Disability and Health Journal, 9*(3), 457–463.

Mitra, M., Long-Bellil, L. M., Smeltzer, S. C., & Iezzoni, L. I. (2015). A perinatal health framework for women with physical disabilities. *Disability and Health Journal, 8*(4), 499–506.

Mitra, M., Parish, S. L., Akobirshoev, I., Rosenthal, E., & Simas, T. A. M. (2018). Postpartum hospital utilization among Massachusetts women with intellectual and developmental disabilities: A retrospective cohort study. *Maternal and Child Health Journal, 22*(10), 1492–1501.

Mitra, M., Parish, S. L., Clements, K. M., Cui, X., & Diop, H. (2015). Pregnancy outcomes among women with intellectual and developmental disabilities. *American Journal of Preventive Medicine, 48*(3), 300–308.

Mitra, M., Parish, S. L., Clements, K. M., Zhang, J., & Simas, T. A. M. (2018). Antenatal hospitalization among U.S. women with intellectual and developmental disabilities: A retrospective cohort study. *American Journal on Intellectual and Developmental Disabilities, 123*(5), 399–411. https://doi.org/10.1352/1944-7558-123.5.399

Mitra, M., Smith, L. D., Smeltzer, S. C., Long-Bellil, L. M., Moring, N. S., & Iezzoni, L. I. (2017). Barriers to providing maternity care to women with physical disabilities: Perspectives from health care practitioners. *Disability and Health Journal, 10*(3), 445–450.

Monsen, K., Sanders, A., Yu, F., Radosevich, D., & Geppert, J. (2011). Family home visiting outcomes for mothers with and without intellectual disabilities. *Journal of Intellectual Disability Research, 55*(5), 484–499. https://doi.org/10.1111/j.1365-2788.2011.01402.x

Mosher, W., Bloom, T., Hughes, R., Horton, L., Mojtabai, R., & Alhusen, J. L. (2017). Disparities in receipt of family planning services by disability status: New estimates from the National Survey of Family Growth. *Disability and Health Journal, 10*(3), 394–399.

Murphy, N. A., & Elias, E. R. (2006). Family home visiting outcomes for mothers with and without intellectual disabilities. *Pediatrics, 118*(1), 398–403.

National Alliance to Advance Adolescent Health. (2019). *Got transition.* GotTransition.Org. Retrieved from https://www.gottransition.org/providers/index.cfm

Neckerman, K. M., Garfinkel, I., Teitler, J. O., Waldfogel, J., & Wimer, C. (2016). Beyond income poverty: Measuring disadvantage in terms of material hardship and health. *Academic Pediatrics, 16*(3), S52–S59.

Nelson, A. (2002). Unequal treatment: Confronting racial and ethnic disparities in health care. *Journal of the National Medical Association, 94*(8), 666–668.

Nosek, M. A. (2016). Health disparities and equity: The intersection of disability, health, and sociodemographic characteristics among women. In *Eliminating inequities for women with disabilities: An agenda for health and wellness* (pp. 13–38). Washington, DC: American Psychological Association. https://doi.org/10.1037/14943-002

Nosek, M. A., Wuermser, L.-A., & Walter, L. J. (1998). Differences in contraceptive methods used by women with physical disabilities compared to women without disabilities. *Primary Care Update for OB/GYNS, 5*(4), 172–173. https://doi.org/10.1016/S1068-607X(98)00076-6

Nosek, M. A., Young, M. E., Rintala, D. H., Howland, C. A., Foley, C. C., & Bennett, J. L. (1995). Barriers to reproductive health maintenance among women with physical disabilities. *Journal of Women's Health, 4*(5), 505–518.

O'Toole, C. J., & Bregante, J. L. (1992). Disabled women: The myth of the asexual female. In *Sex equity and sexuality in education* (pp. 271–279). Albany: State University of New York Press.

Parish, S. L., Mitra, M., Son, E., Bonardi, A., Swoboda, P. T., & Igdalsky, L. (2015). Pregnancy outcomes among US women with intellectual and developmental disabilities. *American Journal on Intellectual and Developmental Disabilities, 120*(5), 433–443.

Pendo, E. (2008). Disability, equipment barriers, and women's health: Using the ADA to provide meaningful access.. *Louis UJ Health L. & Pol'y, 2*, 15.

Powell, R. M., Mitra, M., Smeltzer, S. C., Long-Bellil, L. M., Smith, L. D., & Iezzoni, L. I. (2017). Family attitudes and reactions toward pregnancy among women with physical disabilities. *Women's Health Issues, 27*(3), 345–350. https://doi.org/10.1016/j.whi.2017.01.003

Powell, R. M., Mitra, M., Smeltzer, S. C., Long-Bellil, L. M., Smith, L. D., Rosenthal, E., & Iezzoni, L. I. (2019). Adaptive parenting strategies used by mothers with physical disabilities caring for infants and toddlers. *Health & Social Care in the Community, 27*(4), 889–898. https://doi.org/10.1111/hsc.12706

Rotarou, E. S., & Sakellariou, D. (2018). Depressive symptoms in people with disabilities; secondary analysis of cross-sectional data from the United Kingdom and Greece. *Disability and Health Journal, 11*(3), 367–373. https://doi.org/10.1016/j.dhjo.2017.12.001

Servais, L. (2006). Sexual health care in persons with intellectual disabilities. *Mental Retardation and Developmental Disabilities Research Reviews, 12*(1), 48–56. https://doi.org/10.1002/mrdd.20093

Shepard, C. L., Yan, P. L., Hollingsworth, J. M., & Kraft, K. H. (2018). Pregnancy among mothers with spina bifida. *Journal of Pediatric Urology, 14*(1), 11.e1–11.e6. https://doi.org/10.1016/j.jpurol.2017.08.001

Signore, C. C. (2012). Pregnancy in women with physical disabilities. In *Queenan's management of high-risk pregnancy: An evidence-based approach*, 253–259.

Silvers, A., Francis, L. P., & Badesch, B. (2016). Reproductive rights and access to reproductive services for women with disabilities. *American Medical Association Journal of Ethics, 18*(4), 430–437.

Silverstein, M., Hsu, H. E., & Bell, A. (2019). Addressing social determinants to improve population health: The balance between clinical care and public health. *Journal of the American Medical Association, 322*(24), 2379–2380.

Sinclair, J., Unruh, D., Lindstrom, L., & Scanlon, D. (2015). Barriers to sexuality for individuals with intellectual and developmental disabilities: A literature review. *Education and Training in Autism and Developmental Disabilities, 50*(1), 3–16. JSTOR.

Smeltzer, S. C., Mitra, M., Long-Bellil, L., Iezzoni, L. I., & Smith, L. D. (2018). Obstetric clinicians' experiences and educational preparation for caring for pregnant women with physical disabilities: A qualitative study. *Disability and Health Journal, 11*(1), 8–13.

Stewart, D. E., Robertson, E. O., Dennis, C., & Grace, S. L. (2003). *Postpartum depression: Literature review of risk factors and interventions.* Toronto: University Health Network Women's Health Program.

Streur, C. S., Schafer, C. L., Garcia, V. P., Quint, E. H., Sandberg, D. E., & Wittmann, D. A. (2019). "If everyone else is having this talk with their doctor, why am I not having this talk with mine?": The experiences of sexuality and sexual health education of young women with spina bifida. *The Journal of Sexual Medicine, 16*(6), 853–859. https://doi.org/10.1016/j.jsxm.2019.03.012

Streur, C. S., Schafer, C. L., Garcia, V. P., & Wittmann, D. A. (2018). "I don't know what I'm doing... I hope I'm not just an idiot": The need to train pediatric urologists to discuss sexual and reproductive health care with young women with spina bifida. *The Journal of Sexual Medicine, 15*(10), 1403–1413. https://doi.org/10.1016/j.jsxm.2018.08.001

Tarasoff, L. A., Ravindran, S., Malik, H., Salaeva, D., & Brown, H. K. (2020). Maternal disability and risk for pregnancy, delivery, and postpartum complications: A systematic review and meta-analysis. *American Journal of Obstetrics & Gynecology, 222*(1), 27.e1–27.e32. https://doi.org/10.1016/j.ajog.2019.07.015

Tucker, J., & Lowell, C. (2016). *National snapshot: Poverty among women & families, 2015.* National Women's Law Center. Retrieved from https://nwlc.org/wp-content/uploads/2016/09/Poverty-Snapshot-Factsheet-2016.pdf

van Schrojenstein Lantman-de Valk, H. M. J., Rook, F., & Maaskant, M. A. (2011). The use of contraception by women with intellectual disabilities. *Journal of Intellectual Disability Research, 55*(4), 434–440. https://doi.org/10.1111/j.1365-2788.2011.01395.x

Waldman, H. B., & Perlman, S. P. (2016). Oral health of women with disabilities. In *Eliminating inequities for women with disabilities: An agenda for health and wellness* (pp. 115–132). Washington, DC: American Psychological Association. https://doi.org/10.1037/14943-007

Walsh-Gallagher, D., Sinclair, M., & Mc Conkey, R. (2012). The ambiguity of disabled women's experiences of pregnancy, childbirth and motherhood: A phenomenological understanding. *Midwifery, 28*(2), 156–162.

Wendell, S. (2013). *The rejected body: Feminist philosophical reflections on disability.* New York: Routledge. https://doi.org/10.4324/9780203724149

Wisdom, J. P., McGee, M. G., Horner-Johnson, W., Michael, Y. L., Adams, E., & Berlin, M. (2010). Health disparities between women with and without disabilities: A review of the research. *Social Work in Public Health, 25*(3–4), 368–386.

World Health Organization. (2001). *International classification of functioning, disability and health: ICF.* Geneva: World Health Organization.

Wu, J. P., McKee, K. S., McKee, M. M., Meade, M. A., Plegue, M. A., & Sen, A. (2017). Use of reversible contraceptive methods among US women with physical or sensory disabilities. *Perspectives on Sexual and Reproductive Health, 49*(3), 141–147.

Chapter 11
Aging with a Disability

Philippa Clarke, Erica Twardzik, Clive D'Souza, and Michelle Meade

11.1 Introduction

Every day between 2017 and 2030 approximately 10,000 adults within the United States will turn 65, drastically shifting the age distribution within the population (Wick, 2017). With increased age there will be a greater proportion of adults with acquired visual impairment, hearing loss, osteoarthritis, dementia, and other chronic health conditions. In addition, with medical advances promoting early survivorship and improved disease control, there is a growing population of individuals aging with a disability (Strauss, DeVivo, Paculdo, & Shavelle, 2006). The dual phenomena of global aging coupled with increased longevity for individuals with disabilities creates new challenges for societies striving to meet the needs of populations aging into disability and those aging with disabilities acquired earlier in the life course (Bickenbach et al., 2012; Kaufman et al., 2014; LaPlante, 2014).

P. Clarke (✉)
School of Public Health and Institute for Social Research, University of Michigan, Ann Arbor, MI, USA
e-mail: pjclarke@umich.edu

E. Twardzik
School of Public Health and School of Kinesiology, University of Michigan, Ann Arbor, MI, USA
e-mail: etwardzi@umich.edu

C. D'Souza
Department of Industrial and Operations Engineering, University of Michigan, Ann Arbor, MI, USA
e-mail: crdsouza@umich.edu

M. Meade
Department of Physical Medicine and Rehabilitation, University of Michigan, Ann Arbor, MI, USA
e-mail: mameade@med.umich.edu

© Springer Science+Business Media, LLC, part of Springer Nature 2021
D. J. Lollar et al. (eds.), *Public Health Perspectives on Disability*,
https://doi.org/10.1007/978-1-0716-0888-3_11

11.1.1 Aging with Disability vs. Aging into Disability

The experience of growing older *with* a disability and growing older *into* a disability is likely to be considerably different—in part because of the accumulated inequality experienced by those aging with disabilities in terms of their health, and social and economic standing over adulthood (Clarke & Latham, 2014; Ferraro & Shippee, 2009; Ferraro, Shippee, & Schafer, 2009). Advances in medical care and technology have contributed to an increasing number of individuals living into older age with disabilities acquired earlier in the life course (Bickenbach et al., 2012; Kaufman et al., 2014; LaPlante, 2014).

Although those aging *into* disability and those aging *with* disability may share similar functional impairments, the trajectory of experience across the life course is unique. For example, a deaf individual aging may identify as being a part of deaf culture, where friendships and social support develop throughout the life course as a result of disability identity (Brueggemann, 2013). This cultural identity and shared experience can result in strong social support rooted in a shared functional impairment. This social support group likely has extensive knowledge and expertise on their functional impairment, along with experiences and strategies to overcome environmental barriers that can be shared among the social group. However, someone who develops hearing loss in later life may not have the same level of shared knowledge within their support groups and certainly does not have the same cultural identity as someone within the deaf community. As a result, an older adult aging into disability will have to develop strategies to overcome barriers in a shorter period of time and may obtain advice solely through their medical care provider. This may result in a more isolating experience with hearing loss than among someone who had hearing loss early on in life.

Existing models of "successful" aging in the gerontology literature emphasize independence and good health (Rowe & Kahn, 1997, 2015), but the cumulative effects of living with a physical disability for many years present unique challenges for those aging with a life-long health condition (Minkler & Fadem, 2002; Molton & Yorkston, 2017; Verbrugge & Yang, 2002). The co-occurrence of health conditions associated with aging, along with secondary health problems that develop as a result of the disabling condition (such as pain and fatigue), create distinct health management and accommodation needs for persons aging with disability (Iezzoni, 2014).

People with disabilities are more likely to be obese and are more likely to be sedentary than persons without disabilities (Ferraro & Booth, 1999; Ferraro, Su, Gretebeck, Black, & Badylak, 2002; Stolzle & Fox, 2011). They are more likely to be current smokers and less likely to have seen a dentist in the past year; and they are more likely to experience an unmet medical need due to cost. Qualitative research by Rimmer, Riley, Wang, Rauworth, and Jurkowski (2004) indicates that more than half of adults with disability do not engage in any leisure-time physical activity due to a multifactorial set of barriers in the built and social environment, including economic issues, equipment barriers, negative perceptions and attitudes by persons who are not disabled, and policies and procedures within communities and recreational facilities.

In addition, people with movement-related impairments and mobility limitations are less likely to receive cancer screening and other preventive health services (Chevarley, Thierry, Gill, Ryerson, & Nosek, 2006; Iezzoni, Davis, Soukup, & O'Day, 2002; Iezzoni, McCarthy, Davis, & Siebens, 2000; Ramirez, Farmer, Grant, & Papachristou, 2005), in part due to physical barriers either within or leading up to healthcare facilities (Andriacchi, 1997; Gans, Mann, & Becker, 1993). Given these challenges, adults with disabilities who age into later life are likely to be at a disadvantage with respect to their health than those aging without disabilities. The development of effective strategies to address the unique needs of persons aging with disability, therefore, requires an understanding of the factors operating at multiple levels, from the individual level to the larger societal context.

In this chapter we review key concepts and theoretical frameworks in the disability and gerontological literatures to help guide our discussion on aging with disability. We then go on to use these conceptual frameworks to articulate some of the key issues in public health research on aging and disability, including healthcare access, technology and supports, and the role of community and environmental contexts.

11.2   Key Concepts and Theoretical Frameworks

Disability with aging can encompass a number of health conditions. Some include pediatric onset conditions (e.g., cerebral palsy), while others are acquired conditions that occur sometime after infancy (e.g., post-polio syndrome). Some conditions have a sudden onset (e.g., spinal cord injury), while others occur more gradually (e.g., multiple sclerosis). Disability can result from physical impairments, sensory impairments, or cognitive impairments. The experience of aging with these different conditions is complex and heterogeneous, and we are unable to delve into these differences within the scope of this chapter. But it is important to recognize that different health conditions create a different dynamic for individuals as they age. For example, the gradual onset of conditions may allow for more adaptive and adjustment strategies than for sudden onset conditions. But regardless of the condition, the disablement process is inherently a dynamic interaction between the impairment and the social and environmental context in which the individual is embedded across the life course. The complexity of barriers that exist highlights the importance of developing solutions that operate on multiple levels, including the need for "care coordination" that considers and integrates the many aging, disability and healthcare-related laws, policies, and financing incentives.

Healthy aging is a multifaceted concept associated with (a) enhanced longevity and reduced mortality and morbidity, particularly by preventing (or appropriately managing) secondary and co-morbid conditions and associated adverse events, including ER visits and hospitalizations; (b) achieving assisted autonomy (vs independence) to conduct activities of daily living (Molton & Yorkston, 2017); and (c) participating in meaningful life activities (such as family, social, and community participation and employment) that enhance a sense of purpose and quality of life.

11.2.1 Aging from a Life Course Perspective: Cumulative Advantage and Disadvantage

The study of aging has a long history in social gerontology. Rather than conceptualizing aging as simply "old age," gerontologists have long argued that aging is a *process* that is shaped by social structures over time from birth to death. The age structure of the life course as a system of social statuses has long been theorized and studied in social gerontology (Cain, 1964; Neugarten, 1970; Riley, 1971) and more recently in public health (Kuh, Ben-Shlomo, Lynch, Hallqvist, & Power, 2003). As early as 1964, Leonard D. Cain, Jr., used the term "life course" to "identify, isolate, and systematize a life course, or age status, frame of reference..." (Cain, 1964, p. 273). In this perspective, the life course is seen as an age-graded structure defined by the social organization of status positions and roles (Riley, 1971). These scholars were influential in directing attention to the effects of structured social inequality over the life course as shaped by political and economic interests (Townsend, 1981; Walker, 1981), particularly the role of the state through its control of work, education, and marriage transitions (Mayer, 1997).

In the American context, the life course perspective was heavily structured by work and articulated as having three major stages: education or a "preparation for work" stage, the working or "career" stage, and a "retirement" stage (Cain, 1964; Kohli, 1986). Following childhood and early education, young adults assume major role commitments, and this is increasingly occurring in the late rather than the early 20s (Booth, Crouter, & Shanahan, 1999). This separate life stage, now frequently termed the "developmental" period of adulthood (Arnett & Taber, 1994), is typified by gains in statuses and roles (early career path, marriage, and asset acquisition) with associated economic, health, and social benefits. This is followed by the midlife period of adulthood (typically from age 40 to 55), characterized by the stability of marital and employment roles and the social and economic status they confer. Finally, the later stage of the life course is marked by role exits (retirement and widowhood), declines in function, and decreased sense of control.

The age-structured organization of social status positions and roles is helpful for understanding the challenges faced by those aging with a disability. Since much of public policy concerning the life course is predicated on the assumption that the life course is normatively experienced, departures from it can generate hurdles and barriers. Critical periods of adulthood, such as the developmental period where individuals embark on key social roles, are particularly vulnerable to disruption among those with disabilities. Health problems over childhood and early adulthood are likely to have negative consequences for educational attainment and stable employment (Jin, Shah, & Svoboda, 1995). Delays in entering the career trajectory are considered by society as being "off-time," leading to disadvantages entering stable careers over early to mid-adulthood. The economic and social consequences of unstable career trajectories are well documented in the feminist (McMullin, 2000) and gerontological literatures (Elder, Shannahan, & Clipp, 1994) but are applicable to those aging with disabilities as well.

Engagement in economically productive work roles forms the basis of social and economic policy, and employment is the key mechanism by which individuals can attain health insurance and social security benefits in American society. Research suggests that, at any given time, only about 30% of individuals with severe physical disabilities are employed as compared with 85% of the population of individuals without disabilities (Bureau of Labor Statistics, U.S. Department of Labor, 2016). Individuals with disabilities also receive less compensation and are more likely to be underemployed than the general population (Clarke & Latham, 2014). Because of a fear of being without medical care, a significant percentage of individuals with disabilities who receive public health insurance (e.g., Medicare and/or Medicaid) are concerned about working too many hours and losing their coverage. As a result, individuals with long-term disabilities are less likely to enter into older adulthood with a significant savings and more likely to experience co-occurring challenges of disability and poverty (Clarke & Latham, 2014; Iezzoni, 2014). Thus, delays or limits in educational and employment attainment among people aging with disabilities have reinforcing and reciprocal effects over time.

The concepts of cumulative advantage and disadvantage in the life course perspective refer to the "Matthew Effect," a term coined by Robert Merton and drawn from the gospel of St. Matthew. The verse states: "For unto every one that hath shall be given and he shall have abundance: but from him that hath not shall be taken away even that which he hath" (quoted in Merton, 1968). The Matthew Effect describes how individuals who are already healthy and educated and have a stable income are able to accrue health benefits, more education, better jobs, and even more income over the course of their lives. Conversely, those without higher education are restricted in their access to stable employment and income trajectories, which are perpetuated through fewer health, social, and economic benefits that are reinforced over time. Much of life course research has tended to focus on adolescence and young adulthood as formative periods and crucial determinants of the subsequent adult life one leads (Booth, Crouter & Shanahan, 1999; Arnett & Tabr, 1994). Thus, individuals with disabilities face disadvantages early in the life course which can have long-term consequences for their lives with aging. The development of effective strategies to address the unique needs of persons aging with disability requires an understanding of the factors operating at multiple levels, from the individual level to the larger societal context.

11.2.2   The International Classification of Functioning, Disability, and Health

The World Health Organization's (WHO) International Classification of Functioning Disability and Health (ICF) (WHO, 2001) is a universal framework adopted internationally that can be useful for understanding the dynamics of aging with a disability. The ICF is based on a biopsychosocial model that conceptualizes disability as a process by drawing attention to socio-environmental factors that can interact with underlying impairments and injury factors to impede or enhance a person's ability to engage in activities and participate fully in society. The ICF is a conceptual framework that identifies three levels of functioning: the level of the body (mental, emotional, physiological, or anatomical structures or functions), the level of activities (mobility, self-care, general tasks), and the level of society (participation in life situations). Negative functioning at these three levels is represented by impairments, activity limitations, and participation restrictions. For example, an individual aging with muscular dystrophy may experience pain (impairment in sensory functions) that leads to difficulty in mobility (activity limitations), which may restrict his or her involvement in life situations, such as meeting with close friends or engaging in leisure activities (participation restriction). The ICF also emphasizes the role of environmental factors and personal factors that can impede or enhance a person's functioning. The comprehensive list of environmental factors in the ICF identifies a wide range of potential environmental barriers and facilitators, including technological supports (e.g., assistive devices), social supports and relationships, attitudes and stereotypes, public/private services or policies, and natural and human-made environments. In this context, disability only results if there is a gap between a person's capabilities and the demands created by the social and physical environment).

11.2.3   The Model of Healthcare Disparities and Disability (MHDD)

Emerging research on healthy aging with a physical disability emphasizes the importance of accessible, quality health care and strong, supportive social ties (Krause & Coker, 2006; Molton & Yorkston, 2017). There is also a growing recognition that barriers in the surrounding social and built environment can create challenges for accessing these health and social resources (e.g., physical and transportation barriers, limited access to personal care attendants, and concerns about personal safety) (Iezzoni, 2014; Rimmer, Chen, & Hsieh, 2011). Models of "successful" aging with long-term physical disability must consider the complex interplay among factors at the individual level and factors related to the surrounding social and environmental context (Minkler & Fadem, 2002; Molton & Yorkston, 2017).

The Model of Healthcare Disparities and Disability (MHDD; Meade, Mahmoudi, & Lee, 2015) conceptualizes the interaction of personal and environmental factors as having its own impact on health and functional outcomes. Specifically, the MHDD builds on the ICF while integrating models of healthcare disparities (Smedley, 2006) to explain how a mismatch between personal factors, (including health beliefs and health literacy), and environmental factors, (including organizational structures and policies, the knowledge and attitudes of healthcare providers, and the accessibility of community services and the built environment), results in reduced *affordability, availability, accessibility, acceptability, and accommodation* of health care for individuals with disabilities. These factors can also result in reduced quality and utilization of health care and increased unmet healthcare needs. These deficits, in turn, influence an individual's functioning, activity, and participation. More importantly, the MHDD allows for the recognition of a wealth of *modifiable factors* to improve healthcare access, quality, and outcomes for individuals with disabilities and places responsibility for addressing the disparities with healthcare systems.

For individuals aging with disability, MDHH emphasizes the role and importance of quality health care for the aging population and the multitude of factors which negatively impact access to and quality of care for individuals with disabilities. Among the many issues are the lack of healthcare providers—including geriatricians—with adequate training to provide appropriate medical care to individuals with disabilities, inaccessible clinics and hospitals, and insufficient healthcare funding, which can precipitate bankruptcy when trying to finance the sudden onset of health conditions. Of relevance, the National Academies of Sciences, Engineering, and Medicine recognized challenges in this area (National Academies of Sciences, Engineering, and Medicine, 2016), stating:

> *"The healthcare workforce is a critical component of the supports needed to enable people with disabilities and older adults to maximize their independence and live in the community. However, the required ingredients for this much-needed workforce go beyond making sure there are enough providers; having providers with the right knowledge is also key."*

11.2.4 The Ecological Model of Adaptation and Aging

The ecological model of adaptation and aging (Lawton & Nahemow, 1973) is most often cited by those conducting accessibility and inclusive design research (Iwarsson & Stahl, 2003). This model introduces concepts of "individual competence" or capacity to describe the person and "environmental demand" to define the environment in terms of its design features and space constraints (Lawton & Nahemow, 1973). Informed by an ecological model, the theory of competence-environmental press highlights the dynamic impact of environmental barriers and facilitators depending on the personal and functional capacities of the individual. According to this model, environmental demand is acknowledged as having a differential or varying impact on user performance depending on the users' functional abilities. A key feature of the ecological model is the fit between individual competence and environmental demand. An individual with functional limitations may be challenged by the environment but may, at the same time, experience well-being if they can find a way to adapt to those barriers (Lawton & Nahemow, 1973). Conversely, a lack of coherence or fit in attaining this balance manifests in reduced levels of independence, and physiological and psychological stress (Steinfeld & Danford, 1999).

The practice of universal or inclusive design requires applying knowledge of the interactions between people and their environment across the diverse spectrum of users' abilities and limitations as compared to traditional design approaches that may focus on the typical or average user. By definition, inclusive environments and products are intended for use by the broadest range of users possible, irrespective of age and ability, and with ease, efficiency, and positive social consequences.

11.2.5   *Layering Disability on Top of an Aging and Life Course Framework*

In conceptualizing the health and functioning of individuals living (and aging) with disability, it is useful to think of positive health status as a three-dimensional road or path with defined boundaries or borders. Good health is achievable but narrows with both age and disability severity. Individuals who are younger and those without disabilities have a wider margin of health, and inconsistent health behaviors have less of a negative impact on health. Negative health events, such as hospitalizations and functional decline, are possible but less frequent, and more easily recovered from, in part because the individual has greater reserves of both physical health and (often) social resources upon which to draw. Conversely, older adults and those with more severe impairments have a narrower road (or margin of health) such that more conscious, frequent, and consistent positive health behaviors are required to sustain or regain positive health. For a person with a disability a fall from a wheelchair or a pulled muscle is not a simple event, but can swiftly lead to reduced health and functioning if he or she is no longer able to independently conduct activities of daily living nor maintain positive health behaviors.

With this perspective, both personal and environmental factors influence health status for those aging with a disability. Personal factors include *genetics*, the family history and risk of developing various diseases; *health behaviors*, including diet, exercise, and smoking as well as regular use of preventative care services; *skills* such as the ability to communicate and engage people in problem-solving; and factors such as gender, race, education, and income. *Environmental factors* that influence this process include the people around you, including their knowledge and attitudes, including family, friends, social networks, healthcare providers, and others in positions of authority; the quality of the actual environment, air quality, crime, and water safety; and the accessibility of the built environment, including how easy or hard it is to get around. (Frequently the individual has to deal with an environment that challenges them in ways that it does not do for others).

Moreover, the severity of disability interacts with environmental factors to influence functional outcomes—though not in a linear fashion. For individuals with less severe impairments, personal factors may compensate for the lack of environmental supports or resources to make it possible for them to maintain independence with aging. In contrast, individuals with severe disabilities, such as high-level, complete tetraplegia, do not simply rely on the people, technology, and supports in their environment to enhance functioning; rather, these supports are necessary to conduct basic activities of daily living, including eating, getting out of bed, or even breathing. However, both groups experience significant disadvantage as compared with individuals aging without any disability.

The path of health, then, becomes wider with more protective personal factors and a more supportive environment, and narrower with more negative personal and environmental factors. If the aging process already narrows the path—to greater or lesser degrees depending on resources—then disability creates incremental challenges, narrowing it further and making the maintenance of good health a matter of complexity for someone aging with a disability, or a caregiver (or both).

Take, for example, the general issues of aging. Bones get more fragile, skin less elastic, and social networks decrease as individuals retire and friends either die or move away. Communication gets harder as vision and hearing decline; rates of falls, fractures, and social isolation rise. Declines are not inevitable, but maintaining the same level of functioning takes more effort (e.g., more careful diets, regular exercise, planned time to socialize). If disability is layered on top of this, with its preexisting environmental and physiological challenges with fewer resources, there is an added pressure on often already stressed coping mechanisms. A fall from a wheelchair results in the need for part-time or full-time assistance—whether at home or a nursing home— which reduces control over diet and the ability to regularly perform the exercise and social activities that had previously helped maintain health. Once again, it is not impossible for health to be regained, but it takes more time, effort, and resources for those aging with disability.

11.3   Technology to Support Healthy Aging with Disability

Technology has always played a role in enhancing quality of life for people with disabilities and is especially relevant with aging. Ramps, canes, and glasses help people function in their environments. There is also a growing interest in promoting and leveraging the development of new and more complex and advanced technologies to facilitate the maintenance of health and quality of life of older adults and people with disabilities. There is no doubt that if the goal is to keep individuals in their homes and communities as they age, technology can be designed and implemented to facilitate this goal. Within this process, though, it is critical that the relevant interactions between impairments, personal factors, and environmental factors are understood and planned for upfront rather than attempting to adapt or retrofit solutions later.

To the extent that advanced technologies are proposed as a solution to maintaining health, facilitating community living and enhancing quality of life, it will be critical that these policies and laws address coverage of and/or access to such technologies, even those that may also be considered "general use"—such as tablets to use with health management apps—as opposed to specialized medical equipment.

Moreover, it needs to be considered that socioeconomically disadvantaged census tracts and rural tracts tend to be areas with low broadband adoption and less Internet access (Douthit, Kiv, Dwolatzky, & Biswas, 2015). In a national survey of Americans age 18+ conducted in 2003, only 33% of adults with a disability live in a household with Internet access compared to 60% among those without a disability (Dobransky & Hargittai, 2006). As such, in order for the development of mHealth and connected technology to have an equal chance of benefitting *all* Americans, solutions will have to be found to ensure equal access to informational technologies. Money is often scare for people with disabilities and their family members. As such, it is important to develop new apps and programs that are based upon (and sustained upon) devices that they already have.

For example, Flint, Michigan, is a city of approximately 97,000 people. The population is 60% African American with 41.2% of the population living in poverty, and a median household income is $25,650. People with disabilities comprise 18.1% of the population under 65 years old (from 2013 to 2017). While 70.6% of households in Flint reported having a computer (2013–2017 Census), only 54.5% had a broad Internet subscription. Moreover, among older adults (65 years and older) in Flint, 45% did not have Internet access. These statistics highlight the problems with relying only on informational technology, whether to distribute reliable and timely information or as a sole necessarily component of providing support or assistance. In a recent needs assessment conducted in Flint of older adults, participants noted that timely and reliable information available via television, mail, and the newspaper was critical for obtaining up to date water-related information in 2013 because many older adults did not use the computer nor have computer skills. Online information was not seen to be helpful.

An individual's social network also plays a significant role in the extent that technology is likely to be accepted, utilized, and integrated to assist in maintaining health and enhancing quality of life. For older adults and individuals aging with disabilities, then, it will also be critical to ensure awareness and acceptance of advanced technology not just by peers but also by family members and caregivers; the prior is critical for normalizing use and acting as either facilitators or barriers to use. Use and acceptance of the technology by paid and unpaid caregivers will be important in supporting older adults and individuals aging with disabilities to remain in their homes. The tasks performed by these individuals range from providing emotional support to assisting with practical activities such as home repairs, driving, and shopping, to facilitating problem-solving and planning to providing assistance with personal/intimate care needs such as bathing and toileting.

The goal of keeping older adults and people with disabilities in their homes and communities is also connected with both ensuring access to knowledgeable healthcare providers and facilitating the management of chronic conditions and impairments in home environments. This includes supporting the completion of complex management behaviors. Technology has the potential to continue to influence such outcomes, but its adoption is limited by the degree that people are willing and able to use it as part of their regular activities or workflow. For example, technology can assist with gathering and transmitting data, but knowledgeable providers with the time and appropriate training are still needed to evaluate and make judgments based on that data.

Advanced technologies can play a significant role in assisting to identify risk and tailor or personalize solutions based on defined characteristics or variables. However, in order to optimize outcomes for health and community living, it is important that technology that is developed to enhance health management is able to be readily integrated into the workflow of healthcare providers. To the extent that technology creates or provides data, this information must be useful to physicians or other clinicians, and it has to be quick, it has to be visual, and it has to be available when the person is right in front of them.

Knowledge about the issues and needs of people aging with disabilities and the healthcare providers who work with them is also critical to inform policies which create standards or encourage the use of technology. For example, electronic health records (EHR) were not widely adopted until after the Health Information Technology for Economic and Clinical Health (HITECH) Act was passed in 2009 and connected with funding in 2011. Other policies which supported better health data transfer between various computers and apps and improved data transfer related to patient portals included Fast Healthcare Interoperability Resources (FHIR) and Meaningful Use II. Today, EHRs are an integral component of health care, FHIR is improved, many patient portals and mobile health apps exist, and smartphones are ubiquitous. These resources, however, are not available to all patients, and facilitating access to these technologies to allow for the most effective use of the data is not well-developed. The future of integrating mHealth and EHRs is focused on improving clinical outcomes and delivering value. To do that, barriers for technical integration must be reduced or eliminated, which requires shared patient/clinician cooperative development that is agile and human-centered. Moreover, policy must continue to support the development of accessible health records, patient portals, and apps to promote their integration into the healthcare practice.

11.3.1 Technology Development and Disability/ Impairment-Related Considerations

In the context of health management and quality of life, technology is primarily a facilitator of the underlying activity that the user relies on to get to a certain goal or outcome. What is offered should have an identified need that applies to the individual user involved. In the world of disability and aging, there are many user groups that require different solutions (Beer et al., 2019), which makes it different from developing a piece of technology such as the iPhone, which has, in effect, a generic user. Because of that, personalization is important. The benefits of an app must be designed for the individual, recognizing the unique needs of older adults and those aging with disability. Because technology has to be personalized or tailored, developers need to make decisions and choices based on their knowledge of the end user. Given the percentage of older adults with disabilities and the relationship between level/severity of disability and need for assistance, if technology is going to be seen as a potential solution for assisting this group to maintain health and quality of life while also controlling costs, it is critical that they are part of the key audiences considered up front. As such, knowing about the ways that physical, sensory, cognitive, and psychiatric impairments influence the ability to use and benefit from various technologies is important.

Technological interventions have typically been person-oriented or environmentally oriented. Person-oriented interventions emphasize strategies initiated by a person when the person needs them, for example, using mnemonic techniques to teach street names and locations to a person with topographical disorientation (Davis & Coltheart, 1999) or verbal priming for amnesia (Kapur, Glisky, & Wilson, 2004). Environmentally oriented interventions, which are based on changing the environment, are helpful for people who are unable to learn the independent use of compensatory strategies (i.e., writing a letter by using specialized software and communication interventions like adapted word processors, personal information managers, cueing systems using cellphones).

Physical disabilities most often influence physical interactions with technologies. Impairments of hands, arms, and torso may require that the technology considers if the user needs to physically touch the device/technology and how those motions are perceived. For example, if a user has motor control issues, they may not have the dexterity to perform the quick double tap required of many apps, and so single action mechanics may need to be a basic rule or have assistive logic there that helps with complex operations. For individuals aging with disabilities that involve both physical and cognitive comorbidities, the complexity of developing and sustaining independence can be confounded by motivational factors and specific cognitive impairments. In particular, gross motor ability, manual dexterity, and education level are important determinants of adaptive behavior in this population (Donkervoort et al., 2007). While little is known about the contributions of specific psychological or cognitive factors, there has been compelling research on the role of motivation in adaptive behavior and decision-making. Motivational difficulties, including the ability and/or desire to initiate behavior, can adversely affect learning and executing adaptive behaviors (Tuminello, Holmbeck, & Olson, 2012).

These findings provide evidence of the importance of how user factors may impact the ability of adults aging with and into disability to engage with mHealth. While a discussion of what specific factors to consider or how the types of adaptations to be made given specific impairments is beyond the scope of this chapter, the key issue is that adopting a user-centered approach is critical when developing technological systems for people aging with and into disability. Individuals aging with disability may have a set of unique characteristics (e.g., cognitive impairments, salient symptoms, limited literacy) that affect their ability to engage with the system, and the environment that they may be living in may be not have the infrastructure (e.g., access to electrical outlets for charging, regional wireless access) that many types of technology depend upon.

11.3.2 Transportation Technology

Access to safe, accessible, and useable transportation options is vital to supporting social interactions, community participation, positive health behaviors, and successful aging among people with disabilities. Transportation barriers, however, continue to restrict community participation for adults with disabilities (Goldman & Murray, 2011; LaPlante & Kaye, 2010; Lenker, D'Souza, & Paquet, 2017; National Council on Disability, 2005; Nelson/Nygaard Consulting Associates, 2008). More than half a million people with disabilities cannot leave their homes because of difficulties in accessing transportation (Bureau of Transportation Statistics, 2003). Even when they are able to leave their home, 30% of Americans with disabilities have inadequate access to transportation. Consequently, four times as many people with disabilities as without lack suitable transportation options to meet their daily mobility needs (National Council on Disability, 2005). Lack of transportation was reported as the second most important barrier to unemployment by people with disabilities, preceded only by lack of skills and training. The 2005 White House Conference on Aging ranked transportation options for older Americans to be among the top three priorities facing older adults (WHCOA, 2005). Addressing the needs of older adults and people with disabilities through increased accessible and affordable transportation options is critical for improved access and opportunity for all.

The Americans with Disabilities Act (ADA) requires public transit agencies that provide fixed-route service to provide "complementary paratransit" service to people with disabilities who cannot use the fixed-route bus or rail service because of a disability within 3/4 of a mile of a bus route or rail station, at the same hours and days, for no more than twice the regular fixed-route fare. With reduced ability to drive, problems with accessing the vehicles of family or friends which are unequipped to accommodate wheelchairs, and reduced ability to use public transit, ADA paratransit as a mobility option is essential for reducing dependence and social exclusion. This has become evident through the increased demand and rising costs of providing complementary paratransit. Paratransit use climbed 7% from 2007 to 2010 alone and is 3.5 times more costly than fixed-route transit (Government Accountability Office, 2012).

Technology-mediated ride hailing services such as Uber and Lyft that allow users to book and pay for rides through a smartphone app have certain benefits over public transit, paratransit, or relying on family members for transportation. However, equal access to such services for people with disabilities remains a challenge with high, fluctuating costs (e.g., due to dynamic, congestion pricing schemes) only being one of the issues. There are still stark differences in quality of service experienced by people with disabilities due to factors such as the shortage of accessible vehicles (e.g., ramp equipped vehicles), navigating to precise and accessible pickup locations, access to smartphones and electronic payment methods, and phone apps that might be difficult to use due to a vision or motor impairment or often due to lack of familiarity with accessibility options such as screen reading and wireless Braille compatibility.

In addition, those living in areas with high levels of poverty often have reduced access to public transportation and fewer opportunities for street and sidewalk mobility and physical activity. Curb cuts, ramps, smooth pavement, and barrier-free sidewalks are some of the environmental factors that can enhance independence and social participation among adults with physical and ambulatory disabilities, especially those using wheeled mobility assistive technology. Recognizing that technology is only as useful as the environments in which it operates is essential for supporting independence, health, and civic participation.

Climate and temperature extremes are also related to successful transportation options for people with disabilities. Icy surfaces, snow banks, and snowy/slushy surfaces are the most frequently named barriers to mobility during winter, particularly by those with underlying limitations in physical functioning (Li, Hsu, & Fernie, 2010). Evidence also indicates that snow lodged in wheeled mobility devices forms an obstacle in the wheels and drive mechanisms and decreases the slip resistance of motorized scooters (Tadano, Tsukada, Shibano, Ukai, & Watanuki, 1998).

Automated vehicles (AVs) hold great promise for increasing door-to-door, barrier-free transportation options for people with disabilities and older adults who are more likely to be unable or ineligible to drive (Claypool, Bin-Nun, & Gerlach, 2017; National Council on Disability, 2015). The needs of these diverse user groups must be defined and addressed in the inclusive design of automated vehicle transportation systems. Inclusive design, or universal design, implies the design of technology and systems that accommodate the widest range of potential users, including people with and without disabilities. It is very likely that near-future deployment of level 4 and 5 slow-speed autonomous shuttles (i.e., vehicles capable of performing driving functions without a human operator; Cregger et al., 2018) will serve on-demand, shared rides—called "microtransit"—to solve first mile/last mile gaps and multimodal connection issues by attending to underserved populations and locations and into off-hour travel times when typical transit services are less frequent. Mobility on demand through AVs will vastly increase the reach of public transit and paratransit (or potentially even rendering obsolete our current models of paratransit). Conversely, it is possible that AVs and related robotics and mobility technologies—far from improving independence and inclusion—could introduce new transportation barriers and increase social inequality even further if accessibility is not designed into these systems from the start. Thus, it is imperative that the goals, needs, and priorities of diverse users with disabilities and older adults are defined and addressed in the inclusive design of connected and automated vehicles and transportation systems (Tabattanon, Sandhu, & D'Souza, 2019).

It is worth emphasizing that the impact of AVs goes beyond just automating the task of driving to also include automated and assistive technologies that support safe and independent vehicle ingress/egress, passenger securement, payment, and in-vehicle communication during both routine trips and in emergencies. Allied technologies related to geo-mapping, mobile computing, and robotics will also improve independence and participation for older adults and individuals with vision impairments and/or cognitive impairments such as dementia through apps for orientation and wayfinding, negotiating obstacles and traffic, identifying wheelchair-accessible routes, locating accessible pickup and drop-off points, and safely moving about in their neighborhood (Bayless & Davidson, 2019).

Currently, there are no federal or industry guidelines or evidence-based design tools for accessibility that are specific to driverless AVs. Human factor research is needed to develop and evaluate new accessibility guidelines for AVs, including for low-speed automated shuttles that are increasingly being used in public transit and on-demand mobility (Bayless & Davidson, 2019; Tabattanon et al., 2019). Engagement opportunities and funding mechanisms are needed that encourage researchers, standards agencies, and the transportation industry to work with members and advocates of the aging and disability community in the accessible design and evaluation of AVs and related mobility technologies. Public transit operators, nonprofit organizations, area agencies on aging, and centers for independent living and local communities can benefit from funding and incentives to engage and deploy new mobility technologies and services including AVs particularly in communities that are underserved by other forms of transportation such as public transit. Research is needed to understand the extent to which these new forms of mobility on demand can help adults aging with disability to remain in their homes to age in place, increase independence in mobility in their community, and improve their own health and well-being but also for caregiving family members.

11.4 Environments and Communities to Support Healthy Aging with Disability

There are both overlapping and yet distinctive environmental and community needs to support healthy aging with a disability and aging into disability. This is both a challenge and opportunity for public health professionals to develop strategies that support healthy aging for adults with disabilities. There is a critical need for intentional, proactive creation of environments, communities, and a society that are inclusive of older adults with disabilities, both acquired and early onset.

11.4.1 Aging in Place

To prepare for the challenges of an aging population, there are additional policies and services available that focus on living in the community rather than relying on institutions as the primary axis of care. Healthy People 2020 established a goal to "reduce the proportion of noninstitutionalized older adults with disabilities who have an unmet need for long-term services and supports" (Healthy People 2020 Older Adults Objective (OA-8), n.d.) in order to support community living as people age, commonly known as aging in place. As defined by the Center of Disease Control and Prevention, aging in place represents "the ability to live in one's home and community safely, independently, and comfortably, regardless of age, income, or ability level" (Centers for Disease Control and Prevention, 2009). Interest in aging in place comes from the social and personal benefits of older adults staying within their home. Benefits of maintaining home residence include reduced cost, preserving social connections, increased personal independence, and familiarity with surroundings. For these and other reasons, it is not surprising that 90% of people aged 65 years and older wish to reside in their own homes for as long as possible (Burton, Mitchell, & Stride, 2011).

Aging in place is not a "one-size-fits-all" concept, and the complexity of the dynamic relationship between person and place is reflected by the volume and diversity of published literature on this topic. Gerontological research investigating aging in place began in the 1980s and has expanded as a key area of interest, with nearly 10% of all gerontological published literature in 2010 examining aging in place (Vasunilashorn, Steinman, Liebig, & Pynoos, 2012). In addition, the diversity of topics examining aging in place has expanded to discussing topics such as health and functioning, environment, services, and technology as key players for aging in place (Vasunilashorn et al., 2012). Below we discuss known benefits and common barriers of aging in place.

Aging in place has multifaceted benefits to society and to individuals (e.g., social, emotional, and physical health). Home and community supports have been introduced to promote people living in their homes for as long as possible (Szanton, Leff, Wolff, Roberts, & Gitlin, 2016). Aging in place avoids the costly option of institutional care, which is one reason why health and aging policy makers are in favor of options encouraging aging in place (Kitchener, Ng, Miller, & Harrington, 2006). In addition, policy often communicates the advantages of individual choice, independence, and the maintenance of social support and connections for older adults (Mor et al., 2007). Furthermore, older adults themselves articulate similar benefits and expand to say that aging in place has meaning beyond the physical and social surroundings. The place in which older people have spent their life holds emotional ties to memories within space, recalling past interactions with loved ones, and celebrations of milestones throughout their life course, and the home can be an extension of an older adults' self and identity (Oswald & Wahl, 2005; Wiles, Leibing, Guberman, Reeve, & Allen, 2012). Although there are great benefits to aging in place, older adults face numerous barriers to maintain their home residence.

Maintaining home residence can be especially challenging when faced with life changes such as declining health, widowhood, or loss of income. Previous research has shown that approximately one third of all community dwelling older adults report functional limitations in activities of daily living, which in the absence of a supportive environment can lead to greater challenges with aging in place (Fuller-Thomson, Yu, Nuru-Jeter, Guralnik, & Minkler, 2009). Although there may be community-based services to support the maintenance of home residence, there is a growing population of older adults who do not qualify for publicly funded services and for whom the costs of supportive community-based services are not within their budgetary means (Mutchler, Shih, Lyu, Bruce, & Gottlieb, 2015). This gap in service access can lead to older adults with unmet needs and result in either premature institutionalization or hazardous living environment.

Moreover, the design of homes and communities can serve as a major barrier for aging in place among those aging with disability. Older adults identified that multi-level buildings need an elevator, that all homes have appropriate bathrooms and kitchens, that passages and doorways are large enough to accommodate a wheelchair or walker, and that the housing units have adequate heating and cooling systems (World Health Organization, 2007).

Community factors also play a large role in living and aging with a disability. Outdoor environmental barriers such as poor transportation, discontinuous or uneven sidewalks, curbs, noise, and inadequate lighting can threaten someone's ability to age in place (World Health Organization, 2007). Unfortunately, research about interventions to improve community living outcomes among individuals with disabilities is sparse. More prevalent are studies that predict nursing home placement in the elderly (Luppa et al., 2010). Within this area, research findings suggest that institutionalization is associated with underlying impairments in cognitive and/ or physical functioning combined with a lack of supports and assistance for daily living (Luppa et al., 2010). Interventions that have proven effective in improving community living outcomes appear to apply complex approaches for supporting individuals with disabilities in their home environments. In particular, Beswick and colleagues (2008) found that complex interventions applying geriatric assessment of general older adults and community-based care after home discharge showed an impact on reducing the risk of not living at home as well as on reducing nursing home admissions.

In October of 2015, the Forum on Aging, Disability, and Independence within the National Academies of Sciences, Engineering, and Medicine conducted a workshop to discuss Policy and Research Needs to Maximize Independence and Support Community Living among people with disabilities and older adults (National Academies of Sciences, Engineering, and Medicine, 2016). In particular, the workshop addressed policy and research needs associated with the four focal areas seen as key to supporting community living and maximizing independence: (a) home and community settings, (b) services and supports, (c) workforce, and (d) financing. While the focus of the activity was to obtain a better understanding of the issues rather than offer formal conclusions or recommendations, it nonetheless identified both best practices and gaps in both policy and research.

Among the particular programs and best practices that were discussed in the workshop were the Personal and Home Care Aide State Training (PHCAST) Program and the Geriatric Workforce Enhancement Program (GWEP), both administered by the Health Resources and Services Administration (HRSA). While PHCAST focuses on the training of personal and home care aides, GWEP is focused on primary care systems and connecting them with existing community programs and organizations. At the center of each is the recognition of the specific information, competencies, and resources that are needed to adequately support individuals with disabilities and older adults in a community environment.

11.4.2   Housing Accessibility and Affordability

Stable, quality housing is a cornerstone of health and well-being for all age groups and is a significant social determinant of health. A critical driving force for safe, stable, and quality housing is cost. One third of all adult households aged 50 and older (20 million people) are paying more than 30% of their income for housing; and adults within this group are said to be "housing cost-burdened" (Joint Center for Housing Studies at Harvard University (JCHS), 2014). Shortage of affordable housing can place these households at risk for homelessness. Adults aging with disability can face additional barriers to affordable housing, such as inaccessible housing needing home modifications, rental units that are accessible may have increased demand and price, and the accumulation of risk over the life course and fewer financial resources to draw upon due to the structural and cultural barriers to employment throughout their lives. There are federal policies in place to support affordable and accessible housing for those whom have aged into disability and those who are aging with a disability. Within this section we describe policy to support housing affordability and policy supporting housing accessibility for those aging with disability.

Subsidized housing and increasing the size and diversity of housing are two policy strategies to promote affordability of housing. The Department of Housing and Urban Development (HUD) has a number of programs to support aging in place. Opportunities for subsidizing housing for older adults include housing choice vouchers, Project-Based Rental Assistance (Section 8) program, and public housing options. In addition, there are opportunities for low-income housing tax credits, with a portion of the housing tax credits earmarked for residents over the age of 55 (Kochera, 2006). Beyond just housing assistance, HUD also works to increase the size and diversity of housing available to older adults. Section 202 of HUD constructs housing units to serve low-income elderly households. Low-income elderly households are defined by at least one member over the age of 62 and earning no more than 50% of the area median income. Among eligible households, the average wait list time is a year or longer due to the high demand of Section 202 housing (Vandawalker, Locke, & Lam, 2012).

Federal policy to support accessible and safe housing has developed incrementally over time, where new policies have attempted to fill the gaps of previous legislation. In 1973 the first disability civil rights law was enacted in the United States. Section 504 of the Rehabilitation Act more broadly prohibited discrimination against people with disabilities in programs and activities that receive federal funding and more specifically included policy to support accessible housing (Section 504, n.d.). Within this act at least 5% of federally funded multifamily housing units must be built or rehabilitated so that they are accessible to people with mobility impairments, and nonhousing facilitates must be designed and constructed or altered so that they are accessible to persons with disabilities (Section 504, n.d.). In 1988 the Fair Housing Amendment Act was written into the Civil Rights Act of 1968 (Fair Housing Act and Amendments, 2012). The Fair Housing Amendment Act prohibits discrimination on the basis of disability in housing sales, rentals, or financing (Fair Housing Act and Amendments, 2012). This extension to the Civil Rights Act requires that housing providers must permit reasonable structural modifications and that newly constructed multifamily dwellings with four or more units must provide basic accessibility to people with disabilities (Fair Housing Act and Amendments, 2012). A policy on the horizon is the Inclusive Home Design Act, first introduced to Congress in 2003 (National Council on Independent Living, n.d.). This act is based on a concept of "visitability," where all single-family or owner-occupied housing is designed so that the residence can be visited by those with difficulty with steps or those who use wheelchairs or walkers (National Council on Independent Living, n.d.). The visitability of a home is defined by three basic requirements: (1) "one zero-step entrance," (2) "doors with 32 in. of clear passage space," and (3) "one bathroom on the main floor you can get into in a wheelchair" (National Council on Independent Living, n.d.). This visitability policy is a policy that would benefit the vast majority of society: people moving into their home, an older adult visiting grandchildren, young mothers with a stroller, and those aging with disability. Although this policy did not receive the anticipated traction at the federal level, some local level governments have started to adopt these standards (National Council on Independent Living, n.d.).

11.4.3   Holistic Socio-Environmental Design

There are a multitude of phrases used to describe holistic socio-environmental city design, such as "elder-friendly cities," "child-friendly cities," or "disability-friendly cities." These phrases can become even more specific, such as "dementia-friendly cities," resulting in recommendations that are specific to a functional impairment (Mitchell, Burton, & Raman, 2004). However, these phrases and the meaning behind them have more similarities than differences. The goal of these movements is to create a city that is not for the "average user" but for all users of the space for a diverse set of purposes. Highlighted below are some of the major efforts to create a more holistic socio-environmental design with an aspiration for creating space that is universally designed.

A major development toward a more holistic socio-environmental city was the World Health Organization's (WHO) Age-Friendly Cities Guide (WHO, 2007). Using focus groups with older adults, caregivers, and service providers in 33 cities around the world, the Global Age-Friendly Cities Project developed the Age-Friendly Cities Guide. The guide includes a checklist of 88 features that optimize opportunities for health, participation, and security as people age in urban environments. With input from stakeholders in age-friendly cities, the WHO was able to articulate a comprehensive list of components needed to create age-friendly cities. Eight key topic areas identified within the Age-Friendly Cities Guide include transportation, housing, social participation, respect and social inclusion, civic participation and employment, communication and information, community support and health services, and outdoor spaces and buildings (WHO, 2007). Within each topic area, the guide delves into specific themes within the topic area and data to support the importance of each theme. For example, within outdoor spaces and buildings, the guide describes the importance of benches along a walking route and how a place to rest facilitates outdoor mobility, and lack of places to rest may serve as a barrier. Building off this foundation, AARP has developed an initiative to support holistic socio-environmental communities through its Livable Communities Program.

Endorsed by the WHO's Age-Friendly Communities Program, the Livable Community initiative offers toolkits and how-to guides to assess the "age-friendliness" of local cities and communities. Using local built and social environmental indicators such as housing, transportation, walkable neighborhoods, and destinations, a community can generate a "Livability Index" (AARP Livability Index, n.d.). In addition, AARP administers a community survey to adults age 50 or older asking standardized questions about WHO's domains of an age-friendly cities. These questions include information on housing, outdoor spaces and buildings, transportation and streets, social participation, inclusion, and education opportunities. Lastly, AARP has developed a Network of Age-Friendly States and Communities where they engage elected officials, partner organizations, and local leaders to guide their home community through the age-friendly network's assessment, planning, and implementation resources, and evaluate their progress toward a more holistic socio-environmental community. This program has tremendous reach in the United States, with over 100 million people who live in a community that is enrolled in the AARP Network of Age-Friendly States and Communities.

Focusing on an idealistic age-friendly city, or a one-size-fits-all approach, however, can overlook the heterogeneity of cities and the diverse needs for those aging with disability (Buffel, Phillipson, & Scharf, 2012). A single prescription for an "age-friendly city" or "disability-friendly city" may not be realistic. In addition, the top-down approach of the Age-Friendly Communities model has been critiqued as "producing urban environments *for* people" rather than "developing neighborhoods *with* and *by* older people" (Buffel et al., 2012, p. 609). It may be more effective to leverage the insights and opinions of people aging with disability directly, in order to identify which components of the environment are necessary to meet the needs of the people who inhabit a specific space. This approach directly involves older adults with disability in the development of policies and programs to design local areas that are sustainable (Buffel et al., 2012; Jeste et al., 2016). Participation from the community is vital to ensuring that older adults with disabilities have a say in the development of holistic socio-environmental communities. This can include soliciting participation from community organizations, movements, or planners in a wide range of ways, such as consulting communities on policy development, involving community members throughout the process of policy development, and collaborating or partnering with target populations.

The translation of research findings to improve the socio-environment is most effective when it includes interventions at multiple levels. Based on an ecological model, these levels include the individual (e.g., knowledge, attitudes), interpersonal connections (e.g., family, friends), organizational (e.g., senior centers, hospitals), community (e.g., design, access, connectedness), and public policy (e.g., national, state, local law) (Greenfield, 2012). This multilevel approach can be effective in informing the public and inter-sectoral groups on the importance of the socio-environmental context for healthy aging with disability and how to adapt cities and communities to meet the needs of all people.

11.5   Conclusions

As the population ages and as the number of adults aging with early acquired disability grows, there is a pressing need for public health to integrate aging and disability into its practice and education. In order to meet the needs of this growing and diverse population, the public health workforce needs to be equipped with the tools to understand the differences in the health of those aging into disability and those aging with disability, including the consequences of the cumulative effects of living with a disability over the life course. Knowledge of the resources and supports that can modify the consequences of disability for healthy aging can shape interventions and treatment recommendations. In this chapter we have highlighted research and policy related to the role of healthcare access, transportation, technology, and community environments. These factors should be considered when faced with the challenges of supporting the growing number of Americans aging with and aging into disability.

11.6   Resources for Further Exploration

- "Charting the LifeCourse": A tool kit for learning about the life course perspective: https://www.lifecoursetools.com/
- AARP Livability Index: Great Neighborhoods for all Ages: https://livabilityindex.aarp.org/

References

Andriacchi, R. (1997). The internal medicine perspective. *American Journal of Physical Medicine & Rehabilitation, 76*(3), 17–20.

Arnett, J. J., & Taber, S. (1994). Adolescence terminable and interminable: When does adolescence end? *Journal of Youth and Adolescence, 23*, 517–537.

Bayless, S. H., & Davidson, S. (2019). *Driverless cars and accessibility: Designing the future of transportation for people with disabilities*. Washington, DC: ITS America.

Beer, J. M., Rogers, W. A., Sanford, J. A., Remillard, E. T., Phillips, C., & Campbell, M. (2019). A panel discussion on human factors considerations for persons aging-in-place with disability. *Proceedings of the Human Factors and Ergonomics Society Annual Meeting, 63*(1), 1–5.

Beswick, A. D., Rees, K., Dieppe, P., Ayis, S., Gooberman-Hill, R., Horwood, J., & Ebrahim, S. (2008). Complex interventions to improve physical function and maintain independent living in elderly people: a systematic review and meta-analysis. *The Lancet, 371*(9614), 725–735.

Bickenbach, J., Bigby, C., Salvador-Carulla, S., Heller, T., Leonardi, M., LeRoy, B., ... Spindel, A. (2012). *Bridging knowledge, policy and practice in aging and disability.* Retrieved from Toronto, Canada, http://www.marchofdimes.ca/dimes/images/emails/FICCDAT/Toronto_Declaration.pdf

Booth, Crouter, & Shanahan. (1999). *Transitions to Adulthood in a Changing Economy: No Work, No Family, No Future?* Westport, Connecticut: Praeger

Brueggemann, B. J. (2013). Disability studies/disability culture. In M. L. Wehmeyer (Ed.), *Oxford handbook of positive psychology and disability* (pp. 279–299). New York, NY: Oxford University Press.

Buffel, T., Phillipson, C., & Scharf, T. (2012). Ageing in urban environments: Developing 'age-friendly'cities. *Critical Social Policy, 32*(4), 597–617.

Bureau of Labor Statistics, U.S. Department of Labor. (2016). 17.5 percent of people with a disability employed in 2015. *The Economics Daily*. Retrieved February 10, 2018, from https://www.bls.gov/opub/ted/2016/17-point-5-percent-of-people-with-a-disability-employed-in-2015.htm

Bureau of Transportation Statistics. (2003). *Transportation difficulties keep over half a million disabled at home*. BTS Issue Brief. Washington, DC: US Department of Transportation. Retrieved from https://www.bts.gov/archive/publications/special_reports_and_issue_briefs/issue_briefs/number_03/entire

Burton, E. J., Mitchell, L., & Stride, C. B. (2011). Good places for ageing in place: Development of objective built environment measures for investigating links with older people's wellbeing. *BMC Public Health, 11*(1), 839.

Centers for Disease Control and Prevention. (2009). *Healthy places terminology*. Retrieved October 24, 2019, from https://www.cdc.gov/healthyplaces/terminology.htm

Cain, Leonard D., Jr. (1964). Life course and social structure, pp. 272–309 in Robert E.L.Faris (Ed.), Handbook of Modern Sociology. Chicago: Rand McNally and Company.

Chevarley, F. M., Thierry, J. M., Gill, C. J., Ryerson, A. B., & Nosek, M. A. (2006). Health, preventive health care, and health care access among women with disabilities in the 1994-1995 National Health Interview Survey, Supplement on Disability. *Women's Health Issues, 16*(6), 297–312.

Clarke, P., & Latham, K. (2014). Life course health and socioeconomic profiles of Americans aging with disability. *Disability and Health Journal, 7*(10), S15–S23.

Claypool, H., Bin-Nun, A., & Gerlach, J. (2017). *Self-driving cars: The impact on people with disabilities*. Boston, MA: Ruderman Family Foundation.

Cregger, J., Dawes, M., Fischer, S., Lowenthal, C., Machek, E., & Perlman, D. (2018). *Low-speed automated shuttles: State of the practice* (Report No. FHWA-JPO-18-692). John A. Volpe National Transportation Systems Center, Department of Transportation.

Dobransky, K. and E. Hargittai (2006). The disability divide in internet access and use. *Information, Communication & Society 9*(3): 313–334.

Donkervoort, M., Roebroeck, M., Wiegerink, D., Van der Heijden-Maessen, H., Stam, H., & Transition Research Group South West Netherlands. (2007). Determinants of functioning of adolescents and young adults with cerebral palsy. *Disability and rehabilitation, 29*(6), 453–463.

Douthit, N., Kiv, S., Dwolatzky, T., Biswas, S. (2015). Exposing some important barriers to health care access in the rural USA. *Public Health 129*(6): 611–620.

Elder, Shannahan and Clipp. (1994). When war comes to men's lives: Life course patterns in family, work, and health *Psychology and aging 9*: 5–16.

Fair Housing Act and Amendments. (2012, June 20). Retrieved March 19, 2019, from www.nolo.com, https://www.nolo.com/legal-encyclopedia/content/fair-housing-act.html

Ferraro, K. F., & Booth, T. L. (1999). Age, body mass index, and functional illness. *The Journals of Gerontology Series B: Psychological Sciences and Social Sciences, 54*(6), S339–S348.

Ferraro, K. F., & Shippee, T. P. (2009). Aging and cumulative inequality: How does inequality get under the skin? *Gerontologist, 49*(3), 333–343. https://doi.org/10.1093/geront/gnp034

Ferraro, K. F., Shippee, T. P., & Schafer, M. H. (2009). Cumulative inequality theory for research on aging and the life course. In V. L. Bengston, M. Silverstein, N. M. Putney, & D. Gans (Eds.), *Handbook of theories of aging* (pp. 573–593). New York: Springer.

Ferraro, K. F., Su, Y. P., Gretebeck, R. J., Black, D. R., & Badylak, S. F. (2002). Body mass index and disability in adulthood: A 20-year panel study. *American Journal of Public Health, 92*(5), 834–840.

Fuller-Thomson, E., Yu, B., Nuru-Jeter, A., Guralnik, J. M., & Minkler, M. (2009). Basic ADL disability and functional limitation rates among older Americans from 2000–2005: the end of the decline?. *Journals of Gerontology Series A: Biomedical Sciences and Medical Sciences, 64*(12), 1333–1336.

Gans, B. M., Mann, N., & Becker, B. (1993). Delivery of primary care to the physically challenged. *Archives of Physical Medicine and Rehabilitation, 74*(special issue), S15–S19.

Goldman, J. M., & Murray, G. (2011). *TCRP synthesis 88: Strollers, carts, and other large items on buses and trains.* Washington, DC: Transportation Research Board.

Government Accountability Office. (2012). *ADA paratransit services. Demand has increased, but little is known about compliance.* GAO-13-17. Retrieved from http://www.gao.gov/products/GAO-13-17

Greenfield, E. A. (2012). Using ecological frameworks to advance a field of research, practice, and policy on aging-in-place initiatives. *The Gerontologist, 52*(1), 1–12.

Healthy People 2020 Older Adults Objective (OA-8). (n.d.). Retrieved November 1, 2019, from https://www.healthypeople.gov/2020/topics-objectives/topic/older-adults/objectives

Iezzoni, L. I. (2014). Policy concerns raised by the growing U.S. population aging with disability. *Disability and Health Journal, 7*(1 Suppl), S64–S68. https://doi.org/10.1016/j.dhjo.2013.06.004

Iezzoni, L. I., Davis, R. B., Soukup, J., & O'Day, B. (2002). Satisfaction with quality and access to health care among people with disabling conditions. *International Journal for Quality in Health Care, 14*(5), 369–381. https://doi.org/10.1093/intqhc/14.5.369

Iezzoni, L. I., McCarthy, E. P., Davis, R. B., & Siebens, H. (2000). Mobility impairments and use of screening and preventive services. *American Journal of Public Health, 90*(6), 955–961. https://doi.org/10.2105/ajph.90.6.955

Iwarsson, S. and A. Ståhl (2003). Accessibility, usability and universal design—positioning and definition of concepts describing person-environment relationships. *Disability and Rehabilitation 25*(2): 57–66.

Jin, R., Shah, C., & Svoboda, T. (1995). The impact of unemployment on health: A review of the evidence. *CMAJ, 153*(5), 529–540.

Jeste, D. V., Blazer II, D. G., Buckwalter, K. C., Cassidy, K. L. K., Fishman, L., Gwyther, L. P., ... & Vega, W. A. (2016). Age-friendly communities initiative: public health approach to promoting successful aging. *The American Journal of Geriatric Psychiatry, 24*(12), 1158–1170.

Joint Center for Housing Studies at Harvard University (JCHS). (2014). *Housing America's older adults: Meeting the needs of an aging population.* Boston, MA: AARP Foundation and The Hartford.

Kaufman, D. W., Reshef, S., Golub, H. L., Peucker, M., Corwin, M. J., Goodin, D. S., ... Cutter, G. (2014). Survival in commercially insured multiple sclerosis patients and comparator subjects in the U.S. *Multiple Sclerosis and Related Disorders, 3*(3), 364–371.

Kapur, N., Glisky, E. L., & Wilson, B. A. (2004). Technological memory aids for people with memory deficits. *Neuropsychological rehabilitation, 14*(1–2), 41–60.

Kitchener, M., Ng, T., Miller, N., & Harrington, C. (2006). Institutional and community—Based long-term care: A comparative estimate of public costs. *Journal of Health & Social Policy, 22*(2), 31–50.

Kochera, A. (2006). *Developing appropriate rental housing for low-income older persons: A survey of Section 202 and LIHTC property managers*. Washington, DC: AARP Public Policy Institute.

Kohli, M. (1986). The world we forgot: a historical view of the life course. *Later life: the social psychology of aging*. V. W. Marshall. Beverly Hills, CA, Sage: 271–303.

Krause, J., & Coker, J. (2006). Aging after spinal cord injury: A 30-year longitudinal study. *The Journal of Spinal Cord Medicine, 29*, 371–376.

Kuh, D., Ben-Shlomo, Y., Lynch, J., Hallqvist, J., & Power, C. (2003). Life course epidemiology. *Journal of Epidemiology and Community Health, 57*(10), 778.

LaPlante, M. P. (2014). Key goals and indicators for successful aging of adults with early-onset disability. *Disability and Health Journal, 7*(1), S44–S50. https://doi.org/10.1016/j.dhjo.2013.08.005

LaPlante, M. P., & Kaye, H. S. (2010). Demographics and trends in wheeled mobility equipment use and accessibility in the community. *Assistive Technology: The Official Journal of RESNA, 22*(1), 3–17. https://doi.org/10.1080/10400430903501413

Lawton, M. P., & Nahemow, L. (1973). *Ecology and the aging process*. In C. Eisdorfer & M. P. Lawton (Eds.), *The psychology of adult development and aging* (p. 619–674). American Psychological Association.

Lenker, J., D'Souza, C., & Paquet, V. (2017). Chapter 6: Vehicle design. In A. Steinfeld, J. Maisel, & E. Steinfeld (Eds.), *Accessible public transportation: Designing services for riders with disabilities* (pp. 54–67). Taylor & Francis/Routledge: Boca Raton, FL. ISBN: 978-1-48-223410-7.

Li, Y., Hsu, J., & Fernie, G. R. (2010). Winter accessibility survey results: Inadequate consideration of weather elements in the development of pedestrian facilities. *Gerontechnology, 9*(2), 301.

Luppa, M., Luck, T., Weyerer, S., König, H. H., Brähler, E., & Riedel-Heller, S. G. (2010). Prediction of institutionalization in the elderly. A systematic review. Age and ageing, 39(1), 31–38.

Mayer, K. U. (1997). *Life courses in the welfare state Theoretical Advances in Life-Course Research Status Passages and Risks in the Life Course* W. R. Heinz. Weinheim, Deutscher Studien Verlag 1, 146–158

McMullin, J. A. (2000). "Diversity and the state of sociological aging theory". *The Gerontologist 40*: 517–530.

Meade, M. A., Mahmoudi, E., & Lee, S. Y. (2015). The intersection of disability and healthcare disparities: a conceptual framework. *Disability and rehabilitation, 37*(7), 632–641.

Merton, R. K. (1968). The Matthew effect in science: The reward and communication systems of science are considered. *Science, 159*(3810), 56–63.

Minkler, M., & Fadem, P. (2002). "Successful aging": A disability perspective. *Journal of Disability Policy Studies, 12*(4), 229–235. https://doi.org/10.1177/104420730201200402

Mitchell, L., Burton, E., & Raman, S. (2004). Dementia-friendly cities: Designing intelligible neighbourhoods for life. *Journal of Urban Design, 9*(1), 89.

Molton, I. R., & Yorkston, K. M. (2017). Growing older with a physical disability: A special application of the successful aging paradigm. *The Journals of Gerontology: Series B, 72*(2), 290–299. https://doi.org/10.1093/geronb/gbw122

Mor, V., Zinn, J., Gozalo, P., Feng, Z., Intrator, O., & Grabowski, D. C. (2007). Prospects for transferring nursing home residents to the community. *Health Affairs, 26*(6), 1762–1771.

Mutchler, J. E., Shih, Y. C., Lyu, J., Bruce, E. A., & Gottlieb, A. (2015). The elder economic security standard index™: A new indicator for evaluating economic security in later life. *Social Indicators Research, 120*(1), 97–116.

National Academies of Sciences, Engineering, and Medicine. (2016). *Policy and research needs to maximize Independence and support community living: Workshop summary*. Washington, DC: The National Academies Press.

National Council on Disability. (2005). *The current state of transportation for people with disabilities in the United States*. Washington, DC: National Council on Disability.

National Council on Disability. (2015). *Self-driving cars: Mapping access to a technology revolution* (Publication No. 01656924). Washington, DC.

National Council on Independent Living. (n.d.). *About visitability.* Retrieved March 28, 2019, from https://visitability.org/about-visitability/#history

Nelson/Nygaard Consulting Associates. (2008). *Status report on the use of wheelchairs and other mobility devices on public and private transportation.* Washington, DC: Easter Seals Project ACTION.

Neugarten, B. L. (1970). "Dynamics of transition of middle age to old age." *Journal of Geriatric Psychiatry 4*(1): 71–87.

Oswald, F., & Wahl, H. W. (2005). Dimensions of the meaning of home in later life. In G. D. Rowles & H. Chaudhury (Eds.), *Home and identity in late life: International perspectives* (pp. 21–45). New York: Springer.

Ramirez, A., Farmer, G. C., Grant, D., & Papachristou, T. (2005). Disability and preventive cancer screening: Results from the 2001 California health interview survey. *American Journal of Public Health, 95*(11), 2057–2064.

Rimmer, J. H., Chen, M. D., & Hsieh, K. (2011). A conceptual model for identifying, preventing, and managing secondary conditions in people with disabilities. *Physical Therapy, 91,* 1728–1739.

Rimmer, J. H., Riley, B., Wang, E., Rauworth, A., & Jurkowski, J. (2004). Physical activity participation among persons with disabilities: Barriers and facilitators. *American Journal of Preventive Medicine, 26*(5), 419–425.

Riley, M. W. (1971). Social gerontology and the age stratification of society. The Gerontologist 11, 79–87.

Rowe, J. W., & Kahn, R. L. (1997). Successful aging. *The Gerontologist, 37*(4), 433–440.

Rowe, J. W., & Kahn, R. L. (2015). Successful aging 2.0: Conceptual expansions for the 21st century. *The Journals of Gerontology: Series B, 70*(4), 593–596.

Section 504. (n.d.). *Frequently asked questions.* HUD.gov/U.S. Department of Housing and Urban Development (HUD). Retrieved March 19, 2019, from https://www.hud.gov/program_offices/fair_housing_equal_opp/disabilities/sect504faq

Smedley, B. D. (2006). Expanding the frame of understanding health disparities: From a focus on health systems to social and economic systems. *Health Education and Behavior, 33*(4), 538.

Steinfeld, E. & Danford G. S. (1999). Theory as a basis for research on enabling environments. Enabling Environments, Springer: 11–33.

Stolzle, R. A., & Fox, M. H. (2011). Health disparities among adults with physical disabilities or cognitive limitations compared to individuals with no disabilities in the United States. *Disability and Health Journal, 4*(2), 59–67.

Strauss, D. J., DeVivo, M. J., Paculdo, D. R., & Shavelle, R. M. (2006). Trends in life expectancy after spinal cord injury. *Archives of Physical Medicine and Rehabilitation, 87*(8), 1079–1085.

Szanton, S. L., Leff, B., Wolff, J. L., Roberts, L., & Gitlin, L. N. (2016). Home-based care program reduces disability and promotes aging in place. *Health Affairs, 35*(9), 1558–1563.

Tadano, S., Tsukada, A., Shibano, J. I., Ukai, T., & Watanuki, Y. (1998). Driving tests and computer simulations of electric wheelchairs on snow-covered roads. *JSME International Journal Series C Mechanical Systems, Machine Elements and Manufacturing, 41*(1), 68–75.

Townsend, P. (1981). The structured dependency of the elderly: A creation of social policy in the twentieth century. Aging and Society 1(1), 5–28.

Tuminello, E. R., Holmbeck, G. N., & Olson, R. (2012). Executive functions in adolescents with spina bifida: Relations with autonomy development and parental intrusiveness. *Child Neuropsychology, 18*(2), 105–124.

Tabattanon, K., Sandhu, N., & D'Souza, C. (2019). Accessible design of low-speed automated shuttles: A brief review of lessons learned from public transit. In *Proceedings of the 63rd Annual Meeting of the Human Factors and Ergonomics Society (HFES), Seattle, WA, October 2019* (pp. 526–530). https://doi.org/10.1177/1071181319631362.

Vandawalker, M., Locke, G., & Lam, K. (2012). *Evaluation of the Section 202 Demonstration Predevelopment Grant Program.* Abt Associates and U.S. Department of Housing and Urban Development (p. 2).

Vasunilashorn, S., Steinman, B. A., Liebig, P. S., & Pynoos, J. (2012). Aging in place: Evolution of a research topic whose time has come. *Journal of Aging Research, 2012,* 120952. https://doi.org/10.1155/2012/120952

Verbrugge, L. M., & Yang, L.-S. (2002). Aging with disability and disability with aging. *Journal of Disability Policy Studies, 12*(4), 253–267. https://doi.org/10.1177/104420730201200405

Walker, A. (1981). Towards a political dependency of the elderly: A creation age. *Aging and Society 1*(1), 73–94.

White House Conference on Aging (WHCOA). (2005). The booming dynamics of aging: From awareness to action. In *Report of the 2005 White House Conference on Aging, Washington, DC, December 11–14, 2005.*

Wick, J. Y. (2017). Aging in place: Our house is a very, very, very fine house. *The Consultant Pharmacist®, 32*(10), 566–574.

Wiles, J. L., Leibing, A., Guberman, N., Reeve, J., & Allen, R. E. (2012). The meaning of "aging in place" to older people. *The Gerontologist, 52*(3), 357–366.

World Health Organization (2001). International Classification of Functioning, Disability and Health. Geneva, Switzerland: World Health Organization.

World Health Organization. (2007). *Global age-friendly cities: A guide.* Geneva: World Health Organization.

Chapter 12
Disasters and Disability: Rhetoric and Reality

June Isaacson Kailes and Donald J. Lollar

The health of the public is rarely in more jeopardy than during natural or human-caused disasters. During these events each person or family wants to believe that they will be a high priority for those whose responsibility it is to help the public. Those with sufficient resources are more apt to purchase preparations and other services for emergencies and respond with a semblance of order. Likewise, recovery from these events is often enhanced by strong resources. Unfortunately, those without such resources are less prepared, able to respond, and less able to recover. Reliable data are scarce, but a United Nations report confirms that people with disabilities are disproportionately affected by disasters, with Japan reporting that people with disabilities are four times more likely to die when a disaster strikes (UN, 2013). Public health professionals whether in the public or private sector are those whose mission is to help all citizens prepare, react, and recover from disasters. Unfortunately, the mission and its implementation are too often incongruent. As the frequency, scale, duration, and intensity of the disasters increase, the gap across groups grows wider. Smith and Nataro (2015) answered the question of disparity of impact for people with and without disabilities. The Behavioral Risk Factor Surveillance System data were used to describe emergency preparedness of people with activity limitations, comparing those with limitations who use specialized equipment and people with mental health conditions with people without disabilities. The groups with activity limitations and with mental health conditions were significantly less prepared for emergencies than the groups with limitations using specialized equipment or those without disabilities. Adding the variables of nonwhite, without a partner, female, and living in poverty increased the probability of being unprepared.

J. I. Kailes
Disability Policy Consultant, Pomona, CA, USA

D. J. Lollar (✉)
School of Public Health, Oregon Health & Science University, Portland, OR, USA

© Springer Science+Business Media, LLC, part of Springer Nature 2021
D. J. Lollar et al. (eds.), *Public Health Perspectives on Disability*,
https://doi.org/10.1007/978-1-0716-0888-3_12

This chapter outlines the reported missions of public health agencies regarding one of the most disproportionately impacted populations—individuals and families living with disabling conditions. Beyond the intent of the agencies, however, is the reality of the experiences of this group and how this population must strive to find their way toward preparation, reaction, and recovery to disasters. The chapter will describe the intent, but also the reality, and the steps that must be taken by public health professionals to fulfill the mission toward the most vulnerable. As a basis for discussion, we will define the vulnerable population that is the focus of the chapter.

12.1 Definitions

Kailes and Ender (2007) outlined the shift from the traditional public health definition that used the label "special needs" toward a function-based framework for emergency management and planning. This traditional approach included an array of groups, including people living with disabling conditions, those with mental illness, non-English speakers, pregnant mothers, children, and elderly individuals. Using Census data from 2000, Kailes and Enders calculated that these groups would include almost half of the US population. From this early effort evolved the current focus on function and access. The US Department of Health and Human Services (DHHS) Division for At-Risk Individuals, Behavioral Health & Community Resilience (ABC) defines at-risk individuals as those with access-based and/or function-based needs in times of disaster or emergencies, without regard for diagnostic categories, or labels (DHHS, 2019a, b). These individuals or families are defined as:

Access-based needs: All people must have access to certain resources, such as social services, accommodations, information, transportation, medications to maintain health, safety, and independence.
Function-based needs: Function-based need refers to restrictions or limitations an individual may have that require assistance before, during, and/or after a disaster or public health emergency.

The function-based approach was then operationalized in five areas of need, including communication (C), medical (M), functional independence (I), supervision (S), and transportation (T)—(CMIST). The introduction of this approach provided and still provides a clearer framework for addressing the real concerns of people with disabilities before, during, and after disasters (Kailes & Ender, (2007). This framework was updated by Kailes (2017) so that the CMIST acronym encompasses communication (C); maintaining health (M); independence (I); support, safety, and self-determination (S); and transportation (T).

Communication needs include a broad array of the population who have difficulty hearing, seeing, or understanding, for example, hearing verbal announcements or seeing signs that provide directions for assistance. In addition, individuals and/or families who have limited English language skills, whether speaking or reading, are included. The original medical needs (M) of CMIST have been updated to maintaining health. This change allows a more inclusive approach to health during disasters, moving beyond a purely medical perception of needs. Most individuals living with chronic conditions or disabilities manage their own health or can with some level of support. These needs, however, must be understood by emergency planners. Maintaining independence (I) is crucial for the ongoing stability of the individual and family during emergencies. As planners and responders prepare for their roles, including these needs is important for the overall effectiveness of their preparation and intervention. Awareness of the health interventions is extremely helpful, whether related to medications needed, assistive technology required, equipment to aid mobility or hearing and others, or emotional support. Safety, support, and self-determination (S) is a more inclusive term, beyond the initial focus on supervision. Most individuals do not need supervision, beyond those experiencing dementia, young children, or prisoners. Beyond supervision for the few, self-determination is needed for the many. Self-determination emphasizes that individuals maintain their capacity and right to make their own decisions. While all may not be physically independent, all have the right to be autonomous—to make their own life decisions, even during a crisis. This need is particularly important when disasters separate individuals from family and support staff. Finally, transportation needs are often critical for those with limited mobility. Whether for lack of a vehicle, or being unable to drive, or need for wheelchair accessible vehicles, attention to this need is a crucial element of survival before, during, and after a disaster. This so-evident need, however, is not often a focus for planners who are unfamiliar with or insensitive to these groups (Littman, 2005).

In addition, during emergencies, limitations can exponentially increase when people lose their access to items that protect their health, independence, and safety: hearing aids, glasses, contact lenses, mobility aids, essential medications, healthcare supplies, and healthcare services such as dialysis and chemotherapy. People also acquire new temporary or permanent disabilities resulting from emergencies. This diverse group is a large segment of the population that includes people who experience limitations in behavior, walking, balancing, climbing, seeing, reading, hearing, speaking, understanding, and remembering. Individuals with these limitations are often not recognized or counted in emergencies. Extensive examples of various functional limitations during disasters are provided by Kelman and Stough (2015).

12.2   International Guidance

During the past 15 years, international attention has been focused on inclusion of persons with disabilities during preparation for, response to, and recovery from emergencies and disasters. Beginning with the United Nations Convention on the Rights of Persons with Disabilities Article 11, the public health responsibility for ensuring the safety of this population is clear.

States Parties shall take, in accordance with their obligations under international law, and including international humanitarian law and international human rights law, all necessary measures to ensure the protection and safety of persons with disabilities in situations of risk, including situations of armed conflict, humanitarian emergencies and the occurrence of natural disasters. (United Nations Enable, 2007, p. 10)

In addition, Article 12 of the UN Convention includes the right to equal recognition before the law, particularly related to the capacity of adults with disabilities to engage in supportive decision-making. This section is especially relevant during disasters when people with disabilities must make important decisions about their living arrangements, finances, and medical treatments (UN, 2013). Beyond Articles 11 and 12, the UN document proceeds to outline many of the sections that specifically focus on emergency and disaster issues for people living with disabling conditions, including accessibility (Article 9), living independently and being included in the community (Article 19), freedom of access to information (Article 21), and health (Article 25), as examples.

12.3   US Public and Private Disability Initiatives

There are several agencies and organizations responsible for planning and assisting people with disabilities during emergencies. The US Department of Health and Human Services (DHHS) includes a position of Assistant Secretary for Preparedness and Response (ASPR) whose role is to lead the efforts for medical and public health preparedness for, response to, and recovery from disasters and public health emergencies. The responsibility is to collaborate with hospitals, healthcare coalitions, community members, and state/local/tribal/territorial governments, as well as private partners to improve readiness and response capacity (DHHS, 2019a, 2019b). The DHHS also includes the Division for At-Risk Individuals, Behavioral Health & Community Resilience (ABC) whose vision statement is:

to ensure that the access and functional needs of at-risk individuals, behavioral health, and community resilience are integrated in the public health and medical emergency preparedness, response, and recovery activities of the nation by providing policy leadership, subject matter expertise, and coordination to meet the needs of those most adversely affect by a disaster. (PHE, 2019)

ABC (Division for At-Risk Individuals, Behavioral Health & Community Resilience) follows the 2013 Pandemic and All-Hazards Reauthorization Act focusing its efforts on children, older adults, pregnant women, and persons who may require additional assistance. Examples of the groups include individuals living with disabling conditions, individuals living in institutional settings, individuals from diverse cultures or who are not proficient with the English language, those who are transportation limited, and those who are homeless, along with individuals who have chronic health conditions or may have dependency on pharmaceuticals. To reiterate, these groups aggregated would account for almost half of the US population.   Beyond these populations, ABC is responsible for providing mental health, substance abuse, and stress management services to survivors of a disaster and the responders to a disaster. Finally, this Division is responsible for building the foundation for resilience in communities across the nation. ABC describes this part of their mandate as developing a sustained ability for communities to withstand and recover from whatever adversity may come. This vision is that healthy individuals and families have access to physical and mental health care and know the resources in the community to take care of themselves and others in emergency situations.

A revised Pandemic and All-Hazards Preparedness and Advancing Innovation Act recently became law (Diament, 2019). While the larger law focuses on enhancing the government's ability to respond to natural disasters and public health emergencies, it also establishes a National Advisory Committee on Individuals with Disabilities and Disasters. The committee's intent is that people with disabilities will be included in the planning for preparedness and response in times of disasters.

The US DHHS also includes the Centers for Disease Control and Prevention (CDC). CDC is the public health implementation arm in most counties in the USA. In 2016, CDC and the health departments in all 50 states undertook a review of operational readiness to ensure that life-saving medicines and supplies could reach the right people at the right time (CDC, 2017). CDC's Public Health Emergency Preparedness program provides guidance, technical assistance, and evaluation to state and local public health departments. Six domains of preparedness are provided. These include (a) community resilience to assist in preparing for and recovering from emergencies, (b) incident management focusing on coordinating an effective response to emergencies, (c) information management to make sure people have information to take action, (d) getting medicines and supplies where they are needed, (e) expanding medical services to handle large events, and (f) investigating and identifying health threats.

The US Department of Homeland Security (DHS) houses another agency committed to disaster management—the Federal Emergency Management Agency (FEMA). Originally established to coordinate emergency events integrating numerous agencies, FEMA is now a part of the DHS. FEMA's Office of National Preparedness has the responsibility for helping to ensure that the nation's first responders are trained and equipped to deal with various emergencies.

Finally, the American Red Cross (ARC) is a private organization whose mission is to reduce suffering in the face of emergencies by mobilizing volunteers and private donors. Along with FEMA, ARC has developed a manual to assist individuals and families living with disabling conditions to prepare for disasters. The manual affirms that millions of individuals have physical, sensory, or cognitive impairments, and the manual is geared to help preparations in case of fire, floods, or acts of terrorism.

All of these agencies and organizations present a commitment to serving the totality of the population in times of disasters, including individuals and families with disabilities. The materials and interactions with these authorities suggest the sincere intent to be helpful to these diverse groups. We would suggest that because people with disabilities represent some of the most disproportionally impacted individuals, intent is not sufficient to serve this population.

The chapter has thus far made a case for much closer attention to people with disabilities and others with access and functional needs before, during, and after disasters. Definition of those with specific needs has been provided. An overview of those agencies and organizations responsible for planning and intervening to assist people with disabilities during emergencies has been provided. The next sections of the chapter will address the reality beyond the intent during past disasters. Principles for preparation and intervention and a review of the reality of preparedness and response of agencies during several recent disasters are provided. Finally, this chapter will address needed changes in public health philosophy, policy, and actions that will improve the lives of these large and diverse groups.

12.4   From Intent to Sobering Reality

After the 9/11 disaster in 2001, a study was funded by the CDC that investigated what county emergency planners had implemented to include people with disabilities in their management planning. White and his associates randomly selected 30 counties, cities, parishes, plus a borough in New York City for the study. Each of these had experienced a disaster between 1998 and 2003 (White, 2015). Phone interviews and reviews of counties' plans for emergency management were conducted and reviewed to evaluate the inclusion of people with mobility impairments. The results were threefold:

1. A majority of the managers of the emergency services were not trained in what was called "special needs" populations, including individuals with mobility impairments.
2. Little or no representation of persons with mobility limitations was included in the planning of emergency plans or revisions that may have taken place.
3. A majority of the emergency planners had no notion of how many individuals with mobility limitations lived within the areas for which they were responsible.

A follow-up study by the same group addressed issues after Hurricane Katrina hit the southern coast of the USA. White (2015) describes a study underwritten by the National Institute on Disability and Rehabilitation Research (NIDRR) after this devastating hurricane that hit New Orleans directly. This physical description of major portions of the city was like nuclear fallout. Social networks were all but gone. Many neighborhoods consisted of empty houses block after block. Bicycles, boats, and cars still littered the streets for many months. Wheelchairs were abandoned outside the New Orleans Superdome where many people with disabilities had sought refuge.

In 2008 a report chronicling the response to the Southern California wildfires described cross-cutting issues related to people with disabilities in disasters. These include the assumption that people in disasters can walk, run, see, drive, read, hear, speak, and understand and respond immediately to instructions and/or alerts. Few fiscal resources, except for specified state agencies, are used to identify and address barriers to ensure the safety of all individuals in the state and usually exclude those with disabilities. The report chronicles the response and recovery efforts associated with the wildfires with specific emphasis on communication access, caring for and sheltering a large group of people including those with disabilities, evacuation and transportation problems, and the interaction of non-governmental and advocacy organizations for individuals in long-term care facilities.

Specific evidence of the extreme difficulty experienced by people with disabilities is found in the Executive Summary of the report by Disability Rights North Carolina (DRNC) after the 2018 Hurricane Florence (DRNC, 2019). The organization monitored shelters operated by the American Red Cross to house families displaced by the hurricane. During 47 days DRNC talked with greater than 300 individuals in 26 shelters. In addition, 150 shelter staff and additional service providers were interviewed in 14 counties. Results from interviews and visits to the shelters included these outstanding concerns:

1. Many shelters were inaccessible to individuals with limited mobility, including steep steps to reach their beds or use the bathrooms or other activities of daily living. Some individuals were not allowed to use elevators, thus requiring they wear diapers, a gross loss of dignity.
2. One of the medical shelters that was supposed to allow for care of individuals needing more acute medical care than usual was in a state psychiatric hospital, with issues of poorly functioning heat/air conditioning and plumbing. Additional emotional discomfort for the survivors was the hospital was in an area at risk for flooding and without an adequate emergency evacuation plan.
3. Different shelters had quite varying degrees of services available. Some federal and local agencies served some of the shelters, while others had many fewer services, thereby reducing an individual or family's ability to recover their previous lives.
4. Long-term issues remain, with concerns for many with disabilities about food insecurity, housing, and even drinking water in many areas.

The After Action Report from Hurricane Harvey, a culminating document from the 2018 *Getting It Right Inclusive Disaster Strategies Conference*, highlighted a plethora of difficulties in equal access, including alerts, warnings, and notifications; evacuation problems; sheltering in the most integrated setting; health maintenance and acute medical care; life-saving and life-sustaining goods and services; food and potable water; registering for disaster services including FEMA and state emergency programs; housing; return to school, work, home, and community; and disaster recovery and mitigation investments (Roth, Kailes, & Marshall, 2018). Government agencies failed people with disabilities during disasters affecting Puerto Rico, Houston, and North Carolina.

A 2019 alert from the *Journal of Emergency Management* (McKay, 2019), the too often-seen reality is that people with disabilities often face a clear possibility of placement in long-term care facilities either as preparations are being made or as the disaster is occurring. The results from poor planning, lack of services in a community, and waving legal protections during emergencies allow inappropriate placement to occur and often in facilities with few accessible bathrooms, entrances, access to cooling for medications, and sometimes even electricity to keep life-sustaining and life-saving health devices running. Individuals who are transported to these facilities often become lost to the system, since no records are kept. Conditions are worse than in their previous living setting.

Across these specific disasters, there are many common deficiencies seen in the public response. Key findings from the Disability Rights North Carolina report conclude that federal, state, and local emergency management official are inadequately addressing the needs of people with disabilities during disaster planning. When the state of North Carolina introduced a new position for disasters, Disability Integration Specialists (DIS), the staff provided support for people with disabilities after Hurricane Florence. However, shelter staff need more training to adequately fill their role as helpers. In addition, North Carolina's ongoing failure to invest in accessible, affordable housing was made worse by the hurricane.

Finally, in mid-2019, the Government Accountability Office reported that the Federal Emergency Management Agency is doing poorly in its response and assistance to people with disabilities during disasters, as well as children, senior citizens, and low-income individuals (Rogers, 2019). During testimony before a US House of Representatives Homeland Security Subcommittee on Emergency Preparedness, Response, and Recovery, witnesses reported that people with disabilities and others with access and functional needs are more likely to die or be injured during a disaster due to a lack of planning, accessibility, and accommodations. Problems include access to transportation, medical equipment and health care, and shelters during and after a disaster. In addition, FEMA reduced the number of disability integration staff deployed during disasters, transferring these duties to general FEMA staff. These staff members, as of the report, were not being trained to address the needs of these groups, hence creating a greater risk for a double disaster. FEMA indicated a training course would be available in another year, tempting fate.

Without proper preparation from a community and individual perspective, there will most always be poor response during or after a disaster. Without appropriate training and preparation of responders, there will be inadequate capacity to seek out and assist people with disabilities and others with access and functional needs. The majority of the general population may be served somewhat better, but these groups will suffer greatly.

12.5   Principles for Preparation and Response

1. Preparedness for emergencies begins with communicating information to the population(s) at risk. The overall characteristics of this information is that it be real, specific, and current (Kailes, 2016). The guidelines for producing useful and relevant information include several steps. The relevant information should be developed in partnership with people who live with disabilities—and others with access or functional needs. The term "inclusive" is one that should be in the

vocabulary of any public health professional—not just the word but the understanding of the idea that people with disabilities are an integral part of planning. Public health professionals have for years been clear that any public health programs that affect women, or people of color, or the LGBTQ community will, of course, include representatives of those groups. It is often the case, particularly in disability communities, that information is being developed for, instead of with, them.

2. Respectful listening should occur during the interactions. Often, public health professionals who have little experience with individuals with disabilities focus only on their perceptions of their own role, and only half listen to the folks they are supposed to serve. The inherent disrespect keeps them from "hearing" what is being communicated. This active listening sets the stage for the third principle.

3. Planners can be sure that needs are not overlooked. The content of the information can then take into account varied limitations and suggestions by the affected community members—whether they be activities such as hearing, seeing, moving around, speaking, or cognitive issues, such as remembering, learning new information, understanding instructions, or problem-solving and decision-making.

4. The fourth principle is based on the notion that a large percentage of people with disabilities do not have sufficient resources to prepare easily for emergencies or disasters. Therefore, low- or no-cost solutions are important. A lengthy list of low-cost supplies becomes a high-cost kit! Dividing needed resources into essentials, useful, and personal, for example, helps individuals to know what is absolutely needed in disasters. Bethel, Foreman, and Burke (2011) used BRFSS data that showed people with disabilities, those reporting fair or poor health, or those with three or more chronic conditions were less likely to have even the most essential resources, food, water, flashlight, and radio, even though they were more likely to have a 3-day supply of medications than healthier populations.

5. Specific information should be made available in accessible and usable formats. Of course, the ways for individuals to receive these varied formats, i.e., which agency or organization has the materials, how to contact that organization, and how to request the information in a usable format, are important.

6. It is also important that any resources be backed up by specific links or phone numbers that can fill in the blanks that may occur if a primary source does not work out.

Embedded in these principles is the notion that attending to details is a survival skill when living with disability and functional needs, details that can be easily overlooked without the lived experience. This experience can be communicated by "professional disability advocates" but can also be discussed by average folks in a community who have the chance to tell their story, share their experience, and often suggest creative (to the professionals) ideas. "Drop, cover, and hold" may be helpful to the general population during an earthquake, but individuals with mobility limitations may not be able to complete these movements. Suggesting that one cover their neck and head with their arms or grab a pillow until the shaking stops may be a workable alternative. Uneducated public health professionals may feel very good about suggesting that individuals plan in advance for shelter choices that will work for themselves and their animals. That kind of vague advice does not give information about where or whom to contact, how to know the distance these options are from home, and what transportation is available for getting to them. Medical emergency systems are often suggested resources, but this assumes that first responders are not overwhelmed and that landline phones and cell phones or emails and texts are working—and they sometimes are not. In other words, for almost any suggestion, there are myriad reasons that will often not be helpful, and backups become important to know. HL Mencken said, "for every complex problem, there is an answer that is clear, simple, and wrong." This is too often the case when public health professionals are too cavalier about needs of people with disabilities generally but particularly in times of crisis. People with disabilities and public health workers must be willing to communicate, then cooperate, and then collaborate as they implement the realities of these principles for preparation and response.

12.6 Specific Recommendations for Preparedness and Response

12.6.1 American Red Cross and US Federal Emergency Management Agency (ARC/FEMA, 2019)

These two organizations cooperated to prepare a publication specifically focused on disaster preparation for **individual** people with disabilities. The document is thorough but at times assumes a level of resources not available to a large percentage of people with disabilities. Papers by Smith and Nataro (2015) and by Bethel et al. (2011) provide definitive data showing the difference in preparation for disasters between with and without disabilities, especially when adding poverty as a factor. The ARC/FEMA publication, however, does provide numerous helpful steps that can be taken by the general public but of specific importance for people with disabilities or others with access or functional needs.

The steps in preparation include getting informed, making a plan, assembling a kit, and maintaining both the plan and the kit. As a starting point, one should create a personal support network. This group can help one to identify what resources will be needed in case of an emergency. The network should include the person's relatives, neighbors, friends, family, roommates, and co-workers. The network should include at least three people from any location where the individual spends time. Home, school, workplace, volunteer site, and other places where a person spends time should be included. Second, the individual should determine what they can do independently and with what steps they will need help. Working with a personal network, the individual can answer questions needing answers during a disaster. Questions related to daily living would be included, e.g., what is needed for personal care, including personal care equipment or adaptive eating devices, or what is needed for backup water service and electricity-dependent equipment. A second area of questions relates to getting around, such as accessible transportation (lift or ramp equipped), debris removal from critical paths of travel like sidewalks and ramps, or help with errands getting emergency supplies at public distribution centers or groceries, medications, or barriers to having caregivers get to the individual. Finally, questions about evacuation are crucial. These include exiting a building whether home, office, school, etc., getting help if needed, and evacuation devices for building floors that are not at ground level.

As the answers to relevant questions are addressed, a disaster plan can be completed. This plan should include a meeting with family, personal assistants, and building managers and choosing an outside contact in another city, deciding where to meet, deciding on a communication plan, and defining escape routes and safe places. The ARC/FEMA document provides an extensive list of items that compose a disaster supply kit. For purposes of this chapter, suffice it to say this list of "basics" goes far beyond what might be called "essential" items previously, such as clothing for the season, kitchen and cooking utensils, tools, etc.

12.6.2 After Event Reports from North Carolina and California

Organizations also need to have specific steps before, during, and after disasters. The NC After Event Report outlines helpful changes that have been made since Hurricane Florence. Daily telephone conferences among federal, state, and local governmental units and including disability advocates/representatives are crucial for updating information. Interactive maps and daily updates by the NC Department of Public Safety are another important step. Ensuring continued care of persons with acute medical needs should be met by professionally staff medical disaster centers. Access to pharmacies and medications, along with mental health services, transportation, and personal assistance services, should be available.

Positive outcomes were also found in the 2018 Getting It Right Disability Inclusive Disaster Strategies Conference (2018). Extensive collaboration among stakeholders driven by disability leaders' commitment proved essential after Hurricane Harvey. A hotline among a broad array of stakeholders began with hourly and daily teleconferences. A network for organizing, matching, shipping, and distributing disability-related supplies and assistive devices, along with medical supplies, became more and more refined. When usual resources were having difficulty, Portlight Inclusive Disaster Strategies was able to insert disability experts into those communities needing help during the most dire of conditions.

The California Wildfire After Action Report (Kailes, 2008) highlights the need for state emergency planners to develop and offer guidance to local governments regarding how to recruit qualified individuals with an array of disabilities (vision, hearing, mobility, cognitive, mental health, and others) so that operational policies and procedures can be adequately developed. Establishing a permanent Office of Access and Functional Needs in each state and locality, as possible, should be a goal. That office needs to have responsibility and authority and the resources to implement its mission. Annual funding should also be a part of state directives so that preparation is an ongoing activity rather than merely following the next disaster. In addition, funding through grants or contracts should include a mandate to show how a portion of the funds will be allocated to the inclusion of those with functional and access needs. Encouraging, and even promoting, Community Emergency Response Teams (CERT) that recruit and accommodate people with disabilities that are integrated into other community response units should also be an integral part of any state and/or local planning.

Specific governmental public communications with people with disabilities should include multiple formats so that those with hearing or understanding or vision difficulties have access to critical information. Loudspeakers, door-to-doors, and use of pictographs (signs and symbols) are needed for communication of public warnings, alerts, and notifications. Non-governmental organizations (NGOs) should be included in this approach, including NGOs focusing on people with disabilities. Likewise, media and television information should include qualified sign language interpreters and captions for hard of hearing and deaf individuals. Finally, state emergency planners should ensure that wireless communication devices in their states and local jurisdictions are capable of sending emergency alert notifications to the public. These are but some of the 72 recommendations in the report for governmental and non-governmental organizations to implement on behalf of ensuring safety of the public living with disabilities.

12.7 Directions for Public Health Perceptions, Training, and Data

12.7.1 Perceptions

Throughout this chapter there has been an emphasis on the difference between the intent of public health organizations and the actual implementation. Public health professionals are challenged mightily during times of disaster to attend to the needs of all citizens. The gaps and holes in service are excruciatingly clear and painful. Planning and preparation before an emergency occurs is crucial toward mitigating the impact of such an event. Why, then, are there such gaps and holes in service for people with disabilities? Preparation with this group is more complex than even the general population. Planners are required to be more granular than broad in their approaches. The usual public health approach with any underserved population is to engage members of the group in the planning. Perhaps because the disability community is not as geographically concentrated as with many ethnic or racial groups, communication is more complex. For many public health professionals engaged in emergency planning, this diverse population appears an afterthought. In spite of government civil rights compliance laws and funding for numerous disability-centric organizations, there is often no effort to identify and/or reach out for input, even with the new law authorizing a National Advisory Committee on Individuals with Disabilities and Disasters. It is almost as if there is a fatalistic belief that people with disabilities are unable to interact competently with professionals. Another notion assumes just the opposite—that is, that disability advocates will just create another set of expectations that will be difficult to meet because of the sheer complexity of the needs. These perceptions and expectations create the first and primary direction for public health students, educators, and professionals. Orientation and exposure to people with disabilities is a critical direction. Whatever the perceptions and expectations, actual personal interactions with individuals living with disabilities allow a more realistic understanding of the commonalities we share. This activity is so often attached to other minority groups but appears lacking in public health education and work. This one change in public health education can increase the comfort level of young public health professionals as they move into varied public health positions and functions. Disaster preparation and interventions are especially needful of this orientation.

12.7.2 Training

Training for public health professionals is an evolving activity. As greater awareness and sensitivity develops, there is a greater need for specific, real, and current education about the needs of people with functional needs during disasters. Kailes (2017) has outlined important principles for training, including:

1. Refreshing content and materials frequently
2. Training teams
3. Elevating the importance of exercises
4. Using multi-session reinforced interval learning
5. Putting equal emphasis on just-in-time training
6. Using evaluation methods that measure delivery effectiveness, performance, impact, and outcome

Continual refreshing of disaster content and materials for people with disabilities and others with access and functional needs is the beginning. As technology has advanced, all of us, including public health professionals and people with disabilities, have decreased attention spans, so the methods of teaching and learning have to adapt. Exercises to heighten focus for disasters should be continually revised. In addition, training teams allows continued reinforcement of investment to the mission and helps individual providers maintain appropriate new practices and procedures as they evolve. A part of this team emphasis is the acknowledgment that often when one member of a group attends helpful training, those experiences are not shared with other members of the team upon return from training. This aspect of training is crucial to maintain a clear sense of "team." As more individuals share experiences of training, the exercises themselves are elevated in importance. This is particularly true when exercises may be difficult and require more intense emotional and physical energy. Motivation toward stronger performance is enhanced. A fourth element of training is acceptance of the notion that solid effective training does not occur in a single session, or even 1- or 2-day training events. Repetition is important in learning, especially when the performance will be needed during stressful times. Regular intervals for training allows the public health professionals to more fully integrate the information and actions into their professional behavior, even professional identity. Kailes calls the fifth feature "just-in-time" training. Alongside the actual training should be companion documents that outline seminal competencies in the form of checklists, field operation guides, and aids that reinforce the competencies generated during the training. Consistent teams are the ideal. Unfortunately, professionals and volunteers change jobs, move, or for other reasons change responsibilities. The team may change, but the tangible products can provide the coherence for teams to work together under disaster conditions. Mobile devices, even when energy sources are poor, can provide vital information for helpers in the field. Finally, evaluation procedures are crucial in assessing the effectiveness of the response and outcomes. Evaluating the processes implemented during a response is critical for assessing how the various stages of identification, responses, procedures, and operational steps are handled. Beyond processes, however, outcomes, such as the numbers of individuals who were transported, the accessibility, safety and security of the shelters, and the numbers who were able to maintain medications and assistive devices should become standard data collection. Focusing on satisfaction with the training is quite different than addressing the meaningful and relevant outcomes in the field. Often, the two are not correlated in the way they ought.

12.7.3 Data

Public health relies on data to identify specific problems, their presence, and magnitude. Data addressing the impact of disasters on people with disabilities, never mind the general population, is a serious and neglected issue (CRED, 2018). Event-related direct death rates are counted—drownings, falling objects, and responder heroism. Months of long-term infrastructure damage, however, are not correlated with sustained increases in deaths or increased severity of health conditions. For example, the escalating death toll from the Puerto Rico hurricane shows that many more deaths are occurring now when compared with past disaster years (Kishore et al., 2018). The data have become politicized, but it is clear that infrastructure problems after the hurricane have significantly impacted people with disabilities and others with access and functional needs due to interruption of power for those using life-sustaining equipment; critical supplies such as medications and oxygen; substandard health care for dialysis, chemotherapy, and other infusion therapies;

home health and attendant services; and the operation of long-term care facilities. Deaths, both immediate and long-term, must be counted—for their own sakes but also because these rates influence government spending for disasters.

There is no national event surveillance system for natural disasters, such as extreme weather. Survivors of the World Trade Center disaster are included in a national health registry to follow their health status over time, and there is no system for monitoring the health of the affected population during or after natural disasters (Keim et al., 2019). Keim and his co-authors recommend an "evidence-based national strategy that will effectively measure, manage, and report the effectiveness of public health interventions in terms of measurable health outcomes, such as mortality." Approaches used by the National Traffic and Motor Vehicle Safety Act of 1966 are recommended as a model for disaster strategy. This model combined preventive and response programs, using a system to manage the social factors and risk factors to develop interventions. For disaster events the USA continues to expend most of its energy on the response after the event rather than on prevention. No one government agency has the specific mission to measure and reduce the impact of disasters over time (National Academy of Science, 2016). To implement such a plan, according to Keim et al., there needs to be a national disaster safety administration to develop and enforce national disaster safety standards. In addition, an independent board to investigate disaster-related mortality should be established. Finally, a national center for disaster statistics should be established so that a national database for disaster-related data can be developed.

When data are being considered, identifying varied functional needs and environmental characteristics will be critical for success. The World Health Organization has developed a framework and coding system that directly addresses functional needs and environmental factors affecting individuals. The International Classification of Functioning, Disability and Health (ICF) (WHO, 2001) provides the basic scheme for identifying, even without identifying the individuals, the types of functional limitations, and the environmental factors, barriers, or facilitators that compose a disaster scenario. The ICF addresses the needs identified by CMIST, such as communication, and allows descriptions of both the individual's level of independence and environmental factors such as health needs and transportation. Suffice it to say that the ICF has the potential to provide the basic data needed during disaster planning and response and recovery to clarify gaps as well as strengths in any developing system.

It is clear that such developments would potentially have a great impact on disaster-related efforts affecting people with disabilities. The continuing concern is that, even in this set of recommendations for the general public, people with disabilities will be an afterthought. The chapter has outlined some of the ways in which intent and reality differ regarding emergency planning and emergency services for people with functional and access needs. Public health professionals in the coming years have an opportunity to frame public health preparation, response, and recovery in a new light on behalf of and with people with disabilities.

12.8   Disaster Exercises

Given the principles included in this chapter, how does a public health professional respond?

Planning
A woman recruited for an exercise was turned away when she arrived and was told "we can't use you because you are deaf."

Transportation and Evacuation
Six facilities (2 hundred-bed nursing homes, 3 large group homes with a total of 15 wheelchair users, and 1 large residential independent living facility with 12 wheelchair users and 4 scooter users) need immediate transportation evacuation assistance. All these facilities had an agreement with the same contractor for emergency transportation. However, the contractor could not respond because they were already busy serving another large residential independent living facility.

Safety and Wellness Checks
A bad storm, lasting over 7 days resulted in over two million people sheltering in place. Many roads are not useable by standard vehicles. CPODs (commodity points of distribution) for food and water have opened. Many calls are coming in from those who are unable to get to the CPODs or who will need assistance carrying supplies back to their home. Others have run out of their medications and need a source of power for their disability-related equipment such as mobility devices. Some require power for their life-sustaining devices such as suction equipment and ventilators. Others need transportation to their dialysis, chemotherapy, or infusion therapy appointments.

Shelters
Widespread sudden power outages are causing many calls to 211 from people dependent on life-sustaining devices. Callers want to know what to do and which shelters are close to these callers that are accessible to wheelchair users and have power they can use. Some callers also need evacuation assistance.

You are not able to understand the speech of a man who is in a wheelchair and wants to enter the shelter. He is alone and he is unable to write notes.

A middle-aged man is outside the shelter and appears to be talking to himself in a loud and angry voice. He is scaring some people.

A family of six has been in the shelter for 2 days. On the second day, their 10-year-old starts screaming uncontrollably while lying on the floor pounding his fists. Other shelter residents are upset and complaining, and they are concerned that the child may be ill or being abused.

References

American Red Cross/USDHS Federal Emergency Management Agency. (2019). *Preparing for disaster for people with disabilities and other special needs.* ARC/FEMA. Retrieved May 15, 2019, from www.redcross.org/services/disaster/beprepared/disabiity.pdf

Bethel, J. W., Foreman, A. N., & Burke, S. C. (2011). Disaster preparedness among medically vulnerable populations. *American Journal of Preventive Medicine, 40*(2), 139–143.

Centers for Disease Control and Prevention. (2017). *Preparedness in action.* Retrieved May 16, 2019, from www.cdc.gov/phpr/whatwedo

Centre for Research for the Epidemiology of Disasters. (2018). *EM-DAT: The International Disaster Database.* Retrieved from https://www.emdat.be/index.php

Department of Health & Human Services. (2019a). *About the division for at-risk individuals, behavioral health and community resilience (ABC).* Retrieved from https://www.phe.gov/Preparedness/planning/abc/Pages/about.aspx

Department of Health & Human Services. (2019b). *Saving lives and protecting Americans from 21st century health security threats.* Retrieved from https://www.phe.gove/about/aspr/Pages/default.aspx

Diament, M. (2019, June 26). Trump signs law improving disaster planning for those with disabilities. *Disability Scoop.*

Disability Rights North Carolina. (2019). *Executive summary. The storm after the storm: Disaster, displacement and disability following hurricane Florence*, DRNC, February.

Kailes, J. I. (2008). *Southern California wildfires after action reports.* Pomona, CA: Center for Disability Issues and the Health Professions.

Kailes, J. I. (2016). *Be real, specific, and current: Emergency preparedness information for people with disabilities and others with access and functional needs.* Edition 1.0.

Kailes, J. I. (2017). *Training: Maximizing your ROI.* Retrieved from http://www.disasterstrategies.org/index.php/blog/june-isaacson-kailes/training-maximizing-your-roi

Kailes, J. I., & Ender, A. (2007). Moving beyond "special needs": A function-based framework for emergency management and planning. *Journal of Disability Policy Studies, 17*(4), 230–237.

Keim, M. E., Kirsch, T. D., Alleyne, O., Benjamin, G., DeGutis, L., Dyjack, D., ... Chan, T. H. (2019). The need for a national strategy to assess and reduce disaster-related mortality in the United States. *American Journal of Public Health, 109*(4), 539–540.

Kelman, I., & Stough, L. M. (2015). *Disability and disasters: Explorations and exchanges.* New York: Palgrave/Macmillan.

Kishore, N., Marques, D., Mahmud, A., Kiang, M. V., Rodriguez, I., Fuller, A., ... Balsari, S. (2018). Mortality in Puerto Rico after hurricane Maria. *The New England Journal of Medicine, 379,* 162. https://doi.org/10.1056/NEJMsa1803972

Littman, T. (2005). *Lessons from Katrina and Rita: What major disaster can teach transportation planners.* Retrieved from http://www.vtpi.org/katrina/pdf

McKay, J. (2019). People with disabilities often face "institutionalization" during disasters. *Emergency Management,* 1–7

National Academy of Science. (2016). *Exploring Disaster Risk Reduction Through Community-Level Approaches to Promote Healthy Outcomes. Proceedings of a Workshop—in Brief.* Washington, DC: National Academies Press.

Partnership for Inclusive Disaster Strategies. (2018, January 23). *Getting it Right 2018 National Inclusive Disaster Strategies Conference.* Washington, DC: Partnership for Inclusive Disaster Strategies.

Public Health Emergency. (2019). Division for At-Risk Individuals, Behavioral Health & Community Resilience (ABC). Online https://www.phe.gove/Preparedness/planning/abc/Pages/about.aspx. Accessed January, 2020

Rogers, C. (2019, July 31). How FEMA struggles to help people with disabilities during disasters. *Federal Times.* Retrieved from https://www.federaltimes.commanagmeent/2019/07/31/how-fema-struggles-to-helppeople-with-disabilities-during-disasters/

Roth, M., Kailes, J. I., & Marshall, M. (2018). *Getting it wrong: An indictment with a blueprint for getting it right*. Retrieved from http://disasterstrategies.org/index.phpnews/partnership-releases-2017-2018-after-action-report

Smith, D. L., & Nataro, S. J. (2015). Is emergency preparedness a "disaster" for people with disabilities in the US? Results from the 2006–2012 Behavioral Risk Factor Surveillance System (BRFSS). *Disability and Society, 30*(3), 401–418.

United Nations Office for Disaster Risk Reduction. (2013). UN global survey explains why so many people living with disabilities die in disasters. Online http://www.undrr.org. Accessed January, 2020.

United Nations. (2007). *Convention on the rights of persons with disabilities*. New York: Department of Economic and Social Affairs. Retrieved from www.un.org

White, G. W. (2015). Wheels on the ground: Lessons learned and lessons to learn. In I. Kelman & L. M. Stough (Eds.), *Disability and disaster: Explorations and exchanges* (pp. 159–169). London: Palgrave Macmillan.

World Health Organization. (2001). *International classification of functioning, disability, and health*. Geneva: World Health Organization.

Chapter 13
Law, Benefits, Disability Rights, and Public Health: A Sum Greater than the Parts?

Silvia Yee

13.1 Introduction

Law can be understood as the regulatory environment that affects virtually every facet of contemporary life, from who can practice medicine to when environmental reviews are required and from housing construction requirements to education funding. Law also mediates individual citizens' relationship to one another and the ability to gain access to social, economic, political, and legal institutions (Sarat, 1990). In the healthcare context, law governs how and when public and private healthcare coverage is offered, what services and treatments must be covered, how coverage is maintained, and who may enforce the rules of coverage. For many who do not have disabilities and who have economic resources, as long as law operates in what is perceived as a neutral way and enforces fairness and our ability to make choices, the pervasive presence of law fades into the background of our daily concerns. For people with disabilities, law may actively enable or prohibit choices in a distinctly non-neutral manner. As one author puts it when describing the role that law plays in the lives of individuals who receive public assistance, "Law is, for people on welfare, repeatedly encountered in the most ordinary transactions and events of their lives. Legal rules and practices are implicated in determining whether and how welfare recipients will be able to meet some of their most pressing needs" (Sarat, 1990). Disability does not equate with being on welfare, but there are significant correlations between disability, lower incomes, unemployment, and enrollment in public programs (Fremstad, 2009; MACPAC, 2017). Moreover, the quotation can be aptly applied even to people with disabilities who are not on public assistance given how much people with disabilities may need to call upon the force of law to gain equal access to transportation, schools, jobs, housing, and health care.

S. Yee (✉)
Disability Rights Education and Defense Fund, Berkeley, CA, USA
e-mail: syee@dredf.org

Public health recognizes how our all aspects of our environment affect individual and corporate health. Since the law is such a pervasive influence in our environment, public health needs to consider law critically. There are multiple connections between the operation of law and public health that have varying degrees of impact on people with disabilities. This chapter will focus on three specific levels of connection. First, laws can be explicitly directed at people with disabilities by establishing how disability is defined and what the status of disability means (e.g., having a disability may result in certain actions being required, provide some kind of eligibility for a benefit, or give others particular control over limited or all aspects of one's life). Second, laws can establish parameters for the availability of social determinants of health (SDoH) such as housing, education, employment, physical environment, transportation, and so forth, both generally and with regard to specific population groups and individual categories. Third, laws can explicitly recognize people with disabilities as **subjects** of law and intentionally mediate the access that people with disabilities have to the law itself as a means of achieving life necessities and goals. Section 504 of the Rehabilitation Act of 1973 (Section 504), the Americans with Disabilities Act of 1990 (ADA), the Fair Housing Act, and the Affordable Care Act (ACA, which is somewhat unique) all establish specific ways for people with disabilities, as subjects and rights holders, to directly wield access to law. Medical-legal partnerships, an emerging phenomenon over the past decade or so that embeds attorneys within a medical context such as hospitals so that they can offer aid to patients who need legal assistance to obtain or maintain various services, also exemplify this level of connection between law and public health by recognizing the health space as a critical arena for increasing disabled persons' positive interactions with law and their access to various other SDoH (Lawton & Sandel, 2014; Sandel et al., 2010).

This chapter places the above connections in an historical framework, first using different US benefits laws in Section II and then US disability rights laws in Section III. Readers who are already very familiar with welfare and benefits laws may choose to first proceed to Section III if their main goal is to familiarize themselves with major disability civil rights and non-discrimination laws. However, this chapter and its analysis of how disability and public health-related laws have evolved over time rest on observations and insights that build throughout each section as ordered. At the end of the chapter, there is additional resource information about various federal, state, and local laws that can affect people with disabilities and some questions to promote practical applications of the material covered.

13.2 Laws Addressing Welfare and Benefits

Some of the earliest federal laws on public health in the United States were enacted to control people with disabilities in some way, ostensibly for their own good and sometimes to protect those without disabilities *from* people with disabilities, for example, the National Quarantine Act (Sess. 2, Ch. 66, 20 Stat. 37, 1878).

Historically, US welfare and benefits laws based on health status seem to have evolved from a focus on more specific populations that have, or are perceived to have, unique health needs to more general populations. This speaks perhaps to the gradual growing public acceptance of disability as a normal part of human life (Iezzoni, 2018). If disability is conceived as something that happens to particular population groups living in special circumstances, for example, a hospital network for sick seamen or native Indian tribes ravaged by European diseases during a time of war (Kelton, 2015) or US veterans returning from active duty, then public health goals are likely to be most efficiently supported by legal strategies that emphasize cure and/or containment of an identified population. Over time, more broadly conceived "universal" benefits and public programs such as Social Security and Medicare came into being, but interestingly, these laws did not particularly account well for the presence of people with disabilities among the general population. As laws were amended to enable people with various disabilities to draw on income supports and other services, the laws also became more focused on using definitions and eligibility rules to control access to benefits that were considered attractive enough to incentivize a fraudulent attempt to present with disabilities.

The attitudes toward disability that were prevalent throughout the twentieth century—disability is an unmitigated negative, disability is rare, any episodic disability must be fraudulent, people with disabilities are unemployable, lazy people will fake having disabilities to avoid work—may perhaps underlie the general tendency for universal benefits such as Social Security and Medicare to be entitlement benefits, while population-specific benefits for people with disabilities usually require ongoing appropriation. In some ways, more recent legislative developments since 2016 have seen a resurgence of some of these older attitudes in recent state trends that on the one hand want to preserve entitlement benefits like Medicaid for the "truly disabled" and on the other hand attempt to impose restrictive qualifying conditions and benefit cutoffs for those who are not generally considered "truly disabled" or are thought to be undeserving of free or low-cost healthcare benefits. These legal and policy trends follow decades of social conceptualization that distinguishes between those poor who are considered deserving and those who are not (Moffitt, 2015).

13.2.1 Creation of the Bureau of Indian Affairs Health Division, Forerunner to the Indian Health Service, and Subsequent Legislation

At the beginning of the nineteenth century, the federal government's primary goal in relation to native Indian populations was military control. Nonetheless, public health needs arose as a direct consequence of military interactions with Indian tribes: "As early as 1802 or 1803 Army physicians took emergency measures to curb contagious diseases among Indian tribes in the vicinity of military posts" (U.S. Department of Health and Human Services, 2019). While the 1921 creation of the Bureau of Indian Affairs Health Division, a forerunner to the Indian Health Services (IHS), may not seem to be explicitly connected to disability, the significant historical and ongoing occurrence of disabilities, health conditions, and health/healthcare disparities among native Indian populations warrants a look at the act today as an example of how one set of laws addresses health and racial/ethnic intersections in ways that continue to evolve. In terms of health disparities, adult American Indians and Alaskan Natives (AIAN) are more likely to self-report fair or poor health and have higher incidences of such chronic conditions as diabetes or cardiovascular disease. Equally significant, suicide is the second leading cause of death among AIAN youth and young adults, occurring at a rate one and a half times higher than the national average (Artiga, Ubri, & Foutz, 2017).

The formal transfer of federal AIAN health facilities from the Department of the Interior to the Public Health Services took effect on, rather ironically, Independence Day 1955 (Public Law 83-568, 1954). The June 1955 press release issued by the Department of Indian Affairs at the time recognized the transfer as a move that capped the Department's growing efforts to address AIAN health needs as a broader public and public health matter, beginning with the creation of a Health Division in 1924 with a head who reported directly to the Commissioner of Indian Affairs (U.S. Department of the Interior Indian Affairs, 1955). The ongoing poor status of AIAN health prompted passage of the Indian Health Care Improvement Act (IHCIA) in 1976 to implement and improve federal Indian health facilities and services (Pub. L. 94-437, 1976). The IHS could be considered a permanent part of the federal infrastructure, but the IHCIA was set up to require ongoing periodic reauthorization and annual appropriation of funds for IHS operations every fiscal year. If the funds appropriated are insufficient for the need, IHS services must be rationed. In 2017, 5.6 million non-elderly adults were identified as fully or partially AIAN. According to the 2010 census, AIANs tend to be concentrated in certain states, but only 22% live on tribal lands or reservations while 60% live in metropolitan areas (Office of Minority Health, Health and Human Services, 2018). This is important since most IHS and tribal-operated hospitals and clinics are generally located on or near federal reservations.

The 2010 passage of the Patient Protection and Affordable Care Act (ACA) (42 U.S.C. § 18001 et seq., 2010) included at least two changes that have had a significant impact on AIAN health. First, the ACA included the *permanent* reauthorization of the IHCIA, something which had been proposed in bill form for over a decade but which federal lawmakers had been unable to pass (National Indian Health Board, 2019). Second, the ACA's provision for Medicaid expansion has measurably reduced AIAN uninsurance rates and increased access to care. The federal Government Accountability Office analyzed data from fiscal years 2013 through 2018 to find that the number of patients who reported having health insurance at IHS hospitals and clinics increased on average from 64% to 78%, with the largest increases occurring in states that expanded Medicaid eligibility under the ACA (U.S. Government Accountability Office, 2019). Third-party payments from Medicaid, Medicare, or private insurers can be collected when eligible AIAN persons receive services at IHS facilities and are an important revenue source for

IHS. IHS staff reported using the 51% increase in third-party payments in the report's 5-year period to increase staff recruitment and retention, medical equipment availability, and other on-site services (U.S. Government Accountability Office, 2019). Medicaid was available to AIAN persons even before the ACA and included special eligibility and consumer protection provisions, but factors such as lower employment rates and median incomes among the AIAN population make eligibility expansion in Medicaid especially important for AIAN individuals and families who fall in the gap between traditional Medicaid and employer coverage or AIAN individuals with disabilities who may need a wider array of services and providers than those typically available through IHS (Artiga et al., 2017).

The use of law to address AIAN public health concerns illustrates the push and pull of a complex range of multiple overlapping factors that affect how laws are used to address public health concerns: current social concerns, academic theories, economic concerns, and political battles among various constituencies as well as between federal, state, and local levels of government and within each level. The public health profession may think that once they have clearly pinpointed a problem, supported their findings with data, and recommended feasible policy and legal responses, the way forward should be obvious. Unfortunately, too many other factors can shape the desired new or amended law, which at the least may have to deal with an existing policy infrastructure on the topic area. For example, healthcare reform for people with disabilities must take account of how coverage for long-term care is not legally required except for institutional care under the public Medicaid program. Even if the status quo somehow could be easily reformed, there is the additional reality that most laws gain an accretion of interpretation from court decisions that can also diverge from the assumptions and intentions of some of those who were involved in the original enactment of the law, as well as those who seek to use the law today.

Current research establishes high rates of health and healthcare disparities experienced by AIAN populations. The Centers for Disease Control and Prevention states that three in ten AIAN persons has a disability, the highest rate of any racial/ethnic group, and of those, over 41% smoke and over 40% are obese (Centers for Disease Control and Prevention, 2019), raising questions about access to common health advice and prevention measures. New measures to address health disparities must take place within an existing framework of specialized and segregated Indian Health Services. Innovations to IHS law improved health care to some AIAN persons but did not necessarily reduce the multiple coverage gaps that AIAN persons faced during periods of geographic, financial, and structural family change. Instead, some of the systemic reforms made in the Affordable Care Act, a law that purports to affect US health care generally, resulted in very specific insurance coverage improvements that positively affected AIAN health. The law has, in effect, come full circle, from specialized back to general, but the accretion of the law itself means that AIAN health today is a highly complex field of regulation to navigate for many stakeholders including the federal government, state Medicaid agencies, tribal authorities, and contracting providers.

Two other conceptual legal ideas should be kept in mind throughout this chapter. One is the legal theory of "disparate impact," which is a legal theory of discrimination that relies on establishing evidence of a discriminatory impact on specific groups of a policy that is seemingly neutral on its face. It is introduced here as a concept that is potentially applicable in a reverse form, when a seemingly neutral policy or law has an unequal *positive* impact. That is, public health researchers and scientists **do** need to unearth and document disparate impact as originally conceived as this can support important impact litigation on behalf of plaintiff groups, but the field of public health **also** can consider and document "disparate benefit." As an example, various legal changes wrought under the ACA brought about disproportionate benefits to specific underserved population groups such as AIAN persons or persons with disabilities that have historically experienced, and/or are currently experiencing, health and healthcare disparities (please see Chap. 15 for further information about employment for people with disabilities).

The second concept is similarly borrowed from a groundbreaking analysis that was originally developed to analyze and compare international laws on disability. Professors Theresia Degener and Gerard Quinn, two experts in international law, wrote at the turn of the last millennium about the gradual shift in national and international law from disability laws that focused mostly on welfare and guardianship toward equal opportunity and non-discrimination (Degener & Quinn, 2002). Degener and Quinn (2002) described a paradigm shift away from a status quo in which "disabled persons were depicted not as subjects with legal rights but as objects of welfare, health and charity programs" (Degener & Quinn, 2002). In the United States, we can see a similar trajectory within certain areas of law, even though the United States has had disability civil rights laws for almost half-a-century and enacted the groundbreaking Americans with Disabilities Act (Pub. L. No. 101-336, 104 Stat. 328 (1990), 1990). The need for federal and state welfare, benefits, and public health laws remained before and after 1990, and only in recent years have we seen gradual attempts to recognize non-discrimination and self-direction in benefits laws which have been slow to accept people with disabilities as "subjects" and not "objects" of law. The decade-long history of the IHS laws illustrates this very trend.

13.2.2   Social Security Act (42 U.S.C. §§ 1396 et seq.)

First enacted in 1935, the Social Security Act created a national income insurance system for certain populations, with different groups being added to the operation of the law over time. Many scholars view the Act as both a specific, logical response to the Great Depression and the culmination of a gradual expansion of fifteenth-century "poor laws" inherited from England that narrowly and inconsistently provided minimal monetary relief to "deserving poor" who were deemed morally upright and totally unable to work for legitimate reasons such as old age or disability (U.S. Social Security Administration, 2019a). The original 1935 law in the

United States was groundbreaking in several aspects, conceived as a universal social insurance scheme whereby all employees would be enumerated, contribute, and then eventually be able to draw down on the collected funds when they became elderly and no longer able to earn an income.

The 1935 law was not truly universal, especially with regard to people with disabilities who could lack the employment needed for threshold inclusion in the social insurance scheme. People who did not have traditional employment situations with monetary pay, such as homemakers, were also excluded. There was an attempt to capture persons who were already low income at the point the legislation was signed and who were presumed to be incapable of gainful employment: very low-income "aged blind" were in the original 1935 legislation and the 1950 amendments added very low-income people with disabilities. The 1950s brought a further series of disability-specific amendments in the national social insurance program: a "freeze" on already accumulated benefits for workers who acquired disabilities was enacted in 1954, additional benefits were created in 1954 for workers who became disabled between the ages of 50 and 64 and for disabled adult children, and age restrictions on disability benefits and their dependents were abolished in 1960.

The legislative development of the Social Security Act shows how disability remained something of an afterthought even as the United States attempted to put into place a universal social insurance scheme as a safety net against poverty. Blindness was pervasively associated with inability to work, and people who were blind are in the original law, but other persons with different types of disabilities or the situation of children with disabilities as they age were only considered and added over time. This implies that the model that lawmakers had in mind for the safety net remains a pattern of "able-bodied" Americans, mostly men, who consistently work and support their families until retirement unless they became significantly disabled. When the Social Security Act of 1972 authorized the new program of Supplemental Security Income (SSI), it was to finally consolidate benefits paid to very low-income individuals who were aged, blind, or disabled and streamline the bewildering array of federally administered cash benefits for needy individuals and couples that somewhat haphazardly developed on federal and state welfare benefit rolls over time. A few years after that, the 1980 Amendments to the act formally instituted a more specific gatekeeping roll that required beneficiaries who qualified on the basis of disability to provide medical "certification" of their ongoing eligibility for SSI. While the review process has been further modified over the years, partly to try and mediate the significant employee resources that review required, SSI still requires medical case review of individuals who receive SSI, but the period of review changes depending on whether the disability is classified as one for which improvement is "expected," "possible," or even "not expected" (U.S. Social Security Administration, 2019a, 2019b).

Whether a benefit is characterized as an entitlement or not, benefit recipients are "objects" of the law who have little or no control over the laws that provide access to such necessities of life as income, housing, and health care. Other people set up the rules, other people decide eligibility, other people decide whether the amount is sufficient for your life situation or whether that fact is even relevant, and other people determine if and how you can make a complaint or appeal its outcome. In this context, it cannot be assumed that individuals who are intended recipients under the law in fact receive the benefits for which they are eligible just because the benefits law exists. Nor can it be assumed that everyone who is eligible **equally** benefits from the law, in practice or even in theory. For instance, how a law is administered, whether that is specified in the law or its regulations, or simply left to a de facto matter of written or unwritten policies, has a significant impact on the people who manage to successfully enroll and stay enrolled (or not) in a benefits program (Gustafson, 2011). Moreover, there have been numerous studies at different time periods that establish how complex paperwork and conditional administrative requirements tend to reduce enrollment of people with disabilities in the very public programs that are intended to benefit them (Hahn et al., 2017; Pavetti, Derr, & Martin, 2008). These issues remain highly topical today in light of a January 2018 initiative from the federal Center for Medicare and Medicaid (CMS) that invited states to incorporate work requirements, program limitations, and additional administrative procedures in their Medicaid programs through a Section 1115(b) waiver process (Centers for Medicare and Medicaid Services, 2018) that would allow states to waive some typical Medicaid requirements. Numerous states from Arizona to Kentucky to Utah have applied for CMS approval for at least some segment of their state's Medicaid-eligible population (Grusin, 2019), despite evidence that "red tape and paperwork requirements have been shown to reduce enrollment in Medicaid across the board, and people coping with serious mental illness or physical impairments may face particular difficulties meeting these requirements" (Center on Budget and Policy Priorities, 2019 (revised)). Even if a benefits program purports to make exemptions for people with disabilities, some who should be exempt are inevitably caught up in disenrollment and are disproportionately likely to experience additional administrative delays, penalties, and other interruptions in services.

13.2.3   Titles XVIII and IX of the Social Security Act (Medicare and Medicaid Acts)

Titles XVIII and XIX of the Social Security Act, more commonly known as Medicare and Medicaid, respectively, were signed into law in 1965 as basic health insurance programs for Americans that did not have health insurance. Like social security income payments created 30 years earlier, Medicare was established through a specific payroll tax and primarily conceived as a benefit that would accrue to those over 65 so they would not have to bear on their own, as stated by President Lyndon Johnson, "the problem of costs of illness among our older citizens" (U.S. Social Security Administration, 2019a). Initially, coverage was also quite narrow and primarily limited to costs of hospitalization and doctor visits. Amendments made in 1972 expanded coverage to people under 65 years who required renal dialysis or kidney transplants, as well as people with long-term disabilities; the latter was subject to a considerable waiting period before they could use benefits which was another way to ensure that the disability was long-term (Centers for Medicare and Medicaid Services, 2019). Over the following years, additional benefits such as hospice services for the terminally ill were added to Medicare coverage, people under 65 with amyotrophic lateral sclerosis (ALS) could access Medicare without a waiting period, and access to Medicare services was improved for persons eligible for both Medicaid and Medicare. The next major change to Medicare occurred with the Medicare Prescription Drug, Improvement, and Modernization Act of 2003 (Public Law No: 108-173, 108th Congress, 2003) which allowed Medicare services to be administered and delivered through private health plans and expanded Medicare coverage to include an optional prescription drug benefit that would begin in 2006.

Though the Medicaid act was signed at the same time as the Medicare act, the two laws differed in their intended eligibility population and method of administration, though the development of each law over the decades also reflects similar trends. Medicaid was aimed at specific categories of low-income individuals/families and designed as a "federal-state partnership" with the federal government supplying up to half the costs and a basic framework of federal standards and requirements while each state had considerable freedom to fashion a "state Medicaid plan" that was responsive to "local" conditions and needs. As a result, Medicaid eligibility, benefit coverage, and maintenance rules can differ widely among the states. As in Medicare, Medicaid over the years has seen an expansion of covered population groups (e.g., the broader inclusion of pregnant women and children after the 1972 linking of eligibility to social insurance payments), a wider array of benefits, and increasing use of managed care organizations to deliver public health program services (Using Medicaid to Support Working Age Adults with Serious Mental Illnesses in the Community: A Handbook. A Brief History of Medicaid, 2005). The Omnibus Budget Reconciliation Act of 1981 established a way for states to "waive" certain federal Medicaid requirements and provide personal care assistance and other home- and community-based services to Medicaid-eligible individuals who qualify for an institutional level of care (U.S. Social Security Administration, 2019a), giving people with disabilities and advocates an important way to advocate for community-based services for people with significant chronic disabilities.

We currently live at a time when large national programs such as Social Insurance, Medicaid, Medicare, the Supplemental Nutrition Assistance Program, and Housing and Urban Development (HUD) rental existence have existed for decades. But America is a federal entity where individual states have greater or significant legislative authority over many of the areas that we commonly consider social determinants of health. Health insurance, for example, is primarily a matter of state jurisdiction. However, when the federal government offers states funds to establish a particular program such as Medicaid, then it also has authority to set up a framework of rules and standards for how the program will operate. Both Medicaid and Medicare have seen periods when the federal government, through CMS, has either imposed a greater degree of detailed common program standards and rules **or** has "backed off" and encouraged "state flexibility" and the use of waivers to avoid existing program standards and rules.

The history of the Medicare and Medicaid acts, like the IHS legislation, shows how social insurance laws in the United States originated with general population goals and only came to recognize disability-specific needs over time and often in ways that result in significant coverage gaps arising from the different factors mentioned above. For example, in 1972, younger people with end-stage renal disease (ESRD) were made eligible with a waiting period of only 3 months for Medicare because the condition can quickly lead to known health outcomes that require expensive treatment and make employment difficult or impossible. Roughly 22% of Medicare enrollees purchase private supplemental Medicare insurance or "Medigap" policies to help cover significant co-pays and deductibles which most Medicare enrollees must pay out of pocket (An Analyst in Health Care Financing, 2015). The federal standardization of Medigap policies and increase in consumer protections which took place in the 1980s and 1990s did **not** include individuals under 65 (Center for Medicare Advocacy, 2019). Instead individual states could decide if Medigap insurers had to offer policies to individuals under 65. In 2018, 23 states did **not** mandate this coverage, despite the fact that 43–62% of all individuals in their state with ESRD are under 65 (American Kidney Fund, 2018). That means people under 65 with ESRD can be personally responsible for thousands of dollars in medically necessary lifesaving treatments, even though they have Medicare coverage. California, for example, has a law that requires Medigap insurers to make their plans available to those under 65 who have medical conditions *except for those who have ESRD*, apparently a compromise made between patient groups who wanted guaranteed issue of Medigap policies for people under 65 and insurers who were resistant to covering the treatments needed by ESRD patients (Jaffe, 2016).

Even as there are multiple gaps in law that arise in large part because of a systemic failure to conceive of disability as a natural part of the full range of life experience, we also see an encouraging trend toward recognizing people with disabilities as *subjects* of law and not only objects. This trend can be seen even in the area of health care, benefits, and other laws that directly regulate access to the social determinants of health, though it is most apparent in disability rights laws which will be covered in the next section of this chapter. For example, the 1986 passage of the Employment Opportunities for Disabled Americans Act amended the Medicaid act by permanently authorizing SSI payments and Medicaid eligibility for employed people with disabilities when their earnings exceed maximum eligibility levels but they cannot afford healthcare coverage equal to Medicaid (Pub. L. No. 99-643, 1986). The law necessarily acknowledges the reality of working people with disabilities and the economic and health-related challenge that people with significant disabilities face even after they receive effective education and career opportunities. It may, in fact, be the passage and influence of disability rights laws that have helped infuse concepts such as "person-centered care" and an orientation toward patients as subjects within benefits laws and policies. Nonetheless these concepts can be slow to reach the level of ground-level implementation where disability rights laws similarly encounter resistance to consistent implementation.

13.2.4   Developmental Disabilities Legislation

Benefits or welfare legislation that was developed originally for a population of people with disabilities provides an interesting contrast to how general social insurance law comes to account for disability. The roots of the *Mental Retardation Facilities and Community Health Centers Construction Act of 1963* (Pub. L. No. 88-164, 77 Stat. 282) lie in the medical model's idea at the beginning of the 1960s of what people with developmental disabilities (DD) needed, professional medical expertise and specialized health centers. The main idea was not necessarily to *replace* institutions with community-based services but to *improve* them through improved resources. A 1970 amendment to the law introduced the definition of "developmental disability" for the first time, including some specific diagnostic conditions beyond "mental retardation" that develop before 18 years, and continued the arc of institutional treatment by authorizing state involvement in the construction of institutions and the creation of State Councils on Developmental Disabilities to plan services and support delivery for people with DD (Pub. L. 91-517, 84 Stat. 1316, 1970).

By the mid-1970s, however, DD legislation seemed to take an early step toward recognizing access to law itself as a critical component of health and well-being for people with DD, spurred by the reality that many individuals in this population group face multiple barriers to knowing their rights or enforcing implementation of those rights. As a consequence, the Developmentally Disabled Assistance and Bill of Rights Act (Pub. L. 94-103, 1975) created a set of rights for persons with DD and obligated states that accepted federal financial assistance under the act to establish protection and advocacy programs (P&A) that would advocate for the rights of developmentally disabled individuals and provide them with individual legal and administrative assistance to receive the services assured under federal laws. At the same time, the DD definition was revised again to specify that the listed specific conditions were expected to continue indefinitely and constitute a "substantial" disability. By the 1984 amendments, independence, productivity, and integration were explicitly established as goals within the law (Pub. L. 98-527, 1984). These goals together emphasized developmentally disabled persons' control and choice over their own lives, engagement in work with income, participation in community activities with persons who do not have disabilities, and residence in homes or homelike settings in the community rather than institutional settings. It is interesting to note that these amendments took place 6 years before passage of the Americans with Disabilities Act of 1990 (Pub. L. No. 101-336, 104 Stat. 328, 1990). The 2000 amendments to the DD law also strengthened the P&A agencies in every state by giving them unique access to the records of any individual with DD who is in any residential facility that has received complaints, if the individual either does not have a legal guardian or their guardian is the state. Some P&As have applied this legal investigative power to contemporary issues, such as the treatment of immigrant children and adults with disabilities who have been detained at the southern border of the United States, for example (Fischer, Gonzalez, & Diaz, 2019).

The 2000 amendments saw additional leaps in the development of DD laws which were increasingly both rights-oriented and varied in the services and supports made available for developmentally disabled individuals (Pub. L. 106-402, 114 Stat. 1677, 2000). The critical role of the State Councils on Developmental Disabilities has also crystallized and taken on a character that emphasizes developmentally disabled individuals as subjects of law. The DD Councils had already moved toward a focus on systemic advocacy and deinstitutionalization. These substantive legal changes were now backed up by a legal requirement that DD Council membership had to be one-third composed of persons with DD, one-third composed of parents/guardians of children with DD or relatives of adults with DD who cannot advocate for themselves, and one-third a combination of the first two categories, including at least one adult member who lives in an institution or who represents someone who lives in an institution. The 2000 DD law also appropriated funds for University Centers for Excellence in Developmental Disabilities (UCEDDs), regional research and teaching facilities that provide training and technical assistance on DD to healthcare professionals, as well as direct services and supports to people with DD of all ages and their families.

These newer legal requirements are a meaningful distance from the law that initially focused on funding the construction of segregated state facilities for individuals with DD. The law's motivation has moved from building "better" institutions to helping individuals leave institutions. At the same time, it is worth noting that the relatively comprehensive range of services, supports, research grants, protection of patient rights, and legal advocacy available to people with DD is unique. The current multi-part definition of disability that dates from the 2000 DD law is complex and medically based (Administration for Community Living, 2017). It has moved away from a diagnostic basis, and there is more flexibility for children ages 1–9 years to be diagnosed and therefore eligible for services. However, individuals who have disabilities that manifest after age 22 or who become disabled through an accident, may experience the same significant functional limitations and service needs, economic prospects, level of inaccessibility and discriminatory barriers, and risk of institutionalization but will fall outside of the ambit of the DD laws and their provision of services, supports, and care coordination. The P&A system of legal and administrative representation and technical assistance is the one component of the DD laws that is more broadly available to people with non-DD disabilities through a series of laws that have extended its permissible client base (Children's Health Act of 2000, Pub. L. No. 106-310, 114 Stat. 1101, 2000; Protection and Advocacy for Individuals with Mental Illness Act of 1986, Pub. L. No. 99-319, 100 Stat. 478, 1986; Rehabilitation Act Amendments of 1993, Pub. L. No. 103-73, 107 Stat. 726, 1993).

The deliberate expansion of not only legal rights under the DD laws but the role of attorneys and advocates who are appointed to monitor and aid implementation and enforcement of those rights by people with disabilities is an acknowledgment of law as a social determinant of health, whether that is explicitly stated or not. The myriad services and supports provided to persons with DD and their families under the law, most of which are either directly health-related or are accepted as social determinants of health, such as education, are only paper promises if the rights are unknown and unenforceable once known. Similarly, the best-intentioned laws for improving the health and well-being of people with disabilities cannot function without funding. In this aspect, the federal DD laws are distinguishable from the general Social Security, Medicare, and Medicaid laws which are entitlement laws. The federal and state governments involved are generally obligated to provide stated benefits to everyone who qualifies and applies. That is not the case for the DD law, which requires periodic Congressional appropriations. Funding levels appropriated between 1988 and 2008 remained essentially flat at approximately 170 million in inflation-adjusted 2008 dollars, even as mandates and service coverage have expanded (National Council on Disability, 2011). The final thing to note, in terms of the four factors we noted at the beginning of this chapter, is that the DD law, despite weaknesses of limited funding and wide service and implementation variance among states (National Council on Disability, 2011), is nonetheless a prime example of how federal law can be refined and made increasingly effective and relevant as a tool to further the health and well-being of at least some people with disabilities. This then raises a fundamental question; is the well-being of people with disabilities better served by laws tailored to specific groups of people with disabilities or specific disability-focused issues or by general laws that are drafted, implemented, and enforced in disability-inclusive ways? Which route is more practically and politically viable? Would the answer change depending on the kind of "well-being" that is being addressed?

The next section on disability civil rights laws may not provide the full answer, but it strongly argues the case for emphasizing integration and reasonable accommodation of people with disabilities as a necessary component for achieving laws that benefit people with disabilities.

13.3   Laws Addressing Discrimination

The laws covered in this section are addressed mostly in the chronological order of their passage. They vary in the breadth of their topical coverage, but each has a disability rights approach distinguished by the recognition of individuals with disabilities as subjects of law who have rights that can be enforced by administrative complaints to federal agencies that are given investigative powers and enforcement authority, as well as through purely private lawsuits. The laws single out disability discrimination as a primary barrier for disabled persons and introduced the key concept that *equality could require different treatment* (Mayerson & Yee, 2001). Covered entities that are subject to disability rights law therefore have an obligation to provide physical accessibility, reasonable accommodations, effective communication, and modifications to policies and procedures to ensure equal opportunity and full inclusion of people with disabilities. Each law, below, also gives a federal agency or agencies the authority to develop, enact, and enforce binding regulations that go into significant detail concerning specific standards and requirements under the laws.

13.3.1   Section 504 of the Rehabilitation Act of 1973

As the oldest federal disability civil rights law in the United States, Section 504 of
the Rehabilitation Act of 1973 or Section 504 (Pub. L. No. 93-112, 87 Stat. 394,
1973) prohibits discrimination on the basis of disabilities in programs and activities
that are conducted by the federal government or in public *or* private programs and
activities that receive federal financial assistance. At a little over 70 words, the law's
breadth of coverage is a function of the federal government's breadth of activity and
its deep involvement in funding state and local governments, as well as assisting
individuals who participate in certain activities, such as subsidizing loans to students who attend private colleges. Federal agencies and operations span topical
areas such as transportation, education, health, housing, welfare, criminal and civil
law, civil rights in employment, and the US postal service. Section 504's brevity is
possible because various federal agencies are charged with developing, promulgat-
ing, and enforcing much more detailed regulations that establish non-discrimination
standards and enforcement rights and remedies. This approach, which gives a significant role to agency regulatory action, was carried over to the ADA, even though
that later law was both longer and more detailed than Section 504. The positive
aspects of this approach include the benefit of agency subject matter expertise and
the potential for individuals with lived experience, advocates, and academics to
shape regulations by submitting public comments that agencies are legally required
to read and consider. The negative aspects include court decisions that can narrowly
impose interpretive boundaries on what agency regulations can authorize in light of
what an actual Congressional law says (National Council on Disability, 2001), and
the risk that a given administration will stock federal agencies with political appoin-
tees that are disinterested in consumer advocacy and rights or even in upholding the
legitimate professed goals of the agency.

Much of Section 504's power as "the first disability civil rights law" derives from
its role as a catalyst for the birth of a disability civil rights movement with wide-
ranging political, social, cultural, and legal ramifications that would resonate for
several decades (Pelka, 2012; The Power of 504, 1977). The 5 years that passed
between Section 504's enactment and the implementation and enforcement of the
regulations that brought that law to practical life were marked by increasing protests
and direct action by people with disabilities, culminating in a week-long occupation
of a federal building in San Francisco by disabled people, aided by a wide range of
civil rights allies and advocates. Section 504 is the best-known section of the
Rehabilitation Act in terms of disability civil rights, but other sections of the
Rehabilitation Act were also enacted to ensure equal opportunities for people with
disabilities, particularly in the area of employment. Section 501 requires federal
agencies of the executive branch to provide disability affirmative action and non-
discrimination in employment practices (Pub. L. No. 93-112, 87 Stat. 390, 1973),
and Section 503 requires the same from larger federal government contractors and
subcontractors (Pub. L. No. 93-112, 87 Stat. 393, 1973). Section 508 has become
increasingly important with the ongoing advance of digital electronic and

information technology since it requires technology that is developed, maintained, procured, or used by the federal government to be accessible to people with disabilities, including employees and members of the public (Pub. L. No. 93-112, 87 Stat. 394, 1973).

The next two laws each are good examples of all three ways in which law connects with public health and people with disabilities. Each law is specific to people with disabilities, the laws deal with education and housing, respectively (both of which are widely acknowledged as being a SDoH), and each law follows the civil rights model of recognizing persons with disabilities as subjects of law who have direct access to administrative complaint mechanisms and courts for enforcement. Neither law is particularly explicit about the connections between education, housing, and either public or individual health, but they function to remove barriers that impede people with disabilities from achieving higher levels of education and accessible affordable housing. In that respect, the third law addressed below, the Americans with Disabilities Act (ADA), is similarly intended to remove discriminatory barriers that inhibit people with disabilities from entering mainstream American life on multiple fronts and therefore functions as an indirect way to address disability access to various SDoH. Like the education and housing laws, the ADA's connection with health is mostly unsaid. The final three acts described in this section are more explicit about the connections between discrimination and health as they are topical healthcare laws.

13.3.2   Individuals with Disabilities Education Act

The Individuals with Disabilities Education Act (IDEA) (Pub. L. No. 101-476, 104 Stat. 1142, 1990), renamed from the Education for all Handicapped Children Act of 1975, requires public schools to make available to all eligible children with disabilities a free appropriate public education (FAPE) in the least restrictive environment appropriate to the child's education needs. The FAPE requirement in public education is the core of IDEA since it includes both federal financial assistance to State and local education agencies and the concomitant obligation to ensure that eligible children with disabilities from 3 to 21 years receive special education and related services. The obligation includes developing an Individualized Education Plan (IEP) that meets the needs of individual students with disabilities and requires annual review. IEP development must also follow strict procedural obligations and include the child's teacher(s); the parents (or educational guardian), subject to certain limited exceptions; the child, if determined appropriate; an education agency representative who is qualified to provide or supervise the provision of special education; and other individuals at the parents' or agency's discretion. Under IDEA, the parents of a student with disabilities receive numerous due process rights that are intended to safeguard the child's right to an IEP and FAPE. For example, parents who disagree with a school's proposed IEP and feel they did not receive adequate notice or consideration can request a due process hearing and a review from the state educational agency. Parents can also privately appeal the state agency's decision to state or federal court. In practice knowing how to maintain those rights and when to trigger them can be significant responsibilities for parents, especially parents with limited English proficiency or who work full-time in low-income jobs with limited time to prepare for and attend IEP and service meetings. Due process proceedings and lawsuits take even more preparation time, and advocacy and attorney assistance can be hard to find. IDEA's enforcement and regulatory authority rest with the Office of Special Education and Rehabilitation Services (OSERS) in the US Department of Education.

IDEA intersects with disability health needs in several ways. For example, there is usually considerable overlap between a child's general disability-related healthcare needs and the kinds of special education services or devices recognized in the IEP as essential for educational benefit such as speech therapy or assistive technology. There can also be some overlap in coverage between a school district's special education obligation and a child's Medicaid or private health insurance coverage, but close coordination between school districts and local education authorities and a child's healthcare providers is not common and children can still experience gaps in service needs. It is also important to remember that some children with disabilities will not qualify under IDEA, which applies to 13 specific disability categories and a more general "other health impairments" category. The categories include autism, vision impairments, deafness/hearing impairments, deaf-blindness, intellectual disability, developmental delay, orthopedic impairments, serious emotional disturbance, specific learning disabilities, speech or language impairments, traumatic brain injury, and multiple disabilities. IDEA therefore retains ties with a diagnostic medical concept of disability.

The overlap between IDEA and Section 504 is also worth noting. Public schools receive federal financial assistance, and Section 504's broader definition of disability obligates schools to provide disability-related accommodations and policy modifications so that a child with disabilities will have equal access to educational benefits, even if the child's disability does not fit IDEA's requirements. For example, a student who has asthma, HIV, or another chronic condition may not qualify for special education under IDEA if the condition is medically controlled and the child is achieving excellent grades and getting along well with peers. However, the child could still qualify under Section 504 for an educational plan that ensured equal access to education, by allowing the child to self-modify PE activities outside without penalty when there is poor air quality, for example, or exceed the number of "tardy" times typically tolerated in a given month because of standing morning medical appointments. Any student who qualifies under IDEA would also be protected under Section 504, but the reverse is not true. It also may be helpful, when distinguishing between the two, to recall what advocates often say: special education is a service, not a place. IDEA is not only or necessarily for students who are stereotypically associated with a segregated classroom. At the same time, a disabled student may, for whatever reasons, not seem to require special education services regardless of having a medical diagnosis (DREDF, 2018).

13.3.3   Fair Housing Act

The Fair Housing Act (FHA) has long defined and prohibited housing discrimination on multiple bases such as race, color, religion, sex, familial status, and national origin and, after amendments made in 1988, includes disability as well (Pub. L. No. 100-430, 102 Stat. 1625, 1988). FHA extends beyond housing that receives federal financial assistance to include private housing as well as State and local government housing. Housing discrimination includes treating prospective or current buyers or renters differently because of their disability in the sale or rental of housing or denying housing to a buyer or renter who has a disability or who is associated with an individual with disabilities who intends to live in the residence (i.e., a spouse or child). FHA covers a wide swath of housing activities such as marketing, financing, zone practices, and new construction design.

The FHA also obligates housing owners to make reasonable accommodations in their policies and procedures to ensure that people with disabilities get equal housing opportunities. For example, a building cannot use a "no pets" policy to refuse to rent to someone who uses a service animal related to a disability. However, housing owners must allow, but need not pay for, reasonable access-related modifications of private and common living spaces such as laundry facilities, so that a tenant can equally enjoy the benefits of their housing. New construction of multi-family housing with four or more units must have specific accessible design features in the units and accessible common areas.

Enforcement and regulation-making authority under the FHA lies with the US Department of Housing and Urban Development (HUD). Individual renters, buyers, and housing applicants can file an administrative complaint with HUD or bring a private civil lawsuit. Everyone needs affordable permanent housing, but people with mobility disabilities, persons with mental health disabilities that continue to be highly stigmatized among the general public, and people who use assistance or emotional support animals can find it especially difficult to find housing that provides the physical features and/or policies that allow them to feel secure and fully functional in their own homes. Under the current federal administration, HUD recently proposed a new "Affirmatively Furthering Fair Housing" rule that significantly weakens strong non-discrimination regulations that were first issued under President Obama (Department of Housing and Urban Development, 2020), sending a signal to renters/buyers with disabilities, housing advocates, and landlords that ensuring housing for people with disabilities and other groups that have traditionally faced housing discrimination is not a HUD priority.

13.3.4 Americans with Disabilities Act

The Americans with Disabilities Act of 1990 (ADA) passed Congress close to two decades after Section 504, and the ADA emulates both the breadth of Section 504's topical scope and its model of dividing regulatory and enforcement authority among different federal agencies, but the ADA is still likely the more well-known and most iconic law with regard to disability rights. The ADA indisputably places people with disabilities as subjects at the center of the law and was written and passed through close coordination among the grassroots disability community, specific disability advocacy groups, and elected officials and lawyers with disabilities (Wright & West, 2002). As a civil rights law, the ADA does not address disability benefits laws and does not take a human rights approach that directly recognizes the right of individuals with disabilities to have their needs acknowledged and met. Instead, the law focuses on eliminating physical and procedural barriers that people with disabilities encounter when entering economic, social, and cultural life in the United States and extends Section 504's mandate of non-discrimination from the public sector to the private sector. As a result, purely private, state, and local government entities such as cities, in activities ranging from transportation to retail to telecommunication to simple employment (where there are at least 15 or more employees), must provide a "level playing field" for consumers and employees with disabilities, irrespective of any federal government involvement or funding.

The law is organized in five "titles." The federal Equal Employment Opportunity Commission (EEOC) has regulatory and enforcement authority over Title I which focuses on employment. It is the only title that requires "administrative exhaustion" by requiring employees to first file a discrimination complaint with the EEOC and get permission before bringing a private lawsuit in federal court. Title II governs non-discrimination in state and local government programs and activities and vests regulatory and enforcement authority in the federal Department of Justice (DOJ). Public transportation and state and county/municipal healthcare services are also covered in Title II, with the Federal Transit Administration (FTA) and the federal Department of Health and Human Services (HHS), respectively, holding regulatory and enforcement authority. Title III broadly covers "places of public accommodation," defined as privately owned retail and service establishments, and DOJ primarily holds regulatory and enforcement authority. Private health entities such as "a pharmacy, insurance office, professional office of a health care provider, hospital, or other service establishment" are explicitly listed as public accommodations in the regulations enacted under Title III (28 C.F.R. Part 36. § 36.104). Title IV is specific to telecommunications relay services, and the Federal Communications Commission has regulatory and enforcement authority. Title V has miscellaneous provisions, including ones that prohibit bad behavior linked to disability such as retaliation against disabled persons who try to enforce their ADA rights or discrimination on the basis of being associated with a person with a disability, such as not promoting an employee who has a child with a disability.

One of the most groundbreaking aspects of the ADA is how the law tried to adapt and respond to concepts of disability that were newly developed in areas such as disability studies at the time. The ADA's "three-pronged definition" of an individual with a disability is a person who has a physical or mental impairment that substantially limits one or more major life activities, a person who has a history or record of such an impairment, or a person who is regarded by others as having such an impairment. The third prong encompassed the social model of disability by recognizing that the legal significance of having a disability does not arise purely as a consequence of physiological symptoms or medical diagnosis as one can be disabled by external barriers and how others treat one. Unfortunately, the conceptual breadth of the definition was interpretively difficult for some courts who treated the definition as setting a high evidentiary threshold for plaintiffs, who had to go into court establishing all the things they could *not* do before they could even try to establish the defendant entity's discriminatory behavior. Even now, the ADA does not contain an exhaustive listing of impairments or disabling conditions, but the ADA Amendments Act of 2008 incorporated a list of physiological conditions that, in the context of litigation, has helped some individuals with disabilities to quickly move past the threshold stage of being recognized as a person with a disability so that they could invoke the law and at least get an opportunity to establish the presence of discrimination. Other important conceptual innovations in the ADA include the groundbreaking concepts of "reasonable accommodations" and "reasonable modifications of policies and procedures" which clearly recognized that people with various disabilities were in a different position than non-disabled persons and therefore needed *different treatment* under the law with regard to both physical and non-physical barriers.

Section 504 and the ADA have been interpreted by courts in essentially similar ways since the ADA was enacted, mostly following legal principles developed in detail under the ADA when it comes to a covered entity's obligation to be physically accessible and provide reasonable accommodations, reasonable modifications of policies and procedures, and effective communication. Healthcare providers, hospitals, and managed care organization are to operate in physical spaces that enable people with disabilities to have physical access and freedom to move about and use the entire facility as independently as possible. Covered entities are required to ensure that they meet specified dimensions for such things as doorway widths, sink height, clear pathways of travel, and elevator Braille signage. Reasonable accommodations and modifications of policies and procedures mean that entities must adjust "typical" office policies and procedures so people with disabilities receive equally effective services. For instance, a medical office may typically require patients to independently undress and get on an exam table, but an individual with functional mobility limitations may need assistance to undress or transfer to an exam table, especially one that has a high fixed height. A healthcare provider cannot refuse to serve a person with a disability because its "procedures" don't usually include personal assistance and cannot require the person with a disability to bring their own personal assistant. Similarly, healthcare entities cannot require a person who is deaf or hard of hearing to bring their own interpreter or charge them extra for interpretation services or require someone who is blind to bring an assistant who can fill out forms for them. Rather, healthcare providers are responsible for "effective communication" that can include sign language interpretation for patients with disabilities, written communications in alternate formats such as Braille or large font print, and additional time to accommodate people with speech or developmental disabilities so that they can provide and receive information from providers for themselves. These legal requirements are not unlimited. A covered entity's specific degree of obligation under Section 504 and the ADA will vary somewhat depending on an entity's size and assets, whether it falls under Title II or Title III of the ADA, or if it receives federal funding.

Part of the ADA's innovation lies in how it tackled some unique aspects of disability discrimination and access. The drafters of the law had to find ways to reach barriers and behaviors that were not necessarily driven by active malice so much as misguided pity, stereotype, and ignorant neglect. The law was especially groundbreaking in its definition of disability and conceptualization of disabled persons as central to the invocation and enforcement of the law, but it is nevertheless not particularly instrumental for addressing the health and healthcare disparities that people with disabilities experience throughout their lives. At their core, the ADA and Section 504 address barriers that can be viewed as discriminatory, and courts have interpreted this to include barriers that have a disparate impact on disabled persons without the need for any finding of animus or bad intention on the part of a defendant (Alexander v. Choate, 1985), but US disability rights laws do not proactively guarantee that people with disabilities will receive needed healthcare coverage or will have basic access to income sufficient to meet disability-related needs, accessible housing, education, nutritious food, or other SDoH. The ADA addresses one highly significant barrier that can impede access to available healthcare services and other SDoH, pervasive discrimination, but civil rights law is not easily wielded to address long-standing and problematic systemic, economic, and structural assumptions about disability and chronic conditions that are embedded in something like how quality-adjusted life years (QALYs) are used to evaluate effectiveness of medical treatments (NCD, 2019b), for instance, or how American health care historically values and funds urgent care over long-term care needs, or how Medicaid favors providing institutional long-term care over home- and community-based long-term care (Kaye & Williamson, 2014).

13.3.5   Paul Wellstone and Pete Domenici Mental Health Parity and Addiction Equity Act of 2008 and Genetic Information Non-discrimination Act of 2008

Both the Mental Health Parity and Addiction Equity Act (MHPAEA) (Division C of Pub. L. 110-343, Section 511 and 512, 2008) and the Genetic Information Non-discrimination Act (GINA) (P.L 110-233, 2008) take a non-discrimination approach that recognizes, respectively, individuals with psychosocial or behavioral health disabilities have the right in certain conditions to equal coverage of their health needs and individuals who have the genetic propensity to develop disabilities in the future have the right to be free from workplace and health insurance coverage discrimination. GINA is administered by the EEOC, and, similar to Title I of the ADA, an aggrieved employee may file an administrative complaint for a violation of GINA with the EEOC, which will investigate and either dismiss the case, giving the complainant a right to file a lawsuit within 90 days, or issue a letter of determination and attempt a conciliation. If this conciliation fails, the agency will either file a lawsuit itself or give the complainant permission to file a lawsuit within 90 days.

MHPAEA does not mandate that employment insurance coverage must cover mental health and addiction treatment, but *if* employment coverage offers such treatment, the law requires that treatment to be offered without quantitative or qualitative limitations such as higher co-payments or cost sharing that are more restrictive than coverage of medical/surgical treatment. In theory, MHPAEA is enforced by a range of federal and state agencies, including state departments of health insurance, the federal Health and Human Services Agency, and the federal Department of Labor (Ard, 2017) depending on the type of insurance coverage at play. The parity law does not directly provide for a private right of action, but MHPAEA protections are included in a section of the federal Employee Retirement Income Security Act (ERISA) that does allow beneficiaries to bring a lawsuit once internal insurance appeals have been exhausted. Some states have also established private rights of action for MHPAEA violations. In practice, agency MHPAEA enforcement has been uneven across states and agencies, leaving enforcement responsibility in the hands of consumers who simultaneously may be dealing with mental health crises or unmet addiction treatment needs. Like IDEA and other civil rights-based laws, placing a rights-bearing individual at the center of a law often means making that individual a linchpin of enforcement, which can be simultaneously empowering and extremely challenging for the individual.

Recent widely recognized public health issues in the United States such as rising suicide rates among young adults and the opioid crises highlight a critical need for people of all ages to have access to mental health and addiction services. In this context, MHPAEA's protections assume even greater importance, which also brings its weaknesses into sharp relief. Some states simply fail to aggressively enforce MHPAEA. Private consumers bear a heavy burden to distinguish what kind of coverage they have in relation to ERISA, exhaust internal insurer appeals, and shoulder the costs of needed advocacy or legal assistance (Ard, 2017). Ultimately, MHPAEA does **not** mandate mental health and addiction treatment; it only requires parity when plans already offer such treatment coverage. This is why, with respect to mental health treatment as well as in various other ways, passage of the Affordable Care Act was such a game changer for people with disabilities.

13.3.6   The Affordable Care Act, Including Section 1557

The Patient Protection and Affordable Care Act (ACA) (Pub. L. No. 111-148, 2010) straddles both "welfare" laws and civil rights/non-discrimination laws as characterized above in this chapter. The ACA perhaps also displays most explicitly the three levels of connection between law and public health that this chapter explores. The law does not look like a typical welfare law since it did not primarily establish a new social program of monetary, health, food, or other benefits for a discrete vulnerable or underserved population. Nonetheless, the ACA functionally *acts* as a welfare law in many ways. It establishes new kinds and levels of federal support for existing healthcare benefits and attempts to mandate a kind of universal benefit that folded in different preexisting payers rather than create a new single payer. By including both Medicaid and private payers and outright abolishing private insurance's ability to refuse coverage or charge more on the basis of preexisting conditions, the ACA implicitly espoused a "disability rights" view, one that recognizes disability as a natural part of life and fully includes people with disabilities in the same healthcare system that serves everyone else. The ACA did not transform the US healthcare system so much as hijack it and attempt to impose a new framework of benefits coverage, legal access, and non-discrimination over a highly complex system that crossed multiple public and private programs and entities and federal and state jurisdictions, and recognized sub-populations that experience health and healthcare disparities.

The major programs created under the ACA, Medicaid expansion and the creation of private insurance marketplaces, were intended to ensure affordable healthcare coverage for all Americans, but many of the specific rules enacted to provide a floor of fair comprehensive coverage were of "disparate benefit" to people with disabilities. Persons with various disabilities or chronic conditions who had too high an income or levels of assets could qualify for Medicaid in at least some states under new modified adjusted gross income rules. The guaranteed issue and community rating requirements protect people with disabilities and chronic conditions from private insurers' historically common outright denials and exorbitantly priced coverage. The Essential Health Benefits categories that had to be covered in marketplace plans include mental health and substance use disorder services, habilitation and rehabilitation services and devices, and prescription drugs, three categories that are vitally important for many disabled persons but which private insurers in the individual and small group marketplaces could previously omit from coverage partially or fully.

When the ACA and its regulations directly facilitate consistent and sufficient access to needed health care for people with disabilities, including long-term services and supports in some circumstances, the law addresses the first and second levels of connection between law and public health. The law also has an important non-discrimination provision, however, that is explicitly rights-oriented and holds rights-bearing patients at the center of the law while recognizing discriminatory characteristics that limit patient access to health care. Section 1557 of the ACA establishes a broad non-discrimination requirement on the basis of race, color, national origin, sex, age, or disability that references already existing civil rights statutes, including Section 504, and applies them to heath programs and activities which are federally conducted or that receive federal financial assistance. This is significant on the disability front for several reasons. First, the purely private insurers that participate in the individual marketplaces now fall within the scope of Section 1557 and are subject to a non-discrimination mandate, when previously they had fallen within a regulatory "safe harbor" provision in Title V of the ADA that protected the traditional actuarially based decisions of private insurers (42 U.S.C. § 12201(c), 2012; Blake, 2017). Second, the regulations enacted under Section 1557 by the HHS Office for Civil Rights (OCR) clearly reference benefit design, thereby offering disabled persons, advocates, and attorneys an opportunity to question the plan coverage and exclusion decisions that many courts had deemed out of reach, though how far Section 1557 will ultimately reach remains unclear (Doe v. Mutual of Omaha, 1999) (E.S. et al. v. Regence BlueShield et al., 2018). The final non-discrimination regulation passed by HHS OCR in 2016 pointed out in commentary some examples of plan benefit design that could be considered discriminatory under the rule such as placing all of the drug regimens for a particular condition like HIV/AIDS on the most expensive drug formulary tier, though OCR did not include a larger list of benefit design examples that would be considered de facto discriminatory (45 C.F.R. Part 92, 2016). The 2016 final rule also does not include an explicit reference to intersectional discrimination which could encompass, for example, the multiple barriers or bad behavior encountered by people with disabilities who are of a particular race, ethnicity, age, sexual orientation, or gender identity, though the rule's preamble acknowledges that such discrimination "should" be covered under the provisions of Section 1557 (45 C.F.R. Part 92, 2016). Finally, it should be noted that under the current administration, HHS OCR has put out a proposed 1557 rule that roles back and narrows the scope of the current 1557 regulation (84 Fed. Reg. 27846-27895, 27848, 2019), particularly with regard to prohibiting discrimination on the basis of sexual orientation and gender identity.

The ACA has been highlighted by at least one legal scholar as a unique hybrid law that functions as a civil rights law despite its official and popular characterization as a health law (Roberts, 2013), leading her to the conclusion that integrating substantive protections into a civil rights agenda allows advocates "to address the subtle, second-generation discrimination that perpetuates existing inequalities." Professor Roberts sees the potential for other civil rights groups to use this approach, but it could equally be useful for disability rights advocates and researchers strategizing about how law could be used to shape disability-inclusive SDoH other than healthcare access. Ultimately, the promise of the approach must be tempered by the reality that has already been alluded to in this chapter: the successful achievement of a law cannot be expected to fully resolve complex issues. The actual litigation that has been brought under Section 1557 has seen mixed success when raising the possibility of a new integrated right of action in health care that avoids the substantive and procedural limitations that have developed in the jurisprudence of each individual civil rights act that is referenced in Section 1557 (Doe v. Bluecross

Blueshield of Tennessee Inc., 2019; Rumble v. Fairview Health Services et al., 2015). Even with attempts to use Section 1557 in a perhaps more straightforward application of Section 504 to challenge historically ubiquitous discriminatory benefit design, courts have been uneasy about applying case law to the insurance exclusions and practices that have historically excluded disabled persons (E.S. et al. v. Regence BlueShield et al., 2018) (Schmitt v. Kaiser Foundation Health Plan of Washington, 2018). American case law is built on precedent, and judges may be reluctant to expand long-standing civil rights case interpretations of the limitations of the ADA and Section 504 in the insurance and healthcare arena, without a principled way to control that expansion and on the basis of what is only arguably implied in the wording of Section 1557.

There are some other discrete ways that disability concerns are raised in the ACA that are worth mentioning. Section 4302 mandated specific data collection measures on disability, requiring questions on disability status to be included in federal national data collection efforts such as population health surveys to the extent this could be practically achieved. The section also empowered HHS to collect data such as where people with disabilities receive care, which could help researchers to gain greater understanding into how disability health and healthcare disparities systemically occur. Like most legal provisions, however, funding to implement the mandate requires ongoing appropriations. There was a multi-year appropriation for this section when the ACA was first passed that has now ended, and it is unclear how additional funds could be appropriated to continue funding this data collection. Section 4203 is another important and distinct disability provision in the ACA that required the US Access Board, an independent federal standard-setting entity, to establish guidelines for accessible medical examination and diagnostic equipment. The Access Board engaged in a multi-year process and did achieve consensus on a set of standards that were approved internally, but the standards do not have the force of law unless and until the Department of Justice adopts them into regulation and develops relevant scoping rules so that covered entities of various sizes and types will know how many types of each category of exam and diagnostic equipment must be purchased and available for use. The Community First Choice (CFC) Option is another important program first created under the ACA. It incentivizes states to rebalance their Medicaid state plan by increasing home- and community-based long-term services and supports to eligible beneficiaries with disabilities and maximizing self-direction among Medicaid beneficiaries. The CFC Option is, itself, an example of how civil rights laws can come full circle to influence welfare/benefits laws. *Olmstead v. L.C.* (1999), a 1999 Supreme Court decision interpreting Title II of the ADA and well-known among many in the disability community, squarely characterized unnecessary segregation as discrimination and elevated the right of persons with disabilities to live in their own homes and communities with appropriate health and long-term supports. These are the same disability rights principles that lie behind the development of the CFC Option, even though the option arises as a federal funding mechanism in a health insurance bill.

13.4   Conclusion

In addition to the multiple ways in which the ACA illustrates the connections between law and pubic health which are addressed in this chapter, it can also be used to illustrate one more dimension that is not so much a simple connection between law and SDoH as it is an overarching context for both law and SDoH. The ACA was passed in 2010, but state expansion of Medicaid and the operational start of the federal and state marketplaces did not begin until 2014. In the spring of 2019, a group of consumer representatives in the National Association of Insurance Commissioners (NAIC) initiated a focus group study to try and determine whether consumers could distinguish between the comprehensive insurance products regulated in the marketplaces and the short-term limited duration plans which did not have to meet ACA protections but had been touted by the current administration as cheaper viable insurance alternatives for some people. The focus group members each spent an hour one-on-one with a focus group leader going over a short-term plan and disclosure statement. Most consumers had difficulty in that time understanding what a short-term plan was:

> Consumer confusion is exacerbated by the fact that most consumers have become accustomed to, and now expect, their health insurance to reflect the Affordable Care Act's consumer protections. ... the study underscores that consumers do not expect short-term plans to lack the basic benefit standards, cost-sharing parameters, preexisting condition guarantees, and other features that help insulate consumers from financial harm when they buy an Affordable Care Act plan. (Consumer Representives Appointed to the National Association of Insurance Commissioners (NAIC, 2019)).

Laws are ultimately written, acted upon, and interpreted by individuals who do not exist in a stagnant social or cultural context. Over time there is a powerful "feedback loop" between law and society, with factors such as shortening news cycles and social media acting to speed up how quickly feedback occurs. In 2011, one legal scholar described what he saw as a "dual-track" relationship between law and public health: "law helps structure and perpetuate the social conditions that we describe as 'social determinants,' and (2) law acts as a mechanism or mediator through which social structures are transformed into levels and distributions of health" (Burris, 2011). While the observation is useful, it does not seem to factor in the two-way street of influence between law and social structures. The operation of law can impact what people think about, and expect from, the social structures around them. Access to health, as a practical matter of insurance coverage and as a right, is understood differently by many members of the public after multiple years of the ACA. The ACA, in turn, with its framing of benefit design as potentially discriminatory and an overall approach that emphasized how everyone needs good health care, regardless of disability or any other personal characteristic, may not have been possible without the operation of many years of disability rights laws and the open inclusion of people with various disabilities in all aspects of society. And these influences of law, social change, and increased public awareness of economic and power imbalances, all contribute toward a more rounded and nuanced understanding of what constitutes a SDoH.

13.5   Additional Legal References and Resources of Significance to People with Disabilities

- Help America Vote Act (Pub. L. No. 107-252, 116 Stat. 1666, 2002)
  This law requires the provision of physical and programmatic accessibility in all parts of the voting process, from voter registration and training of poll workers to voting equipment and provisional ballots. Voting is a critical component of civic engagement and impacts how the disabled community is perceived as a politically identifiable group and how disabled persons perceive themselves politically.
- Money Follows the Person and Rebalancing
  The Money Follows the Person Rebalancing Demonstration was first conceived of and passed through the Deficit Reduction Act of 2005 (Pub. L. No. 109-171, 2006) and subsequently reauthorized and further funded through federal appropriations in various laws, including the ACA, and most recently in 2019 legislation. The Demonstration financially incentivizes states rebalancing their Medicaid long-term care options toward home- and community-based supports and away from segregated institutional care that people with disabilities often neither want nor require. Over 75,000 individuals with disabilities have transitioned from institutions back into the community under MFP Demonstration projects as of the end of 2016 (Centers for Medicare and Medicaid Services, n.d.).
- Prenatally and Postnatally Diagnosed Conditions Awareness Act (Pub. L. No. 110-374, 122 Stat. 4051, 2008)
  Technological advances in genetic testing for an increasing number of health conditions and disabilities, in conjunction with entrepreneurial and corporate efforts to commercialize these technologies, and ambitious "rogue" scientific efforts to manipulate and engineer human genetics, have led to multifaceted difficult questions for disability communities, as well as disability rights and reproductive rights/justice advocates (National Council on Disabilities, 2019a). The PPDCAA remains one of the very few laws to exist at this uneasy juncture of individual/community and current/future interests. The bipartisan bill was intended to ensure that families who receive genetic testing results indicating the presence of disability receive current and scientifically accurate information about the physical, developmental, educational, and psychosocial outcomes of living with the genetic condition(s) in question. The proposed law would also require the provision of information about the accuracy of the genetic test and disability service referrals. While the bill quickly passed in Congress, it lost its proposed funding along the way and has subsequently had very limited impact in meeting its goals.
- "Public Charge" Regulations and Immigration Proposals (EO on health insurance)
  The "Inadmissability on Public Charge Grounds" final regulation (84 FR 41292, 41292-41508, 2019) was first proposed by the US Citizenship and Immigration Services, Department of Homeland Security, in 2019 and garnered over 266,000

public comments. Under the rule, health status and the presence of disability play a prominent role in how and when an immigrant can be denied admissibility or permanent residence status. Both the final rule and various other immigration-related proposals such as Executive Orders and requirements for proof of health insurance from immigrants have been challenged through litigation brought by advocacy groups who have raised, among other causes of action, the legality of the regulatory action under the Administrative Procedure Act (Pub. L. No. 404-79, 1946).

- Gun Safety and Violence Proposals Focused on Mental Health
Various federal and state proposals have been advanced over the past several years as the United States has experienced tragic and widely covered incidences of gun-related mass shootings, many involving minors. The shootings, as well as all forms of violence relating to guns including suicide, are themselves a public health issue, but the subsequent public association of such violence with individuals with mental health disabilities raises both a distinct public health issue and disability rights issues, especially when such public associations and perceptions are delinked from actual evidence and behavior.

- State, Local, and Municipal Laws on Various Topics such as Family Laws, Vaccination Requirements, and Zoning Bylaws
Many of the topics that affect the daily lives of people with disabilities, deeply implicating their right and practical ability to attend public schools in their own school district, their right to live in supported housing in their community, and their right to have, raise, and keep their children, for example, fall within the jurisdiction of states rather than the federal government. States establish and maintain family law courts, local school districts often have the right to set their own vaccination requirements, and municipalities commonly establish zoning and construction restrictions. While Title II of the ADA does in theory cover all of these entities, in practice, state and local governments in particular are not automatically "self-policing" in their substantive and procedural adherence to disability non-discrimination.

- Convention on the Rights of Persons with Disabilities
This groundbreaking international law on the rights of disabled persons was made possible, in part, by the example of the ADA, which is the first national domestic law on disability rights to be widely recognized among other nations. The CRPD itself is a unique melding of ADA-style disability civil rights as processed through the broader lens of human rights and is readily available online through United Nations sites that also carry it in various languages as well as disability-accessible versions.

13.6 Questions

- How would you characterize, in your own words, the relationship between public health research and demonstrating a need for either a new law or modifying an existing law? What are other considerations that you could address in addition to research?
- Name three ways in which you or your family have experienced the law's connections with public health or the social determinants of health, as outlined in this chapter?
- What are examples of the kind of research that you could undertake if you wanted to support a law to proportionally increase Medicaid funding for home- and community-based services and supports for people with disabilities in your state? Would you want your research, and therefore the law, to cover all people with disabilities, or would you try to target a specific subgroup, by age or by other racial, ethnic, or gender characteristics? Would your research design and thesis change if your goal is to have legislation that directed private insurers to cover home- and community-based services as an integral part of health insurance?
- Do you think the health and wellness needs of people with disabilities are best achieved through specific legislation that primarily focuses on people with disabilities, whether broadly or as specific subgroups, or by legislation that explicitly recognizes disability and people with disabilities within a generally applicable law?
- How can you incorporate the concerns of people with disabilities into the range of your current research interests?

References

Administration for Community Living. (2017). *History of the DD Act Administration for Community Living*. Retrieved January 30, 2020, from https://acl.gov/about-acl/history-dd-act#ftn7

Alexander v. Choate, 469 U.S. 287. (1985).

American Kidney Fund. (2018, February 2). *Medigap and ESRD*. Retrieved January 30, 2020, from https://www.kidneyfund.org/advocacy-blog/medigap-and-esrd.html

Americans with Disabilities Act of 1990, Pub. L. No. 101-336, 104 Stat. 328 (1990). (1990, July 26).

Analyst in Health Care Financing [author name redacted]. (2015, June 24). *Medigap: A primer*. Washington, DC: Congressional Research Service. Retrieved January 30, 2020, from https://www.everycrsreport.com/reports/R42745.html

Ard, J. P. (2017). An unfulfilled promise: Ineffective enforcement of mental health parity. *Annals of Health Law, 26*, 70–85.

Artiga, S. U., Ubri, P., & Foutz, J. (2017, September 7). *Medicaid and American Indians and Alaska natives*. Kaiser Family Foundation. Retrieved January 30, 2020, from https://www.kff.org/medicaid/issue-brief/medicaid-and-american-indians-and-alaska-natives/

Blake, V. (2017). *Rethinking the Americans with disabilities Act's insurance safe harbor*. MDPI Open Access Articles. Retrieved from https://www.mdpi.com/2075-471X/6/4/25/htm

Burris, S. (2011). From health care law to the social determinants of health: A public health law research respective. *University of Pennsylvania Law Review, 159*, 1649–1666.

45 C.F.R. Part 92. (2016). *Nondiscrimination in Health Programs and Activities*. Final Rule, 81 Fed. Reg. 31465.

Center for Medicare Advocacy. (2019, November 24). *Medigap*. Retrieved January 30, 2020, from https://www.medicareadvocacy.org/medicare-info/medigap/

Center on Budget and Policy Priorities. (2019 (revised), March 14). *Taking away Medicaid for not meeting work requirements harms older Americans*. Retrieved January 30, 2020, from https://www.cbpp.org/research/health/taking-away-medicaid-for-not-meeting-work-requirements-harms-older-americans

Centers for Disease Control and Prevention. (2019, October 25). *Adults with disabilities: Ethnicity and race*. Retrieved January 30, 2020, from https://www.cdc.gov/ncbddd/disabilityandhealth/materials/infographic-disabilities-ethnicity-race.html

Centers for Medicare and Medicaid Services. (2018, January 11). *1115 Community Engagement Initiative*. Retrieved January 30, 2020, from https://www.medicaid.gov/medicaid/section-1115-demo/community-engagement/index.html

Centers for Medicare and Medicaid Services. (2019, August 5). Centers for Medicare and Medicaid Services. Retrieved December 10, 2019, from https://www.cms.gov/About-CMS/Agency-Information/History/index

Centers for Medicare and Medicaid Services. (n.d.). *Money follows the person*. Retrieved January 28, 2020, from https://www.medicaid.gov/medicaid/long-term-services-supports/money-follows-person/index.html

Children's Health Act of 2000, Pub. L. No. 106-310, 114 Stat. 1101. (2000).

Degener, T., & Quinn, G. T. (2002). A survey of international, comparative and regional disability law reform. In M. L. Breslin & S. Yee (Eds.), *Disability rights law and policy: International and National Perspectives* (pp. 3–125). Leiden: Brill-Nijhoff.

Department of Housing and Urban Development. (2020, January 14). *Affirmatively Furthering Fair Housing Proposed Rule*. Fed. Reg. 6123-P-02. Retrieved January 30, 2020, from https://www.regulations.gov/document?D=HUD-2020-0011-0001

Developmental Disabilities Assistance and Bill of Rights Act of 2000, Pub. L. No. 106-402, 114 Stat. 1677. (2000).

Developmental Disabilities Assistance and Bill of Rights Act, Pub. L. No. 98-527, 98 Stat. 2662. (1984).

Developmental Disabilities Services and Facilities Construction Amendments of 1970, Pub. L. No. 91-517, 84 Stat. 1316. (1970).

Developmentally Disabled Assistance and Bill of Rights Act, Pub. L. No. 94-103, 89 Stat. 486. (1975).

Disability Rights Education and Defense Fund (DREDF). (2018, September). *A Comparison of ADA, IDEA, and Section 504*. Disability Rights Education and Defense Fund (DREDF). Retrieved January 29, 2018, https://dredf.org/legal-advocacy/laws/a-comparison-of-ada-idea-and-section-504/

Doe v. Bluecross Blueshield of Tennessee Inc., No. 18-5897. (6th Circuit 2019).

Doe v. Mutual of Omaha 179F.3d 557. (7th Circuit 1999).

E.S. et al v. Regence BlueShield et al., No. 2:17-cv-01609. (W.D. Wash., 2018, September 25).

Fed. Reg. 27846-27895, 27848. (2019, June 14). *Nondiscrimination in Health and Health Education Programs or Activities, Notice of Public Rulemaking*.

Fischer, A. J., Gonzalez, P., & Diaz, R. (2019, March). *There is no safety here: The dangers for people with mental illness and other disabilities in immigration detention at GEO Group's ICE Adelanto Processing Center*. Retrieved January 30, 2020, from https://www.disabilityrightsca.org/system/files/file-attachments/DRC_REPORT_ADELANTO-IMMIG_DETENTION_MARCH2019.pdf

FR 41292, 41292-41508. (2019, August 14). *Inadmissability on Public Charge Grounds*.

Fremstad, S. (2009). *Half in ten: Why taking disability into account is essential to reducing income poverty and expanding economic inclusion.* Center for Economic and Policy Research. Retrieved from http://cepr.net/publications/reports/half-in-ten

Genetic Information and Non-Discrimination Act of 2008, Pub. L. No. 110-233. (2008, May 21).

Grusin, S. (2019, December 16). *Section 1115 Waiver Tracking Chart.* National Health Law Program. Retrieved January 30, 2020, from https://healthlaw.org/wp-content/uploads/2019/12/1115-Track-Chart-w-Heading-December-16-2019.pdf

Gustafson, K. S. (2011). *Cheating welfare: Public assistance and the criminalization of poverty.* New York: New York University Press.

Hahn, H., Pratt, E., Allen, E., Kenney, G., Levy, D. K., & Waxman, E. (2017, December). *Work requirements in social safety net programs: A status report of work requirements in TANF, SNAP, Housing Assistance, and Medicaid.* Urban Institute. Retrieved January 30, 2020, from https://www.urban.org/sites/default/files/publication/95566/work-requirements-in-social-safety-net-programs.pdf

Iezzoni, L. (2018, January 19). *Compounded disparities: Health equity at the intersection of disability, race, and ethnicity.* Disability Rights Education and Defense Fund. Retrieved December 15, 2019, from https://dredf.org/wp-content/uploads/2018/01/Compounded-Disparities-Intersection-of-Disabilities-Race-and-Ethnicity.pdf

Indian Health Care Improvement Act, Pub. L. No. 94-437. (1976).

Individuals with Disabilities Education Act, Pub. L. 101-476, 104 Stat. 1142. (1990).

Jaffe, S. (2016, February 4). *Buying supplemental insurance can be hard for younger Medicare beneficiaries.* California Healthline. Retrieved January 30, 2020, from https://californiahealthline.org/news/buying-supplemental-insurance-can-be-hard-for-younger-medicare-beneficiaries/

Kaye, H. S., & Williamson, J. (2014). Toward a model long-term services and supports system: State policy elements. *The Gerontologist, 54*, 754–761.

Kelton, P. (2015). *Cherokee medicine, colonial germs: An indigenous Nation's fight against smallpox, 1518–1824.* Norman: University of Oklahoma Press.

Lawton, E. M., & Sandel, M. (2014). Investing in legal prevention: Connecting access to civil justice and healthcare through medical-legal partnership. *Journal of Legal Medicine, 35*, 29–39.

MACPAC. (2017). *People with disabilities.* Medicaid and CHIP Payment Access Commission. Retrieved January 30, 2020, from https://www.macpac.gov/subtopic/people-with-disabilities/

Mayerson, A. B., & Yee, S. (2001). The ADA and models of equality. *Ohio State Law Journal, 62*, 535–554.

Moffitt, R. A. (2015). The deserving poor, the family, and the U.S. welfare system. *Demography, 52*, 729–749.

National Association of Insurance Commissioners (NAIC) Consumer Representatives. (2019, July 29). *New consumer testing shows limited consumer understanding of short-term plans and need for continued state and NAIC action.* Georgians for a Healthy Future. Retrieved January 29, 2020, from https://healthyfuturega.org/ghf_resource/new-consumer-testing-shows-limited-consumer-understanding-of-short-term-plans-and-need-for-continued-state-and-naic-action/

National Council on Disabilities. (2019, October 23). *Genetic testing and the rush to perfection.* Bioethics and Disability Report Series. National Council on Disabilities. Retrieved January 30, 2020, from https://ncd.gov/publications/2019/bioethics-report-series

National Council on Disability. (2001, August 17). *The Sandoval ruling.* National Council on Disability. Retrieved January 30, 2020, from https://ncd.gov/publications/2001/Aug172001

National Council on Disability. (2011, February 14). *Rising expectations: The developmental disabilities act revisited.* National Council on Disability. Retrieved December 15, 2019, from https://ncd.gov/publications/2011/Feb142011#toc24

National Council on Disability. (2019a). *Bioethics and Disability Report Series.* National Council on Disability. Retrieved from https://ncd.gov/publications/2019/bioethics-report-series

National Council on Disability. (2019b, November 6). *Quality-adjusted life years and the devaluation of life with a disability.* Bioethics and Disability Report Series. National

Council on Disability. Retrieved January 30, 2020, from https://ncd.gov/publications/2019/bioethics-report-series

National Indian Health Board. (2019, November 11). *Brief history of the Indian Healthcare Improvement Act*. Tribal Health Reform Resource Center. Retrieved January 30, 2020 from https://www.nihb.org/tribalhealthreform/ihcia-history/

Nondiscrimination in Health Programs and Activities; Final Rule. 45 C.F.R. Part 92 at 31, 376. (2016, May 18).

Office of Minority Health, Health and Human Services. (2018, March 28). *Profile: American Indian/Alaska native profile*. U.S. Department of Health and Human Services Office of Minority Health. Retrieved January 30, 2020, from http://minorityhealth.hhs.gov/omh/browse.aspx?lvl=3&lvlid=62

Olmstead v. L.C., 527 U.S. 581. (1999).

Patient Protection and Affordable Care Act, Pub. L. No. 111-148, 124 Stat. 149. (2010).

Paul Wellstone and Pete Domenici Mental Health Parity and Addiction Equity Act of 2008, Division C of Pub. L. No. 110-343, Sections 511 and 512. (2008, October 3).

Pavetti, L., Derr, M., & Martin, E. S. (2008, Feburary). *Assisting TANF recipients living with disabilities to obtain and maintain employment: Conducting in-depth assessments 2*. U.S. Department of Health and Human Services, Administration for Children and Families. Retrieved January 30, 2020, from https://www.acf.hhs.gov/sites/default/files/opre/conducting_in_depth.pdf

Pelka, F. (2012). *What we have done: An oral history of the disability rights movement*. Amherst, MA: University of Massachusetts Press.

Protection and Advocacy for Individuals with Mental Illness Act of 1986, Pub. L. No. 99-319, 100 Stat. 478. (1986).

Pub. L. No. 100-430, 102 Stat. 1625. (1988, September 13). *Fair Housing Amendments Act of 1988*.

Pub. L. No. 107-252, 116 Stat. 1666. (2002, October 29). *Help America Vote Act*.

Pub. L. No. 109-171. (2006). *Deficit Reduction Act of 2005*.

Pub. L. No. 110-374, 122 Stat. 4051. (2008). *Prenatally and Postnatally Diagnosed Conditions Awareness Act*.

Pub. L. No. 111-148, 124 Stat. 119. (2010).

Pub. L. No. 404-79. (1946, June 11). *An Act to improve the Administration of Justice by prescribing fair administrative procedure*.

Pub. L. No. 83-568. (1954, August 5). *An Act to the maintenance and operation of hospital and health facilities for Indians to the Public Health Service, and for other purposes*.

Pub. L. No. 88-164, 77 Stat. 282.

Pub. L. No. 93-112, 87 Stat. 390. (1973).

Pub. L. No. 93-112, 87 Stat. 393. (1973).

Pub. L. No. 93-112, 87 Stat. 394. (1973).

Pub. L. No. 99-643. (1986, November 10). *Employment Opportunities for Disabled Americans Act*.

Public Law No: 108-173, 108th Congress. (2003, December 8). *Medicare Prescription Drug, Improvement, and Modernization Act of 2003*.

Rehabilitation Act Amendments of 1993, Pub. L. No. 103-73, 107 Stat. 726. (1993).

Rehabilitation Act of 1973, Pub. L. No. 93-112, 87 Stat. 355. (1973, September 26).

Roberts, J. L. (2013). Health law as disability rights law. *Minnesota Law Review, 97*, 1963–2035.

Rumble v. Fairview Health Services et al., No. 0:2014cv02037. (D. Minn., 2015, March 16).

Sandel, M., Hansen, M., Kahn, R., Lawton, E., Paul, E., Parker, V., … Zuckerman, B. (2010). Medical-legal partnerships: Transforming primary care by addressing the legal needs of vulnerable populations. *Health Affairs, 29*(9), 1697–1705.

Sarat, A. (1990). "…The Law Is All Over": Power, resistance and the legal consciousness of the welfare poor. *The Yale Journal of Law & the Humanities, 2*, 343–379.

Schmitt v. Kaiser Foundation Health Plan of Washington, C17-1611RSL. (W.D. Wash, 2018, February 27).

Sess. 2, Ch. 66, 20 Stat. 37. (1878, April 29). *An Act to prevent the introduction of contagious or infectious diseases into the United States*.

The Power of 504. (1977). *San Francisco, California, U.S.A.: Disability Rights Education and Defense Fund.*

U.S. Department of Health and Human Services. (2019, November 7). *Chapter 3—Indian Health Program.* Indian Health Service, The Federal Program for American Indians and Alaska Natives. Retrieved January 30, 2020, from https://www.ihs.gov/ihm/pc/part-1/p1c3/

U.S. Department of Human Services, Office of The Assistant Secretary for Planning and Evaluation. (2005, January 24). *Using Medicaid to support working age adults with serious mental illnesses in the community: A handbook. A brief history of Medicaid.* U.S. Department of Human Services, Office of The Assistant Secretary for Planning and Evaluation. Retrieved January 30, 2020, from https://aspe.hhs.gov/report/using-medicaid-support-working-age-adults-serious-mental-illnesses-community-handbook/brief-history-medicaid

U.S. Department of the Interior Indian Affairs. (1955, June 26). *Indian Health Services to be transferred July 1.* U.S. Department of the Interior Office of Public Affairs. Retrieved January 30, 2020, from https://www.bia.gov/as-ia/opa/online-press-release/indian-health-services-be-transferred-july-1

U.S. Government Accountability Office. (2019, September 3). *Facilities reported expanding services following increases in health insurance coverage and collections.* U.S. Government Accountability Office. Retrieved January 30, 2020, from https://www.gao.gov/products/GAO-19-612

U.S. Social Security Administration. (2019a, November 16). *Historical background and development of social security.* Social Security Administration. Retrieved January 30, 2020, from https://www.ssa.gov/history/briefhistory3.html

U.S. Social Security Administration. (2019b, November 19). *Benefits planner: Disability—Your continuing eligibility.* Social Security Administration. Retrieved from https://www.ssa.gov/planners/disability/work.html

U.S.C. § 12201(c). (2012).

Wright, P., & West, J. (2002). When to hold 'Em and when to fold 'Em: Lessons learned from enacting the Americans with disabilities Act. In *Disability rights law and policy: International and National perspectives* (pp. 393–411). Ardsley, NY: Transnational Publishers.

Chapter 14
The Interrelationship of Health Insurance and Employment for People with Disabilities

Jean P. Hall

14.1 A Brief History of American Health Insurance

As most Americans are probably aware, the American health insurance system, with its reliance on private, employer-based coverage, is rather unique compared to systems in other industrialized nations. What many Americans may not realize, however, is the profound effect this American insurance system has had on the health and employment of people with disabilities throughout the past half century.

The origins of modern health insurance can be traced back to Chancellor Otto von Bismarck in 1880s Germany. The Chancellor recognized that the health of workers was critical to a strong economy (Social Security Administration [SSA], n.d.-e) and instituted numerous social insurance programs, including statutory health insurance. Originally, this program was instituted only for wage earners and included payment for medical services and lost wages during sickness. By the 1930s, virtually all European countries had some form of government-mandated universal health insurance system. These programs were seen to maintain incomes, productive effort, and political allegiance of the working class. The USA, however, took a different path. Any form of government-run health insurance was strongly opposed in the early twentieth century by newly formed private insurers and by the American Medical Association (Shapiro & Field, 1993). At the same time, a series of events during and after World War II led to the firm entrenchment of an employer-based system in this country. In 1943, the US War Labor Board ruled that employer contributions to employee health insurance did not count as wages, giving employers a way to attract employees during a time with wage freezes and employee shortages. The number of people covered by employer-paid health insurance tripled

J. P. Hall (✉)
Department of Applied Behavioral Science, Institute for Health & Disability Policy Studies
and Research & Training Center on Independent Living, University of Kansas,
Lawrence, KS, USA
e-mail: jhall@ku.edu

© Springer Science+Business Media, LLC, part of Springer Nature 2021
D. J. Lollar et al. (eds.), *Public Health Perspectives on Disability*,
https://doi.org/10.1007/978-1-0716-0888-3_14

during this time. Then, in 1954, the USA determined that employer contributions to health insurance were tax deductible to employers, again greatly increasing the number of employers who opted to provide private health insurance as a means to attract employees (Shapiro & Field, 1993).

These developments largely ingrained the employer-based health insurance system in the USA for working-age adults and also the association between the ability to work and having health insurance. At the same time, however, there was a growing recognition that the costs of health care contributed to high rates of poverty for elderly Americans. In 1965, under the Johnson administration, Congress passed Titles XVIII (Medicare) and XIX (Medicaid) of the Social Security Act, to provide two public health insurance programs:

- Federal hospital insurance for the elderly and optional outpatient insurance for the elderly *Medicare Parts A and B*
- State-managed health insurance for the poor—*Medicaid*

The final passage was driven partly by movements for social justice and partly by increases in poverty among the elderly, pressure on states to care for the poor, and empty hospital beds. Medicare was cast as an employment entitlement or as a reward for having worked and contributed over time (in 1972, Medicare eligibility was extended to adults under age 65 with permanent disabilities who had a work history). Medicaid was seen as a means-tested welfare entitlement to protect society's most vulnerable members and as a way to help states assume a greater share of the welfare burden (as opposed to counties and cities). As Wilbur Mills, then-Chair of the House Ways and Means Committee noted, "It became increasingly clear to me as I studied the programs that a Medicare hospital insurance program for the aged alone was not sufficient to meet the many medical needs of the aged, blind, and disabled or the mothers and children receiving aid for dependent children. With Wilbur Cohen's help, we developed what eventually became Medicaid (Title XIX) and Medicare" (Moore & Smith, 2005).

14.2   How This System Affects Employment for People with Disabilities

This history of health insurance has largely resulted in a two-tiered system of coverage, with most working-age adults and their families obtaining private health insurance through an employer and most elderly Americans, people with disabilities, and families living in poverty obtaining coverage through the government programs of Medicare and Medicaid. Implementation of various parts of the Affordable Care Act from 2010 through 2014 changed this dynamic somewhat, allowing states to expand Medicaid eligibility to childless adults and establishing health insurance marketplaces where individuals can purchase private health insurance. This uniquely

American insurance structure has many implications for the health and employment of people with disabilities.

First, it is important to understand that having health insurance is essential for the well-being of people with disabilities. A recent study indicates that healthcare costs for this population range from three to seven times that of people without disabilities (Kennedy, Wood, & Frieden, 2017). Paying these costs out of pocket would be impossible for most. Next, it is important to understand that the most common pathway to health insurance coverage for American adults—full-time employment—is often not possible for people with disabilities. For the minority of people with disabilities who do access health insurance through an employer or through a family member's employer, many find that the coverage does not include needed services, such as personal assistance, or that out-of-pocket costs such as deductibles, coinsurance, and co-pays are still prohibitively high (Kennedy et al., 2017).

As a result of inability to access employer-based insurance, or the inadequacy of that coverage, many people with disabilities have few alternatives to applying for federal disability benefits in order to obtain Medicare or Medicaid for affordable and comprehensive health insurance coverage. This situation has been dubbed "health insurance motivated disability enrollment" (HIMDE) (Kennedy & Blodgett, 2012), whereby people with disabilities apply for disability benefits not so much for the cash assistance but to obtain critically needed health insurance coverage. As will be seen, this coverage comes at a substantial cost in terms of morale and future employment. Essentially, people with disabilities are trapped into living in poverty and un- or underemployment in order to access adequate health care. In turn, living in poverty can contribute to poorer health, perhaps resulting in an even greater need for comprehensive health insurance and a lifetime reliance on public benefits (e.g., Krahn, Klein Walker, & Correa-De-Araujo, 2015).

14.3   The Application Process for Federal Disability Benefits

In the USA, eligibility for Medicare and Medicaid on the basis of disability is directly tied to eligibility for federal disability benefits. People with disabilities can access federal cash assistance through two separate programs administered by the Social Security Administration: Social Security Disability Insurance (SSDI; Title II of the Social Security Act) and Supplemental Security Income (SSI; Title XVI of the Social Security Act). SSDI, as the name implies, is an insurance program for people who have worked, their spouses, or adult children. It is funded through payroll taxes under the heading of OASDI: Old Age, Survivors, and Disability Insurance. If a worker contributes enough to this system over his or her life, he or she will receive Social Security retirement or "Old Age" benefits. If he or she dies before reaching retirement age, his or her survivors are entitled to benefits. And, finally, if he or she acquires a disability before reaching retirement age, he or she is entitled to cash payments via Disability Insurance. In some situations, his or her spouse or adult children can also access Disability Insurance through the worker's contributions. SSI, on the other hand, is a means-tested cash assistance program for aged, blind, or disabled individuals who have little (if any) income and assets less than $2000 ($3000 for a couple).

In order to qualify for either SSDI or SSI on the basis of disability, an individual must go through the Social Security Administration's (SSA) disability determination process. Essentially, the individual must prove, and continue to prove, that he or she is "too disabled" to work at a gainful level. For purposes of Social Security, this decision is "all or nothing," in that a person cannot be determined partially disabled and therefore eligible for partial benefits. For an adult to be determined disabled, he or she must demonstrate an "inability to engage in any substantial gainful activity (SGA) by reason of any medically determinable physical or mental impairment(s) which can be expected to result in death or which has lasted or can be expected to last for a continuous period of not less than 12 months" (SSA, n.d.-b).

Generally speaking, the disability determination process follows five steps, reviewing:

1. The applicant's current work activity (if any)
2. The severity of his or her impairment(s)
3. Whether his or her impairment(s) meets or medically equals a listing in the Blue Book
4. The applicant's ability to perform his or her past relevant work
5. His or her ability to do other work based on age, education, and work experience

As noted, any current work activity must result in earnings below the substantial gainful activity level (SGA), defined in 2019 as earning $1220 or more per month for non-blind disabled SSDI or SSI applicants and $2040 for blind SSDI applicants (SSA, 2019d). If a person is earning SGA or above, he or she is not considered disabled and is therefore ineligible for cash benefits and associated health insurance programs. In 2019, federal poverty level for a single adult was $1041 per month (US Department of Health and Human Services [HHS], 2019), meaning that earnings of less than $200 per month above poverty level make one ineligible for disability benefits.

If a person passes the earnings test, the disability determination process then considers whether or not his or her condition is severe and whether it meets various benchmarks compiled in the SSA's Blue Book, a listing of impairments and the medical criteria for determining if they can be considered disabling (SSA, n.d.-c). Finally, the process considers the type of work the person has performed in the past, whether he or she can reasonably perform that work now, and, if not, whether he or she can reasonably learn to do new work. All other things being equal, this last criterion makes it somewhat more likely that a person acquiring a disability later in life will receive a disability determination because there is less expectation of learning how to do entirely new work for an older person.

Notably, only about 36% of applications for federal disability are approved based on the initial application (SSA, 2011). Individuals can choose to appeal the initial decision, but the process can be lengthy and challenging. In 2019, the average wait time for an administrative appeals hearing was more than 500 days, down from more than 600 days in 2017 (SSA, 2019c). Indeed, thousands of people die each year while waiting for a hearing (McCoy, 2017). Overall, about 45% are approved from initial application through exhaustion of all appeal efforts (SSA, 2019c). The determination process can be quite taxing, as applicants are required to provide often extensive medical documentation and may need to attend multiple hearings. At the same time, the process requires that they have limited income over the entire appeals period, perhaps approaching—and in some cases exceeding—2 years of time. Once a person receives a disability determination, he or she can then begin receiving SSDI or SSI payments. If eligible for SSI, payments begin immediately; if eligible for SSDI, the individual must wait for 5 months before payments begin. Note, however, that even after going through this lengthy and onerous process, people receiving a federal disability determination are required to undergo a continuing disability review (CDR) every 3–7 years to demonstrate that they continue to have a disabling condition and to review their income and resources to assure they do not exceed allowed amounts (SSA, 2019b).

14.4   SSDI and Medicare

As noted, people who have a sufficient work history to qualify for SSDI can begin collecting cash payments 5 months after receiving their disability determination. Generally, a person must have worked a total of 40 quarters to qualify for SSDI, but this number can be lower for individuals who acquire a disability when young (SSA, n.d.-a). The average monthly benefit amount for SSDI beneficiaries in 2019 was about $1235 (SSA, n.d.-f), but this amount can be much lower for people who are younger and have not paid as much into the program when they acquire a disability and higher for people with long work histories and/or higher-paying jobs. For younger people, especially, the SSDI cash benefit may put their income at or below federal poverty levels.

Twenty-four months after their cash benefits begin (and 29 months after their initial disability determination), SSDI beneficiaries begin to receive Medicare coverage. Thus, these individuals may have been in the application/appeal process and waiting period for Medicare for 4 years or more before their Medicare coverage begins. Historically, thousands of people died each year during the official 24-month Medicare waiting period (e.g., Riley, 2004), and about one-third had no health insurance at all as they waited (Cubanski & Neuman, 2010). This situation may have improved somewhat since implementation of coverage expansions under the Affordable Care Act, which may make marketplace coverage available to some. Note that individuals who qualify for Medicare on the basis of having end-stage renal disease or amyotrophic lateral sclerosis (ALS) are not required to undergo the 24-month waiting period.

Medicare coverage, when obtained, falls into several different categories with varying costs to the individual. Medicare Part A (inpatient) coverage has no premium for individuals who have paid payroll taxes, and Part B (outpatient) coverage has an income-based monthly premium, starting at $136/month in 2019. Medicare Part D (pharmacy) has an average monthly premium of $33. Medicare beneficiaries typically pay a 20% co-pay for services, with no limits or caps on their out-of-pocket spending. Beneficiaries also have the option of enrolling in private Medicare Advantage plans (Part C) instead of Parts A, B, and D, with varying premiums and costs. A discussion of the advantages and disadvantages of each type of plan is beyond the scope of this chapter, but research has shown that people with disabilities disenroll from Medicare Advantage plans at a higher rate than other Medicare beneficiaries (Jacobsen, Neuman, & Damico, 2015). All forms of Medicare provide generally comprehensive coverage for inpatient and outpatient services. No form of Medicare, however, covers long-term services and supports, such as personal assistance in the home, that many people with disabilities need. Thus, while Medicare can be lifesaving for people with disabilities, it still may not meet all of their needs. And, for people with disabilities younger than 65, Medicare coverage remains contingent on having a disability determination via the SSA continuing disability review process, including having employment below the substantial gainful activity (SGA) level. Such a determination can be lost for a variety of reasons, which may result in disincentives to gainful employment for many enrollees, as explained below.

14.5   SSI and Medicaid

People who do not have sufficient work histories to qualify for SSDI may qualify for SSI, as may people receiving very low SSDI payments. Because SSI is a means-tested entitlement program, recipients must have very limited income and resources. Currently, the resource limit for SSI is $2000 for an individual and $3000 for a couple. This cap applies to any cash assets, savings or checking accounts, life insurance policies, land, savings bonds, and other personal property other than one's home, household goods, and one vehicle (SSA, 2019f). Note that these limits have not changed since 1989 (Center on Budget and Policy Priorities, 2019). In 2019, the federal benefit rate or monthly SSI payment was $771 for an eligible individual and $1157 for an eligible individual with an eligible spouse (SSA, 2019e). While some states supplement this amount, the amounts are usually still quite low.

Once a person becomes eligible for SSI, he or she is generally eligible for categorical Medicaid coverage as well. In many states, Medicaid eligibility is automatic for those who receive SSI, whereas other states require a separate application for Medicaid coverage but use SSI rules for eligibility. Nine states, however, use Section 209(b) of the Social Security Act to impose disability or financial eligibility standards that are more restrictive than the federal SSI rules (Feng et al., 2019).

Medicaid is a health insurance program jointly funded by states and the federal government and administered by states. States have wide latitude in the design and management of their programs so long as they meet federal minimum coverage requirements, including inpatient services, outpatient services, and nursing facility services (Rudowitz, Garfield, & Hinton, 2019). Interestingly, prescription drug coverage is not federally required, but all states currently include it. Currently, non-emergency medical transportation (NEMT) to medical appointments is also a required service for non-expansion Medicaid programs, though there have been efforts in the Trump administration to change this coverage to be optional (Medicaid and CHIP Payment and Access Commission [MACPAC], 2019a). Such transportation is not typically covered by private insurance plans and can be extremely important in supporting people with disabilities in accessing care (Hall, Kurth, Gimm, & Smith, 2019). Also of critical importance to people with disabilities, state Medicaid programs have the option of operating home- and community-based waiver programs, which provide additional supports such as case management, attendant care, and respite care—services that empower people with disabilities to live in their communities rather than in institutions. Nationally, about 4.6 million people with disabilities and seniors rely on these waiver services to maintain their independence (Musumeci, Chidambaram, & O'Malley Watts, 2019b). Unfortunately, more than 700,000 additional individuals are on waiting lists for these waiver programs (Musumeci, Chidambaram, & O'Malley Watts, 2019a).

As with SSDI, people receiving SSI must undergo continuing disability reviews periodically over time to assure that they continue to meet disability, income, and resource requirements. Accumulating assets in excess of $2000 for an individual can cause him or her to lose eligibility for SSI and, consequently, Medicaid. As noted, low-income individuals with disabilities who qualify for SSDI and Medicare may also dually qualify for SSI and thus Medicaid (Musumeci, 2017). Currently, more than four million Americans with disabilities under age 65 are dually eligible for both Medicare and Medicaid (Medicare Payment Advisory Commission & Medicaid and CHIP Payment and Access Commission, 2018). These individuals tend to be sicker and poorer than other Medicare beneficiaries, and Medicaid plays an important role in off-setting their out-of-pocket costs and covering long-term services and supports not covered by Medicare (Musumeci, 2017). For these individuals, loss of a disability determination could mean loss of both Medicare and Medicaid benefits.

14.6 Addressing Systemic Disincentives to Employment for People with Disabilities

14.6.1 SSI, SSDI, Medicaid, and Medicare

As has been shown, a federal disability determination is directly tied to a person's inability to work at a substantial level. At the same time, obtaining a disability determination is essential for people with disabilities to gain access to critically needed health insurance through Medicare and Medicaid. As far back as 1986, the National Council on Disability (NCD, 1986) cited fear of losing healthcare benefits through Medicare or Medicaid as one of the major policy issues impeding employment for people with disabilities. Indeed, historically, less than one half of 1% of people on the federal SSDI and SSI programs ever left the rolls and returned to work (Ticket to Work and Work Incentives Improvement Act of 1999 [TW-WIIA], § 2(a)(8)). As one participant at an NCD Town Meeting in 1994, during the time of the attempted Clinton health reform effort, noted:

> ...I face a protracted and intense struggle to obtain the health care I need every day to stay alive. Since 1985, every decision that my wife and I have made about family life, employment or education has been weighed against my need for access to life-sustaining drugs, tests and treatment. (NCD, 1994)

The Social Security Administration offers some programs to allow individuals receiving disability benefits to engage in employment or save money toward employment-related goals, which are summarized in its annual "Red Book" publication (SSA, 2019a). However, many of these programs are limited in scope and not well-utilized. One more widely used program is the 1619(a) and (b) program that allows SSI recipients to earn more and maintain Medicaid coverage, but they must still have assets limited to less than $2000 if single and $3000 if married and fewer than 5% of SSI enrollees utilize this program (SSA, 2019a; VCU Work Incentives Planning and Assistance, 2018).

An important piece of legislation to address the issue of keeping health insurance coverage when returning to work was passed in 1999 in the form of the Ticket to Work and Work Incentives Improvement Act (TW-WIIA, 1999). The "Ticket to Work" portion of the law refers to a voucher or "ticket" available to SSDI and SSI beneficiaries to use in obtaining a variety of vocational services and supports from a network of providers in order to prepare them for work and assist in finding employment. Importantly, ticket users are exempt from continuing disability reviews while using the ticket and making "timely progress" toward substantial employment (SSA, n.d.-g). Unfortunately, the ticket program focuses on full-time employment outcomes and requires a sustained minimum earnings level for participants before service providers will be paid, meaning that many people with disabilities who are unable to work full-time may not be able to fully take advantage of the program (SSA, n.d.-d).

The Work Incentives Improvement portion of the law directly addresses some of the disincentives to employment created by the possible loss of access to public health insurance when beneficiaries increase their income. Indeed, the law notes, "For individuals with disabilities, the fear of losing health care and related services is one of the greatest barriers keeping the individuals from maximizing their employment, earning potential, and independence" (TW-WIIA § 2(a)(7)). Under this part of the law, one important change was to allow SSDI beneficiaries who earned more than SGA after a trial work period to maintain their Medicare coverage for 93 months, extending the previous limit of continued Medicare coverage of 39 months (VCU Rehabilitation Research and Training Center, n.d.). Another extremely important part of the legislation was the option for states to create Medicaid Buy-In programs that allow people with disabilities to earn more and, based on their income, "buy-in" to continued Medicaid coverage via a monthly premium. The law also gives states choosing this option the flexibility to raise the income limits for Medicaid eligibility (up to 450% of federal poverty level), disregard some earned and unearned income, and—unlike the 1619(a) and (b) programs—raise asset limits and exempt certain assets. The Medicaid Buy-In option allowed under TW-WIIA expanded a more limited option that had been made available to states in the Balanced Budget Act [BBA] of 1997 (BBA of 1997). States could also use demonstration waiver programs to expand Medicaid eligibility to working people with disabilities (NCD, 2015). Medicaid Buy-In programs currently operate in 45 states (Kaiser Family Foundation [KFF], 2019).

Research into Medicaid Buy-In programs indicates that they can play a strong role in providing people with disabilities options to work at levels that meet their individual needs while maintaining access to critically needed Medicaid coverage (Hall, Kurth, & Hunt, 2013; NCD, 2015). Importantly, Buy-In programs that allow participants to accumulate assets above the regular SSI limits have greater enrollment, and research has shown that participants who have assets above that limit self-report better mental and physical health and overall quality of life (Hall, Kurth, & Averett, 2016; NCD, 2015). The ability to accumulate more cash assets provides people with disabilities greater financial stability and allows them to deal with emergencies that might otherwise disrupt their employment, such as car repairs. Moreover, the ability to accumulate assets provides a cushion for periods of unemployment and provides an incentive to work more and save more to eventually be able to leave federal assistance and insurance programs completely (Hall et al., 2016; NCD, 2015). A quote from a Medicaid Buy-In participant in Kansas reflects this idea:

> I became quadriplegic in 1985 after being involved in a car accident. *Working Healthy* [the Kansas Medicaid Buy-In] is probably one of the most important programs that have been implemented to help people with disabilities get back to work and become productive citizens. In 2007 I graduated with my Master's degree and was wondering how I was going to ever pay for my student loan. If it was not for *Working Healthy*, I would not be employed and able to pay for my student loans, house payment, and other things I enjoy. I am now making a house payment for something that I will eventually own. My house payment is around $540 a month and I have three bedrooms. Before I got my house I was living in a Section 8 housing one room apartment and the government was subsidizing $740 a month for this. I was getting food stamps and other government subsidies before *Working Healthy*. I now have a full-time job, a home, and I am able to be a productive citizen, and not rely on the government for all those expensive subsidies. (Hall, 2010)

14.6.2   Other Barriers to Employment

Even as programs such as Medicaid Buy-Ins allow people with disabilities to increase employment income and accumulate assets, they may find that their eligibility for other assistance programs such as housing assistance, food stamps, or energy assistance is lost (Hall, 2004). While such losses can be seen as a positive change on the path to independence, lack of linkages between various assistance programs means that a small gain in income can trigger a larger net loss in the value of benefits, such as housing assistance, perhaps resulting in an inability, or at least strong disincentive, to continue employment.

Another systemic barrier to employment is conflicting or negative advice from medical and rehabilitation professionals. Participants in one state's Medicaid Buy-In program reported that service providers often discouraged them from working or working more in the belief that doing so would jeopardize their benefits and/or exacerbate their disabilities (Hall et al., 2013). In actuality, the same study found better physical and mental health, lower rates of smoking, and lower medical costs among Medicaid enrollees with disabilities who were working, even among those working only part-time. From a public health perspective, both of these findings are extremely important. Public health workers should be aware of the positive health benefits of employment and of programs that can support employment for people with disabilities and the importance of adequate health insurance for this population. As we will see, various provisions of the Affordable Care Act have broadened access to health insurance for people with disabilities and, in turn, provided more opportunity to pursue employment.

14.7 How the Affordable Care Act Affects People with Disabilities

Though not specifically targeted at people with disabilities, the Affordable Care Act of 2010 (ACA) has the potential to address many of the historical barriers to health insurance and employment experienced by this population. In particular, the law's prohibition of denials of coverage on the basis of pre-existing conditions, prohibitions on annual and lifetime coverage caps, required coverage of essential health benefits, and requirement to allow children to remain on a parent's policy are extremely important. In addition, the availability of subsidized coverage through the marketplace and the option for states to expand Medicaid eligibility have also been critical in increasing the number of people with disabilities who have insurance (Hall, Shartzer, Kurth, & Thomas, 2017; Kennedy et al., 2017). Each of these facets of the law is discussed in more detail below.

14.7.1 Prohibition of Exclusions Based on Pre-existing Conditions

A groundbreaking feature of the Affordable Care Act is the requirement that plans sold through the marketplace cannot exclude applicants on the basis of having a pre-existing condition. Prior to the ACA, private insurers routinely denied coverage to hundreds of thousands of Americans with such conditions each year. In fact, their business models were built on processes to more effectively identify and refuse coverage for people with pre-existing conditions (Waxman & Stupak, 2010). Thus, before the ACA, access to individual insurance coverage for people with disabilities was extremely limited. In many cases, the only way for people with any existing condition to access such coverage was through a state-based high-risk pool, which operated in 35 states. These pools generally charged very high premiums, tended to have very limited coverage, and imposed significant cost sharing for enrollees (Hall, 2017). As such, they rarely provided the comprehensive coverage and affordable access to care needed by many people with disabilities.

14.7.2   Prohibition of Annual and Lifetime Caps on Coverage

As noted, people with disabilities have average healthcare costs several times higher than those of the general population. Historically, many health insurers imposed annual or lifetime limits on the dollar amount of services their plans covered. Therefore, it was not unusual for a person with a disability to have health insurance but still have very high costs in any particular year not covered by his or her plan or to reach a lifetime limit and no longer have any services covered by the plan. The ACA addresses this issue by prohibiting annual and lifetime dollar caps on coverage (HHS, 2017). The prohibition on caps applies to all essential health benefits (see below) and to both employer-based coverage and individual plans, giving people with disabilities some assurance against catastrophic out-of-pocket costs.

14.7.3   Coverage of Essential Health Benefits

Having access to insurance is an important first step, but, as noted previously, private health insurance coverage has not always met the greater healthcare needs experienced by many people with disabilities. For example, pre-ACA, insurers often covered rehabilitation services that were intended to *restore* function after an illness or injury but rarely covered habilitation services that many people with disabilities need simply to *maintain* function. Under the Affordable Care Act, all private, non-employer-sponsored individual and small-group health insurance plans, including those offered through the marketplace, must cover a list of ten essential health benefits, including:

1. Ambulatory patient services (outpatient services)
2. Emergency services
3. Hospitalization
4. Maternity and newborn care
5. Mental health and substance use disorder services, including behavioral health treatment

6. Prescription drugs
7. Rehabilitative and habilitative services and devices
8. Laboratory services
9. Preventive and wellness services and chronic disease management
10. Pediatric services, including oral and vision care

Section 1302 of the Affordable Care Act specifically directs that when determining essential health benefits, the HHS Secretary shall "(B) not make coverage decisions, determine reimbursement rates, establish incentive programs, or design benefits in ways that discriminate against individuals because of their age, disability, or expected length of life; (C) take into account the health care needs of diverse segments of the population, including women, children, persons with disabilities, and other groups" (Patient Protection and Affordable Care Act, n.d.). Prior to the ACA, insurance companies routinely excluded benefits that might be used by higher-cost enrollees, including people with disabilities, at least in part to discourage their enrollment (Rosenbaum, Teitelbaum, & Hayes, 2011). While the ACA's essential health benefits do not include personal assistance services, the required inclusion of habilitation services and devices, as well as other needed services such as behavioral health and prescriptions, is a major gain for people with disabilities.

14.7.4   Coverage of Children to Age 26

Yet another feature of the ACA that supports access to coverage without impoverishment for people with disabilities is the law's requirement that insurance plans with coverage for dependent children be made available to children until they reach their 26th birthday (US Department of Labor, n.d.). This requirement has resulted in increased insurance coverage and improved access to care for young adults with chronic conditions and disabilities (Huang & Porterfield, 2019). Importantly, availability of insurance through their parents also gives young adults with disabilities some flexibility in their employment, including working part-time and still having access to insurance (Amuedo-Dorantes & Yaya, 2016).

14.7.5   Subsidized Coverage Through the Marketplace

As noted previously, people with disabilities were rarely able to purchase individual (non-employer-sponsored) health insurance prior to the ACA due to their pre-existing conditions. The ACA radically changed availability of such coverage and also its affordability by its establishment of health insurance marketplaces. Coverage through the marketplace is available to any US citizen or legal resident who does not have access to affordable insurance through an employer (affordable insurance is defined as costing less than 9.86% of a person's income) and who is not eligible for any public insurance coverage. Importantly, marketplace coverage is also available to a person if his or her employer offers insurance that does not meet minimum coverage standards in the form of actuarial value, as well (KFF, 2018).

Affordability of marketplace coverage for people with lower incomes is addressed through two forms of subsidies: premium subsidies and cost sharing subsidies. Premium subsidies take the form of tax credits and are available on a sliding basis to people with incomes between 100% and 400% of federal poverty level (138–400% in states that expanded Medicaid coverage; KFF, 2018). Cost sharing subsidies are available on a sliding basis for people with incomes from 100% to 250% of FPL who enroll in a "silver" plan in the marketplace. These subsidies are provided through the insurers and help to offset the costs of deductibles, co-pays, and co-insurance, limiting total out-of-pocket costs to income-adjusted maximums (KFF, 2018).

People with disabilities who have private insurance are more likely than people without disabilities to have obtained it through the marketplace (Kennedy et al., 2017). They can access this form of coverage whether they are working or not and can do so without having to undergo any sort of disability determination process. The coverage will include all of the essential health benefits as required by the ACA described earlier.

14.7.6   Medicaid Expansion

Perhaps one of the most important ACA programs for people with disabilities has been the Medicaid expansion. Unlike categorical Medicaid, which is only available to certain categories of people including those with disabilities, the elderly, and parents and children, eligibility for Medicaid expansion coverage extends to working-age adults regardless of disability or parental status (MACPAC, 2019b). States cannot set their own state-specific disregards, deductions, or assets rules for this coverage. Rather, all states are required to use only a person's modified adjusted gross income (MAGI) as determined by the IRS to determine financial eligibility for expansion coverage. Under these rules, anyone with income up to 133% of FPL, with a 5% disregard that makes the effective cutoff 138%, is potentially eligible. Unlike with categorical Medicaid, *no asset or resource limits are imposed*, so people do not have to restrict savings to maintain eligibility. Importantly, states are also required to have a single portal through which people can apply for marketplace coverage and Medicaid, so that if they are not eligible for the marketplace, they will be informed of their eligibility for Medicaid.

With regard to coverage, states are allowed to offer "alternative benefit plans" (ABPs), which can be different from their traditional Medicaid benefits, but still must include all ten of the essential health benefits. In reality, the great majority of states have chosen to align their Medicaid expansion benefits with their traditional Medicaid benefits for administrative simplicity (MACPAC, 2019b; Rosenbaum et al., 2015). Moreover, people with special medical needs, including many people with disabilities, are exempt from alternative coverage and must be able to access the traditional Medicaid services in their states (Gettens, Henry, & Himmelstein, 2012; MACPAC, 2019b).

When originally passed, the ACA required that Medicaid eligibility be expanded in all states to all adults with incomes up to 138% FPL, regardless of disability or parental status. This requirement was struck down by the US Supreme Court in 2012 in the *National Federation of Independent Business (NFIB) v. Sebelius* ruling, and Medicaid expansion effectively became optional for states to implement. Since that time, many states have opted to expand their programs, but, as of late 2019, 14 states still have not. This situation of some states expanding Medicaid and some not has provided researchers with the opportunity to compare the experiences of people with disabilities in both settings with regard to having insurance coverage and engaging in employment.

One series of studies used data from the Health Reform Monitoring Survey to examine the experiences of people with disabilities living in Medicaid expansion states versus those living in non-expansion states (Hall et al., 2017; Hall, Shartzer, Kurth, & Thomas, 2018). First, this research found that people with disabilities living in Medicaid expansion states were significantly less likely to be uninsured than those living in non-expansion states, reinforcing the importance of the availability of expanded Medicaid in obtaining health insurance for this population. Second, and perhaps more importantly, the research found that employment rates increased for people with disabilities in expansion states and decreased in non-expansion states. Moreover, the rates of people with disabilities who reported not working due to a disability significantly decreased in Medicaid expansion states (Hall et al., 2018). This finding might indicate that people with disabilities living in expansion states were no longer going through a disability determination process to establish being too disabled to work because such a determination is not needed to access Medicaid expansion coverage. In fact, a study in 2017 found a similar trend when examining rates of applications for SSI in Medicaid expansion states versus non-expansion states: SSI applications in expansion states declined by more than 3% while increasing in non-expansion states (Soni, Burns, Dague, & Simon, 2017). At the same time, research has shown that when people with potentially disabling chronic conditions have access to comprehensive health insurance coverage, they are less likely to consider the need to apply for federal disability assistance (Chapman, Hall, & Moore, 2013).

These findings strongly suggest that severing eligibility for comprehensive health benefits from eligibility for cash assistance programs supports efforts of people with disabilities to enter employment and avoid being trapped in a life of poverty. While it is true that income eligibility for Medicaid expansion coverage is capped at 138% FPL, that amount is still considerably higher than SSI income and, in many cases, SSDI income. Moreover, expansion eligibility does not impose resource or asset tests, allowing people with disabilities to accumulate savings to address emergency expenses and save for items to improve their employability, such as reliable transportation or high-speed Internet access. Finally, as people with disabilities earn more, they have the option of transitioning to subsidized marketplace coverage, for which no pre-existing condition exclusions can be applied.

14.8   Implications for Public Health

As members of a health disparity population, people with disabilities face many barriers to improved health. As has been demonstrated here, the historical structure of the American public health insurance system with its connection to cash assistance programs which are tied to an inability to work has contributed to the impoverishment and limited employment of this population for many years. The Affordable Care Act has begun to address this situation in several ways. Availability of subsidized health insurance not tied to full-time employment and not subject to exclusions for pre-existing conditions through the marketplace has made private coverage available to many people with disabilities. In addition, availability of expanded Medicaid coverage without the requirement of a disability determination and without asset and resource caps has made it possible for people with disabilities to work and accumulate assets while maintaining eligibility for coverage that is essential to their health and well-being.

Because employment is associated with improved health (Chiu et al., 2015; Hall et al., 2013; Ross & Mirowsky, 1995), public health programs have an obligation to assure that people with disabilities continue to have access to health insurance that can support their employment efforts. Currently, federal flexibility given to states in how they administer and oversee health insurance via Medicaid and other programs has resulted in very large disparities from state to state in rates of health insurance coverage and access to care (Collins & Lambrew, 2019). Public health workers in states without Medicaid expansion, for example, can work to support expansion efforts in their states that would support work efforts by people with disabilities. Moreover, the Trump administration has been successful in expanding availability of ACA non-compliant plans that may not cover all essential health benefits and may exclude people with pre-existing conditions from coverage (Jost, 2019). Public health workers can raise awareness of the problems with these plans and assure that people have adequate information to enroll in coverage that meets their needs.

Finally, at this writing, the fate of the Affordable Care Act is uncertain, and an upcoming presidential election has resulted in numerous proposals to change how health insurance is provided. Any potential changes to the current system must be monitored for their possible effects on people with disabilities. In the meantime, public health workers should also be aware of community resources, such as Centers for Independent Living, that support marketplace/Medicaid expansion enrollment and provide guidance on disability and community programs that provide additional employment supports. Ultimately, government savings through decreased reliance on federal cash assistance programs by people with disabilities, greater tax revenue from their increased employment, and healthcare savings due to their improved health should all make additional resources available to communities to address other public health issues of concern, helping to improve outcomes for all. As one participant in the Kansas Medicaid Buy-In program suggested, "We are trying to better our life. We don't want to be labeled as living on [welfare]...We want to be a working member of society and...living the American dream" (Hall, 2003).

Resources for Additional Information
American Association on Health and Disability, https://www.aahd.us/
Kaiser Family Foundation, https://www.kff.org/
National Council on Disability, https://www.ncd.gov/
The Commonwealth Fund, https://www.commonwealthfund.org/
The Social Security Administration, https://www.ssa.gov/

References

Amuedo-Dorantes, C., & Yaya, M. E. (2016). The impact of the ACA's extension of coverage to dependents on young adults' access to care and prescription drugs. *Southern Economic Journal, 83*(1), 25–44.

Balanced Budget Act of 1997. Pub. L. 105-33.

Center on Budget and Policy Priorities. (2019). *Policy basics: Supplemental security income.* Retrieved from https://www.cbpp.org/research/social-security/policy-basics-supplemental-security-income

Chapman, S. L., Hall, J. P., & Moore, J. M. (2013). Health care access affects attitudes about health outcomes and decisions to apply for social security disability benefits. *Journal of Disability Policy Studies, 24*(2), 113–121.

Chiu, C. Y., Chan, F., Edward Sharp, S., Dutta, A., Hartman, E., & Bezyak, J. (2015). Employment as a health promotion intervention for persons with multiple sclerosis. *Work, 52*(4), 749–756.

Collins, S. R., & Lambrew, J. M. (2019). *Federalism, the Affordable Care Act, and health reform in the 2020 election.* Retrieved from https://www.commonwealthfund.org/publications/fund-reports/2019/jul/federalism-affordable-care-act-health-reform-2020-election

Cubanski, J., & Neuman, P. (2010). Medicare doesn't work as well for younger, disabled beneficiaries as it does for older enrollees. *Health Affairs, 29*(9), 1725–1733.

Feng, Z., Vadnais, A., Vreeland, E., Haber, S., Wiener, J., & Baker, B. (2019). *Analysis of pathways to dual eligible status.* Retrieved from https://aspe.hhs.gov/basic-report/analysis-pathways-dual-eligible-status-final-report

Gettens, J., Henry, A. D., & Himmelstein, J. (2012). Assessing health care reform: Potential effects on insurance coverage among persons with disabilities. *Journal of Disability Policy Studies, 23*(1), 3–13.

Hall, J. P. (2003). People with disabilities share their early experiences. In *Working Healthy Policy Brief. Number 2.* Lawrence, KS: University of Kansas. Retrieved from https://ihdps.drupal.ku.edu/publications/early-enrollee-experiences

Hall, J. P. (2004). Policy issues for Working Healthy and other states' Medicaid buy-ins: The good, the bad, and what remains to be seen. *Working Healthy, 6.* Retrieved from https://ihdps.drupal.ku.edu/publications/policy-issues-affecting-buy-ins

Hall, J. P. (2010). *Working Healthy: Medicaid participants earning more & costing less.* Retrieved from https://ihdps.drupal.ku.edu/sites/ihdps.drupal.ku.edu/files/docs/WHlegislativeRecept01_13_09.pdf

Hall, J. P. (2017). High-risk pools: An illusion of coverage that may increase costs for all in the long term. *Annals of Internal Medicine, 167*(3), 200–201.

Hall, J. P., Kurth, N. K., & Averett, E. P. (2016). Asset building: One way the ACA may improve health and employment outcomes for people with disabilities. *Journal of Disability Policy Studies, 26*(4), 252–256.

Hall, J. P., Kurth, N. K., Gimm, G., & Smith, S. (2019). Perspectives of adults with disabilities on access to health care after the ACA: Qualitative findings. *Disability and Health Journal, 12*(3), 350–358.

Hall, J. P., Kurth, N. K., & Hunt, S. L. (2013). Employment as a health determinant for working-age, dually-eligible people with disabilities. *Disability and Health Journal, 6*(2), 100–106.

Hall, J. P., Shartzer, A., Kurth, N. K., & Thomas, K. C. (2017). Effect of Medicaid expansion on workforce participation for people with disabilities. *American Journal of Public Health, 107*(2), 262–264.

Hall, J. P., Shartzer, A., Kurth, N. K., & Thomas, K. C. (2018). Medicaid expansion as an employment incentive program for people with disabilities. *American Journal of Public Health, 108*(9), 1235–1237.

Huang, J., & Porterfield, S. L. (2019). Changes in health insurance coverage and health care access as teens with disabilities transition to adulthood. *Disability and Health Journal, 12*(4), 551–556.

Jacobsen, G. A., Neuman, P., & Damico, A. (2015). At least half of new Medicare advantage enrollees had switched from traditional Medicare 2006–2011. *Health Affairs (Millwood), 34*(1), 48–55.

Jost, T. S. (2019). *The past and future of association health plans.* Retrieved from https://www.commonwealthfund.org/blog/2019/past-future-association-health-plans

Kaiser Family Foundation. (2018). *Explaining health care reform: Questions about health insurance subsidies.* Retrieved from https://www.kff.org/health-reform/issue-brief/explaining-health-care-reform-questions-about-health/

Kaiser Family Foundation. (2019). *Medicaid eligibility through buy-in programs for working people with disabilities.* Retrieved from https://www.kff.org/other/state-indicator/medicaid-eligibility-through-buy-in-programs-for-working-people-with-disabilities

Kennedy, J., & Blodgett, E. (2012). Health insurance–motivated disability enrollment and the ACA. *New England Journal of Medicine, 367*(12), e16.

Kennedy, J., Wood, E. G., & Frieden, L. (2017). Disparities in insurance coverage, health services use, and access following implementation of the affordable care act: A comparison of disabled and nondisabled working-age adults. *Inquiry: The Journal of Health Care Organization, Provision, and Financing, 54*, 0046958017734031.

Krahn, G. L., Klein Walker, D., & Correa-De-Araujo, R. (2015). Persons with disabilities as an unrecognized health disparity population. *American Journal of Public Health, 105*(S2), S198–S206.

McCoy, T. (2017, November 20). 597 days. And still waiting. *The Washington Post.* Retrieved from http://www.washingtonpost.com

Medicaid and CHIP Payment and Access Commission. (2019a). *Medicaid coverage of non-emergency medical transportation.* Retrieved from https://www.macpac.gov/publication/medicaid-coverage-of-non-emergency-medical-transportation/

Medicaid and CHIP Payment and Access Commission. (2019b). *Medicaid expansion to the new adult group.* Retrieved from https://www.macpac.gov/subtopic/medicaid-expansion/

Medicare Payment Advisory Commission & Medicaid and CHIP Payment and Access Commission. (2018). *Beneficiaries dually eligible for Medicare and Medicaid.* Retrieved from https://www.macpac.gov/publication/data-book-beneficiaries-dually-eligible-for-medicare-and-medicaid-3/

Moore, J. D., & Smith, D. G. (2005). Legislating Medicaid: Considering Medicaid and its origins. *Health Care Financing Review, 27*(2), 45.

Musumeci, M. (2017). *Medicaid's role for Medicare beneficiaries.* Retrieved from https://www.kff.org/medicaid/issue-brief/medicaids-role-for-medicare-beneficiaries/

Musumeci, M., Chidambaram, P., & O'Malley Watts, M. (2019a). *Key questions about Medicaid home and community-based services waiver waiting lists.* Retrieved from https://www.kff.org/medicaid/issue-brief/key-questions-about-medicaid-home-and-community-based-services-waiver-waiting-lists/

Musumeci, M., Chidambaram, P., & O'Malley Watts, M. (2019b). *Medicaid home and community-based services enrollment and spending.* Retrieved from https://www.kff.org/medicaid/issue-brief/medicaid-home-and-community-based-services-enrollment-and-spending/

National Council on Disability. (1986). *National disability policy: A progress report*. Retrieved from https://ncd.gov/progress_reports/February1986

National Council on Disability. (1994). *Making health care reform work for Americans with disabilities*. Retrieved from https://ncd.gov/publications/1994/July1994

National Council on Disability. (2015). *Home and community-based services: Creating systems for success at home, at work and in the community*. Retrieved from https://ncd.gov/publications/2015/02242015

Patient Protection and Affordable Care Act. (n.d.). Pub. L. 111-148.

Riley, G. F. (2004). The cost of eliminating the 24-month Medicare waiting period for Social Security disabled-worker beneficiaries. *Medical Care, 42*(4), 387–394.

Rosenbaum, S., Mehta, D., Dorley, M., Hurt, C., Rothenberg, S., Lopez, N., & Ely, S. (2015). *Medicaid benefit designs for newly eligible adults: State approaches*. Retrieved from https://www.commonwealthfund.org/publications/issue-briefs/2015/may/medicaid-benefit-designs-newly-eligible-adults-state-approaches

Rosenbaum, S., Teitelbaum, J., & Hayes, K. (2011). The essential health benefits provisions of the Affordable Care Act: Implications for people with disabilities. *The Commonwealth Fund, 1485*(3), 1–16.

Ross, C. E., & Mirowsky, J. (1995). Does employment affect health? *Journal of Health and Social Behavior, 36*, 230–243.

Rudowitz, R., Garfield, R., & Hinton, E. (2019). *10 things to know about Medicaid: Setting the facts straight*. Retrieved from https://www.kff.org/medicaid/issue-brief/10-things-to-know-about-medicaid-setting-the-facts-straight/

Shapiro, H. T., & Field, M. J. (Eds.). (1993). *Employment and health benefits: A connection at risk*. Washington, DC: The National Academies Press.

Social Security Administration. (2011). *Outcomes of applications for disability benefits*. Retrieved from https://www.ssa.gov/policy/docs/statcomps/di_asr/2011/sect04.html

Social Security Administration. (2019a). *2019 Red Book*. Retrieved from https://www.ssa.gov/redbook/

Social Security Administration. (2019b). *Continuing disability reviews*. Retrieved from https://www.ssa.gov/ssi/text-cdrs-ussi.htm

Social Security Administration. (2019c). *Information about Social Security's hearings and appeals process*. Retrieved from https://www.ssa.gov/appeals/

Social Security Administration. (2019d). *Substantial gainful activity*. Retrieved from https://www.ssa.gov/oact/cola/sga.html

Social Security Administration. (2019e). *SSI federal payment amounts*. Retrieved from https://www.ssa.gov/oact/cola/SSI.html

Social Security Administration. (2019f). *Understanding Supplemental Security Income SSI resources—2019 edition*. Retrieved from https://www.ssa.gov/ssi/text-resources-ussi.htm

Social Security Administration. (n.d.-a). *Benefits planner: Disability | How you qualify*. Retrieved from https://www.ssa.gov/planners/disability/qualify.html

Social Security Administration. (n.d.-b). *Disability evaluation under Social Security*. Retrieved from https://www.ssa.gov/disability/professionals/bluebook/general-info.htm

Social Security Administration. (n.d.-c). *Disability evaluation under Social Security: Listing of impairments—Adult listings*. Retrieved from https://www.ssa.gov/disability/professionals/bluebook/AdultListings.htm

Social Security Administration. (n.d.-d). *Informing beneficiaries of the goals of the Ticket program: Employment, benefits reduction and self-sufficiency*. Retrieved from https://yourticket-towork.ssa.gov/Assets/yttw/docs/information-center/resource-documents/program-resources/Informing-Beneficiaries-Goals-of-TTW.pdf

Social Security Administration. (n.d.-e). *Otto von Bismarck*. Retrieved from https://www.ssa.gov/history/ottob.html

Social Security Administration. (n.d.-f). *Selected data from Social Security's disability program*. Retrieved from https://www.ssa.gov/oact/STATS/dib-g3.html

Social Security Administration. (n.d.-g). *Ticket to work: Frequently asked questions.* Retrieved from https://yourtickettowork.ssa.gov/about/faqs.html

Soni, A., Burns, M. E., Dague, L., & Simon, K. I. (2017). Medicaid expansion and state trends in Supplemental Security Income program participation. *Health Affairs, 36*(8), 1485–1488.

Ticket to Work and Work Incentives Improvement Act of 1999. Pub. L. 106-170.

US Department of Health and Human Services. (2017). *Lifetime & annual limits.* Retrieved from https://www.hhs.gov/healthcare/about-the-aca/benefit-limits/index.html

US Department of Health and Human Services. (2019). *Poverty guidelines.* Retrieved from https://aspe.hhs.gov/poverty-guidelines

US Department of Labor. (n.d.). *Young adults and the Affordable Care Act: Protecting young adults and eliminating burdens on businesses and families FAQs.* Retrieved from https://www.dol.gov/agencies/ebsa/about-ebsa/our-activities/resource-center/faqs/young-adult-and-aca

VCU Rehabilitation Research and Training Center. (n.d.). *Extended Medicare provisions.* Retrieved from https://vcurrtc.org/resources/printview.cfm/319

VCU Work Incentives Planning and Assistance. (2018). *Understanding 1619(b).* Retrieved from https://vcu-ntdc.org/resources/WIPA_OtherResources/Understanding%201619(b)%20 2018.pdf

Waxman, H. A., & Stupak, B. (2010). *Coverage denials for pre-existing conditions in the individual health insurance market.* Retrieved from https://oversight.house.gov/sites/democrats.oversight.house.gov/files/documents/Memo-Coverage-Denials-Individual-Market-2010-10-12.pdf

Chapter 15
Public Health, Work, and Disability

Kathleen Sheppard-Jones and Vivian Lasley-Bibbs

15.1 Introduction

In the United States, society places high value on employment. One of the first questions posed when meeting someone is, "What do you do?" It is widely understood that the expected response is to be related to one's line of work. People largely identify who they are based on the job they have. Work is also considered important. The role of employee is one that our culture values (Osburn, 2007). While it is clear that people are motivated to work for a variety of reasons, whether it be for economic self-sufficiency, having an overall sense of purpose, contributing to the world, or simply providing for one's family, one expectation remains the same. As youth exit secondary school, seeking employment or training for employment through continuing education is considered the next step into adulthood. Working is what we do.

We also know that there are greater numbers of people living with a variety of physical and mental impairments in the United States. Estimates and proportions vary widely, but people are living with lifelong disabilities that were previously associated with much shorter life expectancies. Additionally, as people age, they find themselves getting age-related disabilities that they previously did not live long enough to acquire. Advances in our society's technological capabilities also lead to increasing incidence of disabilities that were previously considered unsurviveable. We have also seen an increased incidence of certain disabilities, like autism. Whether there are more people with autism or simply that the diagnosis of autism is increasing has been debated. However, Americans are also experiencing poorer health

Preparation of this chapter was also partly funded by the United States Department of Labor, Office of Disability Employment Policy in the amount of $3.5 million under Cooperative Agreement No. OD-32548-18-75-4-21. This document does not necessarily reflect the views or policies of the U.S. Department of Labor, nor does mention of trade names, commercial products, or organizations imply endorsement by the U.S. Government.

K. Sheppard-Jones (✉)
Human Development Institute, University of Kentucky, Lexington, KY, USA
e-mail: kjone@uky.edu

V. Lasley-Bibbs (✉)
Office of Health Equity, KY Department of Public Health, Frankfort, KY, USA
e-mail: Vivian.Lasley-Bibbs@ky.gov

© Springer Science+Business Media, LLC, part of Springer Nature 2021
D. J. Lollar et al. (eds.), *Public Health Perspectives on Disability*,
https://doi.org/10.1007/978-1-0716-0888-3_15

outcomes that result in disabling conditions, such as diabetes and obesity (Leslie, Sheppard-Jones, & Bishop, under review). These poor health outcomes can also be seen when stratified by race and gender.

There are yet other emerging disabilities, such as opioid use disorder (OUD), that have implications not only for the current generation but for the next. It is estimated that approximately 10% of people who use an opioid will develop an OUD (National Institute on Drug Abuse, 2018). Babies are being born to mothers with OUD and experiencing neonatal abstinence syndrome (NAS). As these children grow, they are needing early childhood interventions and subsequent educational and social supports in school to succeed. As such, the CDC has coined the national situation as an epidemic (CDC, 2017), and huge investments into state level responses that enforce, deter, treat and promote the recovery of OUD. It is estimated that well over two million Americans have an OUD (CDC). In 2018 alone, $420 million have been granted to four states to develop multisystems change interventions.

For these reasons, it has become apparent that the "face" of disability in the United States is changing. Disability is a multifaceted concept that cuts across race, culture, sex, and socioeconomic status. With rates of disability of roughly one in five Americans experiencing one, it is unrealistic to think about disability as something that happens to someone else. If you do not have a disability yourself, you have friends and family who do. You will also, most likely, experience a disability as you age. In fact, the percentage of people with disabilities in the United States is expected to double in less than 20 years (National Governors Association, 2012). The history of disability and work is further described later in this chapter. Policy changes largely arose through grassroots efforts of people with disabilities, families and champions. This "nothing about us without us" emphasis has been ongoing in the disability rights movement. Therefore, when considering employment and disability, it is critical that people with disabilities be included in the conversation—not only as participants but as leaders to help drive change and shape the dialogue. This is so important if we are to help change existing cultural attitudes that often pose greater barriers than the disability itself.

Employment is a pivotal indicator for other life outcomes—having a job is itself linked to a higher quality of life, a sense of self-worth, and greater levels of self-determination (Antosh et al., 2013) and is a key factor in breaking the cycle of poverty for individuals with disabilities (Nye-Lengerman & Nord, 2016). Not only do people with disabilities want to work, but we must recognize this often overlooked heterogenous population of 10.7 million people as a viable and valuable component of the talent pipeline who are not only helping employers in meeting their goals but also helping to grow and maintain a strong economy (Accenture, 2018). Inclusive workplaces combat stereotypes about disabilities and foster innovation, productivity, and positive work environments (Accenture, 2018).

A lack of participation in the workforce has been identified as a public health crisis. Household economic instability results in disparities across life outcomes including health, community integration, and economic self-sufficiency (Smart, 2016). For people with disabilities, disparities in employment represent perhaps the most significant of many economic disadvantages. This is seen in increased likelihood of dropping out of school, increased likelihood of living in poverty, decreased likelihood of being employed, and decreased likelihood of having private health insurance coverage (Houtenville & Boege, 2019). Equally troubling is decreased quality of life that is operationalized through self-reported lower life satisfaction, fewer relationships with people who are not family or paid supports, decreased community participation, and decreased autonomy and decision-making authority. These structural and instructional inequities are heightened for people who are racially diverse (National Academies of Sciences, Engineering and Medicine, 2018).

Historically, public health considers the presence of a disability a failed outcome (Lollar, 2008). Sickness absence in the workplace is also a public health issue (Workplace Health Promotion). However, an understanding of the relationship between disability and work over time indicates cultural shifts that are occurring at a societal level, spurred on by legislative advances and advocacy efforts driven by the disability community. Additionally, our understanding of work and disability is also influenced by the way that we define disability. As we talk about disability, it's important to find a common language.

The medical model of disability is a deficits-based model. Using this lens, the individual is considered to have a defect that is in need of repair. As such, professionals are necessary to provide the needed interventions and to help to make the person as whole as is possible. The medical model supposes that a person with a disability is less than complete. The deficit is seen as innate to the individual, and therefore, the person is in some way considered "abnormal." The problem lies within and is not an issue of others. The medical model seeks to provide a cure using medical care.

Legislation began to change the way that disability was framed. For the purposes of disability and work, the Americans with Disabilities Act (ADA) of 1990 provides a solid starting point from the perspective of employees and employers. The ADA and its subsequent amendments serves as anti-discrimination law for people with disabilities. It is considered civil rights legislation. Titles of the Act specifically address requirements in employment related to hiring and employing people with declared disabilities. The ADA defines a person with a disability as someone who (1) has a physical or mental impairment that substantially limits one or more major life activities, (2) has a record of such an impairment, or (3) is regarded by others as having a disability. Major life activities include a broad array of actions, such as caring for oneself, performing manual tasks, seeing, hearing, breathing, eating, sleeping, walking, standing, lifting, bending, speaking, learning, reading, concentrating, thinking, communicating, operations of major bodily function, and working.

The World Health Organization (WHO) further expands on the defined elements of disability. The WHO definition includes impairment and activity limitation but adds restriction in participating in daily activities, like working, engaging in social or recreation activities, and getting health care. It's important to note that both the ADA and WHO recognize the inability to work to be disabling. If we further appraise the WHO definition, we are effectively creating a social model of disability in which disability can be considered a collection of conditions that are created by the social environments. Using a social model, people have physical or mental impairments, but the disability itself occurs only within the context of society. As an example, a person may have a mobility impairment, but that in and of itself isn't disabling. If that person is not able to get into a building to get to work, the impairment then becomes a disability. This is far different than other models of disability. The social model of disability is at the opposite end of the spectrum from the medical model of disability. Using a social model, a person becomes disabled by lack of accessibility of the physical environment or from society's response to the person.

From a public health perspective, employment is a social determinant of health. Yet optimum health is considered a requirement in order to participate in work. Thus, the distinction of health and disability is an important one. Is it possible to be healthy and to have a disability, or is disability an outcome that occurs in the absence of good health? The World Health Organization (WHO) defines disability as an impairment that limits activity and results in restricted participation in daily activities. Daily activities can include accessing health and preventive care, social activities, and work. Further, the International Classification of Functioning, Disability and Health (ICF) serves as the WHO framework that is used to assess the relationship between health and disability. As such, the WHO recognizes the complex and contextual nature of disability.

15.2 Disability and Work

15.2.1 History of Rehabilitation

The medical model was certainly informative for rehabilitative services for people with disabilities. In fact, the term rehabilitation can be considered "the restoration of a person with disabilities through appropriate training." The field of rehabilitation has experienced growth and shifts over time. In the early 1900s, sheltered workshops gained popularity, as a way to give people with disabilities purpose. Sheltered workshops were a congregate, segregated model of work, primarily associated with people with disabilities all working together, who would earn money based on a piece rate. If you worked in a sheltered workshop, that was the end of the career line. It was a way to offer a means of employment for people who had very low expectations from others. However, rehabilitation of people with disabilities in the United States was seen as a necessary societal response for veterans of wars who experienced injury on the battlefield.

Recognition of the importance of work for people with disabilities largely began following World War I and the passage of the Rehabilitation Act. Soldiers who survived war injuries and returned home needed to transition back to a civilian life that now included a service-connected disability. The Rehabilitation Act created the vocational rehabilitation program, a federal-state partnership with the intent of assisting wounded veterans to obtain a meaningful activity, primarily through work.

The law subsequently included non-veterans with the same goal of assisting people with disabilities in returning to employment and the workforce (Patterson, 2018; Switzer, 2003). Advances in technology and medicine have led to greater numbers of people requiring and benefitting from rehabilitative medical and social services. Sheltered workshops in the 1950s began shifting to a model of work readiness, in which some people transitioned to employment outside of the workshop. The primary impetus for this was the Rehabilitation Act amendments of 1954 and World War II. Veterans returning from this war wanted to return to work, but the sheltered workshop model was not what they sought. This proved to be an opportunity for people with intellectual and other significant disabilities as well.

As the population ages and chronic health conditions increase, the rate of disability is on the rise (WHO, 2018). The passage of the Rehabilitation Act of 1973 and subsequent adoption of the 1990 Americans with Disabilities Act (ADA) saw a shift in focus as people with disabilities became recognized as a minority group that had attained civil rights protections. Discrimination on the basis of disability was now illegal, in employment and in community living. Further shifts away from segregated, subminimum wage sheltered employment to models of supported employment within the community began to grow.

Also during this time, people with disabilities formed powerful advocacy groups led by people with disabilities, spurring on social change in ensuring access to work and independent living for all. Notable leaders with disabilities of the time include Ed Roberts, Judy Heumann, and Justin Dart. More recently, the 2014 Workforce Innovation and Opportunities Act (WIOA) has mandated that greater emphasis be placed on students and youth with disabilities. This effort to improve post-school outcomes is intended to create a smoother transition for youth with disabilities as they exit high school and further align education and state rehabilitation programs (these systems are further discussed later in this chapter).

Because of historical inequities in treatment of people with disabilities, specificity in defining employment is required. To be considered competitive and integrated, employment may be full- or part-time work for which an individual is compensated at a rate of not less than minimum wage, and that can be state or federal, whichever is higher. The rate of pay must be comparable with the rate of pay people without disabilities are being paid for the same type of job. As an example, a company would not be able to pay a nondisabled person $14 an hour for a customer service representative job and a disabled person $12 an hour for the same job, if experience and education levels are the same.

Another important element of competitive and integrated employment is that the employees with disabilities must be able to interact with the nondisabled employees or have that opportunity to interact with nondisabled employees just like they would at any other workplace. This does not include the supervisors who are required to interact or any service providers who interact; it has to be other nondisabled people on the worksite. And as appropriate, employees with disabilities must have the opportunity for advancement that is expected by those without disabilities. To be competitive and integrated in employment, it's not enough for people with disabilities to have jobs. What is needed are careers affording persons with disabilities the opportunity to move up the career ladder just like any employee would be expected to do. People grow professionally through career advancement. Given this, public health professionals should be considering how people with disabilities will advance within the field and how to ensure programs that target employees take into account that an employee with a disability will not be static in the infrastructure of an organization.

The field of public health has long recognized the impact that employment has on quality of life and the related negative mental and physical health repercussions that accompany unemployment (Linn, Sandifer, & Stein, 1985). The culture of the work environment, job tasks, compensation, and stability of the position all can impact worker health (U.S. Department of Health and Human Services, 2018). For people with disabilities, work contributes to both physical and mental health (Rueda et al., 2011; Saunders & Nedelec, 2014). Conversely, lack of engagement in the workforce is connected to poorer health outcomes for a variety of populations.

15.2.2   Unfulfilled Opportunities

While the strides made in legislation set the stage for success in the employment arena, people with disabilities still experience gaps in employment. In 2017, the employment rate for people without disabilities was 76.5% versus 35.5% for people with disabilities (Bureau of Labor Statistics, 2018). This represents a gap of 41% that shows a slight decrease from the 2016 employment rate of 41.4%. However, the gap has remained relatively consistent for the previous decade, with a low of 39.5% found in 2008 (Houtenville & Boege, 2019). Related data also provide a snapshot of national earnings. For full-time workers (defined as working more than 35 h weekly over 50 weeks annually), employees with disabilities earned $40,353 per year, as opposed to $45,449 earned by employees without disabilities. This is a gap of $5096 in median earnings (Houtenville & Boege, 2019).

Another measure of the employment outlook for people with disabilities comes when examining the results of the transition process from school to work. We know that young adults with disabilities face multiple challenges in obtaining successful post-school outcomes. In a National Longitudinal Transition Study-2 report, Wagner, Newman, Cameto, Levine, and Garza (2006) found that for former students with disabilities, 70% had engaged in paid employment since leaving high school, though only 40% were employed at the time of interview—clearly unfavorable to the 63% employment rate of their peers without disabilities. This further reinforces the employment gaps seen across all ages. In recognition of the need for improved post-school outcomes, the Administration for Community Living began the Partnerships in Employment State Systems Change grant program (PIE) as a project of national significance. The grants prioritize employment as an expectation for youth with the most significant disabilities by identifying, developing, and promoting efforts to improve employment outcomes (Administration for Community Living, 2019). One PIE state (KentuckyWorks, n.d.) highlights the following evidence-based practices as crucial to successful post-school outcomes for students with intellectual disabilities, autism, and multiple disabilities:

1. A critical focus on student self-determination—Students' ability to direct their own lives and to make important decisions related to their career goals (Holub, Lamb, & Bang, 1998) has been strongly related to positive post-school outcomes for students (Shogren, Wehmeyer, Palmer, Rifenbark, & Little, 2015; Wehmeyer & Palmer, 2003). Moreover, students *can* be taught to evidence higher levels of self-determination through carefully designed instruction (Wehmeyer, Palmer, Shogren, Williams-Diehm, & Soukup, 2013).
2. Community-based vocational training as an integral part of transition services with an emphasis on paid employment while in high school—Community-based vocational evaluation and job training, and especially paid employment while still in school, have been well documented in achieving positive post-school outcomes for youth with significant disabilities (Carter, Austin, & Trainor, 2012; Lobianco & Kleinert, 2013; Test, 2012).
3. Enhanced parent and family expectations—Parental expectations *are* changeable and are influenced by how well their son or daughter is doing at that specific point in time (Doren, Gau, & Lindstrom, 2013), as well as *teacher and other professional* expectations. Parental expectations are also affected by perceptions (and misperceptions) of the impact of wages upon government benefits (e.g., Supplemental Security Income, Medicaid).
4. Importance of communicative competence—In a study across 15 states and 39,837 students, Towles-Reeves et al. (2012) found that approximately 10% of high school students with significant disabilities did *not* have a formal means of symbolic communication.
5. Interagency collaboration, including Vocational Rehabilitation (VR) and both state and local developmental disability agencies, is well documented in achieving positive post-school outcomes for youth with disabilities (Test, 2012; Winsor, Butterworth, & Boone, 2011). Coordination that includes adult service providers is also mandated as part of a student's individualized transition planning.

While students with disabilities reflect only one segment of the disabled population, they reflect the aptitudes and skills attained through secondary school preparation. As such, students with disabilities represent an important component of the talent pipeline for employers, now and into the future (Whitehouse, Ingram, & Silverstein, 2016).

15.2.3 Employment First

While great legislative progress has been made in the employment arena for people with disabilities, pervasive barriers still remain. Many states have passed legislation or have executive orders in place that establish Employment First principles. The Employment First movement is one that recognizes that people with disabilities should have the opportunity for career advancement, with fair wages in employment that is meaningful (APSE, 2019). This is of significant importance to people with disabilities, but also benefits employers by having access to talented employees. Taxpayers also benefit because public funds that are used to support people with disabilities in segregated programs are lessened, while tax revenues increase as a result of earned income (Whitehouse et al., 2016).

Employment First represents a substantial paradigm shift in the way systems approach disability. It considers employment to be the preferred option for people with disabilities and presupposes the notion that everyone can work. Employment First language also emphasizes that real work for real wages is the first step in ending the cycle of poverty and dependence that often exists for people with disabilities (APSE, n.d.). Most recently, Alaska, New Hampshire, and Maryland represent the first states that have repealed legislation allowing work for subminimum wages.

Additionally, because Employment First opens the door to higher expectations and commensurate pay, it also can provide a mechanism for employer-provided health insurance plans. As has been discussed in this text, health insurance and the access to health care that it brings can be a strong motivator for people with disabilities. Health insurance benefits enable the maintaining of one's health status and warding off of secondary conditions (that can be more disabling than a person's disability). It is well-known that the health of workers is improved when the employee has health insurance. This is particularly important for workers with disabilities. The national APSE organization consists of interdisciplinary members. State chapters build Employment First capacity and policy and work with businesses to strengthen employment opportunities (APSE, n.d.). Working with state APSE chapters and becoming a member can provide public health students and professionals with additional resources and connections related to inclusive employment.

15.3 Systems Involved in Employment Engagement for People with Disabilities

For persons with disabilities, a variety of systems may be encountered when engagement in the workforce is undertaken. These systems can be generic or disability related. The workforce system, healthcare system, education system, and social services systems may all have implications for employment outcomes for people with disabilities. The interaction between systems can create disincentives if policies are not in alignment.

15.3.1 Workforce System

The workforce system exists at the federal, state, and national level. The ultimate role of the system is to connect employers and the talent pipeline (i.e., workforce). When the workforce system is operating well, future needs of businesses are identified and the pool of available workers has the skills required to fill those needs. This requires that the workforce system operates in concert with other community-level systems, including schools and social services. At the state level, One-Stop Career Centers (also known as American Job Centers) exist to make linkages between job seekers and employers. As the name implies, One-Stop Career Centers are intended to address various needs for both prospective employees and employers, from entering the workforce or learning new skills to finding qualified workers. One-Stop Career Centers house state vocational rehabilitation (VR) agencies. VR agencies have a mission to assist people with disabilities in getting and maintaining employment.

15.3.2 Healthcare System

The healthcare system can serve to promote or hinder employment for people with disabilities. Costs of health care are more likely to keep people with disabilities from accessing needed services (CDC, n.d.). Also, accessibility of health care, particularly in rural settings, may not meet the needs of patients who have disabilities, thus necessitating more travel. Furthermore, a lack of training that includes cultural competency and implicit and unconscious bias related to disabilities may decrease practitioner perceptions of being able to successfully work with disabled people. The healthcare system can also hinder people with disabilities from succeeding in employment through low expectations of employment as an outcome. If healthcare professionals do not believe jobs are important or meaningful for patients with disabilities, scheduling of appointments can interfere with the patients' work schedules.

15.3.3 Social Services System

The social services system can vary in structure and location at the state level. From a federal perspective, social services include interventions and services that are intended to "improve the well-being of individuals, families, and communities" (U.S. Department of Health and Human Services, 2018). Programs include Temporary Assistance for Needy Families (TANF), Supplemental Nutrition Assistance Program (SNAP), and Head Start. The Social Security Administration (SSA), as discussed in Hall's chapter of this text (Chap. 14), includes Supplemental Security Income (SSI) and Social Security Disability Insurance (SSDI), both of which provide a gateway to health coverage. Disincentives to seeking employment for people with disabilities are often found in the fear of losing social security benefits and subsequent medical care coverage.

15.3.4 Education System

With regard to education, the Individuals with Disabilities Education Act (IDEA) mandates that students with disabilities have a transition plan in place for exit from secondary school. The federal law requires a transition plan by age 16, though some states opt to begin transition planning earlier, recognizing that more time may be needed for a successful transition. The planning team, which include the student as the central member (and ideally as the team leader), along with school personnel, family, and others who are integral to the plan, meet to develop, review, and assess progress in meeting the transition plan objectives and, ultimately, the blueprint for employment and independent living. See Box 15.1 for an example of how multiple systems must work together if successful employment outcomes are to be attained.

Box 15.1 Systems Involved in Obtaining Employment for a Student with a Disability

Sam is an 18-year-old student with an intellectual disability. He is preparing to graduate from high school and become employed. At school, Sam has a transition team (as mandated by the Individuals with Disabilities Education Act) who have assisted him in learning about jobs and exploring different career clusters. He has received pre-employment transition services around self-advocacy so that he can be more confident when interviewing for jobs. These services are funded through the state Office of Vocational Rehabilitation. Sam and his family also learned about supported decision-making. They are using this model instead of pursuing guardianship for Sam.

Sam has been meeting with a peer counselor at the local Center for Independent Living (CIL). The CIL provided him with information about Supplemental Security Income (SSI) and Sam and his family decided that he would pursue work instead of applying for SSI benefits. He has received transportation training and become more comfortable using the bus. Sam thinks that using the fixed route bus system will be more reliable than the area paratransit taxi system. Though the paratransit option means he would be picked up at his residence, his experience has been that the rides are often late. He does not want to be late for his job, wherever that may be. Sam is fortunate to be able to be on his family health insurance plan, at least for a few more years. It will be important for him to have a job that will provide health insurance benefits in the future.

15.4   Healthcare Model of Disability Related to Work

Work status has long been described from a medical lens. When a person experiences an injury or illness, his or her return to work is determined upon medical release from a healthcare professional. This makes healthcare providers serve as the gatekeeper for workforce participation. If physicians and other health professionals do not promote a return to work as soon as medically feasible, chances are that the employee will not pursue return to work. However, if we want to improve health and reduce health disparities, we must recognize the role employment plays as an important social determinant of health. The role and impact of medical professionals cannot be understated. Use of a health equity lens recognizes the importance of employment as a vehicle where no one is "disadvantaged from achieving this [health] potential because of social position or other socially determined circumstance" (Health Equity, n.d.-a).

15.5   Public Health Role in Return to Work/Stay at Work

Each year, millions of workers experience on and off the job injuries, illnesses, or medical conditions that remove them from the workforce (Ben-Shalom, 2016; Rubin, Roessler, & Rumrill, 2016). These work disabilities are disruptive at the individual and societal level. Workers may move from short-term to long-term disability benefits, culminating at the federal disability Social Security Disability Income (SSDI) rolls, often never returning to the workforce (Strauser, 2014). This negatively impacts the economic outlook for employers who are faced with employee turnover arising from vacant positions, lost productivity, and resulting decreased output. The main driver of the cost of disability to employers and to society as a whole is the number of days, weeks, months, and years that workers lose to disability. Unemployment for Americans with disabilities is also a public health crisis that creates household economic instability and results in disparities affecting life outcomes including health, community integration, and economic self-sufficiency (Smart, 2016).

Employers have a financial interest in returning injured and ill workers to their jobs as soon as possible and maintaining workers with disabilities, with on-the-job accommodations, to reduce turnover, which is widely acknowledged as the most costly personnel expense for today's employers. Avoidable turnover can cost employers up to 33% of a worker's annual salary that is spent in the process of interviewing, onboarding, and training to hire a replacement if that worker leaves (Otto, 2017).

In 2018, eight states were funded to develop model demonstration projects that aim to prevent the development of long-term work disability through early, coordinated health and employment-related services with emphasis on public health. This effort, to develop a network that keeps workers in the workforce following injury or illness, is titled Retaining Employment and Talent After Injury/Illness Network (RETAIN). Successful collaborations created through RETAIN include workforce development entities, healthcare systems, and other systems level partners. The ultimate goals of this effort are:

1. To increase employment retention and labor force participation of people who acquire or are at risk of sustaining work disabilities.
2. To reduce long-term work disability among project participants, as measured by enrollment in Social Security Disability Insurance (SSDI) and Supplemental Security Income (SSI).

Federal workers' compensation laws provide protections and processes that are aimed at helping those who have incurred job-related injuries. However, there is not a similar system in place for non-occupational illnesses and injuries. This is notable because these occur eight times more often than on-the-job issues and result in hundreds of thousands of workers receiving state or federally funded benefits (Neuhauser, 2016). This negatively impacts workers, employers, and communities. Below, we present a model that includes opportunity for public health involvement at multiple points of the intervention process.

For a worker experiencing an injury or illness, a myriad of decision points can make the difference in deciding whether to return to work or exit the workforce. As soon as is medically feasible, early intervention to assist in navigating medical and other important decisions is critical. Early intervention services include:

Case management—Process of planning, assessment, and coordination between a return-to-work coordinator and injured employee can help the person to develop and work toward getting back on the job. This includes coordination of health and employment services through development of a return-to-work plan that supports the person in staying at work or returning to work.

Job analysis—Process of collecting information about the responsibilities, tasks, skills, and environment for a particular job. Job analysis information can be particularly helpful if the person cannot return to the current job, because it is a way to identify those skills that can be transferred to another position.

Assistive technology (AT) evaluation—Devices or products that improve functional capabilities are considered assistive technology. Assistive technology can be used to improve worksite accessibility in a variety of ways, from office layout and computer access to vehicle modifications and compensatory strategies to perform job tasks. Each state receives federal funding to operate state AT programs that include device loans and training.

Peer support—An injury or illness can be a time when a person feels particularly isolated and alone. With disrupted routines, roles, and uncertainty of what the future may bring, it can be especially helpful to connect with someone who has undergone similar life experiences. Ideally, trained peer support specialists provide knowledge, information, and social and emotional supports. Centers for Independent Living, an outcome of the Independent Living movement, are found around the country and include peer support as a core service.

Follow along support—Ongoing check in with the employee to ensure that the return-to-work plan is on track and to provide additional referrals or updates to the plan, as individually determined.

Social support services referral—The most important aspect of return to work. For many American workers, when employment is interrupted due to injury or illness, there is no monetary safety net. The injury or illness may not be as disruptive as the inability to pay the mortgage and the electric bill or buy groceries.

Another substantial element of RETAIN includes employer and healthcare engagement. A major component of this effort includes providing training to employers and healthcare providers. Research shows that most people are better off working and experience improved quality of life, enhanced physical conditioning and mental health and alertness with less relapse or re-injury, and improved patient satisfaction. Keeping an employee engaged in work reduces the impact on a person's family and reduces the likelihood of developing secondary conditions that can delay or complicate recovery (Schultz, Chlebak, & Stewart, 2016).

There are several areas where public health can have meaningful involvement. The training component of RETAIN can benefit from the expertise and community engagement of public health. For example, pain management is considered an important element in successful return to work/stay at work. Alternatives to opioid use can be well delivered through public health programming. In addition, community health workers (CHW) are well suited to be part of the RETAIN team. The CHW is defined as "a frontline public health worker who is a trusted member of and/or has an unusually close understanding of the community served. This trusting relationship enables the worker to serve as a liaison/link/intermediary between health/social services and the community to facilitate access to services and improve the quality and cultural competence of service delivery" (Community Health Workers, 2019). Therefore, the CHW can serve as a link between health care and the community (APHA, 2019). The CHW can also provide advocacy and informal counseling and make referrals for needed social supports (APHA, 2019). This provides an additional catchment for employees who are out of the workplace and in need of social supports during the interim.

Involvement in RETAIN can enhance understanding of supports and resources, including assistive technology and universal design, that can benefit people with disabilities across public health programming. Assistive technology is an individualized solution to enhancing capabilities. Universal design provides another approach that considers how to develop programs, resources, and environments that maximize accessibility for all. We further describe universal design below.

15.6   Universal Design Approach

Universal design (UD) is design that is usable by all people, to the greatest extent possible, without the need for adaptation or specialized design (Story, Mueller, & Mace, 1998). UD began as a way to incorporate design elements in architecture that would be accessible to a diverse set of users (Story et al., 1998). It uses the concept of human factors design, which is design that accommodates the widest possible range of bodies. This idea benefits all people, and particularly people with disabilities. As such, universal design has been recognized as a way to make products, resources, and environments usable by the widest array of people. The UD definition can serve as a response to the WHO definition of disability related to participation restrictions. Within an employment context, the degree of UD that is created in an environment depends on the degree to which it accommodates the widest array of employees and potential employees possible. Universal design concepts dovetail with Healthy People 2020's goal of creating environments that promote good health for all and are particularly practical in the work environment.

Principles of universal design include:

1. Equitable Use—The design appeals to all people and avoids stigmatizing people. Example—the main exterior entrance to a building that includes a ramp, enabling access for all people.
2. Flexibility in Use—The design provides options in methods of use. It is adaptable to the user and can be used at the pace of the user. The design allows for accuracy. Example—a sign that includes text and Braille.
3. Simple and Intuitive Use—The design is easy to use regardless of previous experience. The design accommodates all language abilities. Example—large elevator buttons that light up when pressed.
4. Perceptible Information—The design presents necessary information using images, speech, or tactile guidance. Example—thermostats that provide information using pictures and audibly.
5. Tolerance for Error—The design minimizes and warns of hazards or errors and provides features that promote safety. Example—a double cut door lock that allows a key to be inserted in either direction.
6. Low Physical Effort—The design allows for use with minimal fatigue. The user can remain in a body-neutral position and does not need to repeat an action multiple times. Example—a shower that includes bench seating.
7. Size and Space for Approach and Use—The design provides enough room for all users, either standing or seated to approach, reach, and manipulate. The design provides built-in accommodations. Example—wide door openings on exterior entrances to buildings.

The principles of UD that address accessibility of physical spaces have been further extended to include information sharing, for if the physical structure of a building is accessible to all but transportation resources are only available to people who can read at a tenth grade level or who do not use a screen reader to access information, a smaller subset of individuals will be able to utilize the accessible building. Maximizing UD principles across physical environments, infrastructures, and communications is critical to maximizing the potential of all people (World Health Organization, 2011). Also known as universal design for learning or universal design for instruction, the principles include multiple means of representation, expression, and engagement (Burgstahler, 2009). Just as UD principles benefit the broadest array of people, so does universal design for learning (UDL), through flexibility, reduction of barriers in conveying information, and intentionality of design at the outset. Though universal design for learning might imply its value lies in education, UDL principles transfer across domains and environments. Employing UDL can enhance communications and help to promote improved information sharing.

Universal design principles bring many benefits to the workplace. The Americans with Disabilities Act (ADA) ensures that reasonable accommodations be provided in the workplace for employees with disabilities. A reasonable accommodation is:

> any change to the application or hiring process, to the job, to the way the job is done, or the work environment that allows a person with a disability who is qualified for the job to perform the essential functions of that job and enjoy equal employment opportunities. Accommodations are considered "reasonable" if they do not create an undue hardship or a direct threat. (ADA National Network, n.d.)

However, through the use of universal design, some accommodations may not be needed because accessibility has been considered a priority at the outset (Sanford, 2016). This does not mean that the idea of accommodations in the workplace is not necessary, but rather that if an environment is highly accessible from the outset, a broader array of people will be able to succeed in that environment. In addition, there is no stigma associated with perceived favoritism that can occur if a worker has concerns about negative coworker attitudes. Universal design also addresses issues of an aging workforce. In fact, when using a lens of universal design, public health can influence and improve participation of people with disabilities across all facets of the discipline, not just employment. Though the concept of UD is not a new one, it provides an equitable lens for public health professionals to employ across programs and areas of emphasis. As such, UD can provide practical strategies for public health professionals to enhance policies, procedures, and programs; ultimately this equitable approach enables the field of public health to better promote good health for everyone.

15.7   Conclusion

The perception of disability has changed over time. No longer can the label of disability be considered a failed outcome. In fact, presence or absence of disability can be considered contextual and domain specific. People experience disability in many different ways, and an impairment that is disabling in one environment may not be disabling in another. Additionally, as veterans with service-connected disabilities enter the workforce, as people age into having disabilities, and as people continue to work past the historical age of retirement, there is a greater need for education around how workforce can be inclusive of all people. Public health can help to lead that dialogue.

A great deal of work remains to be done in order to make strides if employment outcomes are to improve for people with disabilities. The expectation of work as the preferred outcome for all people with disabilities is necessary. This must happen at the earliest ages. CDC initiatives promoting early interventions have been instrumental in connecting families and people with disabilities to needed services and supports from the youngest ages. However, as children with disabilities grow into adults, the collaboration and support of public health in assisting people to remain healthy not only in their communities but more specifically in the workplace further enhance public health for all.

Further, an understanding of the complex benefits system that can serve as a disincentive to employment is also imperative. As has been described in Hall's chapter on Health Insurance and Employment in this text (Chap. 14), the Medicare and Medicaid programs that are intended to ensure medical coverage to Americans with disabilities can actually become a barrier to entering the workforce. For many families, the idea of possibly exceeding an earned income threshold that could lead to disenrollment of health insurance as a result of working is not a risk worth taking. Therefore, it is important to have access to benefits specialists who can help disentangle the myths and realities of the impact of employment on healthcare benefits. In the majority of situations, it is better to work than to not work.

Given that approximately 20% of the US population has at least one disability and that people with disabilities experience lower socioeconomic status, public health must engage, actively listen, and provide an often-necessary voice for people with disabilities in an effort to increase community participation. This can be particularly challenging, given that the majority of public health training programs don't include people with disabilities as part of public health programs or include course content around health and disability (AUCD, 2019). Not gaining competencies around disability will mean that a major population is ignored.

Ultimately, our world benefits from having a workforce that is inclusive of people with disabilities. Diversity of experience and in approach to problem-solving benefits employers. Inclusion in employment benefits people with disabilities. As the numbers of people who experience disability continue to grow and evolve, recognizing the value of people with a variety of impairments in all aspects of community life is also a social justice issue. Social justice allows for equal access to not only wealth but other opportunities and privileges. People with disabilities should have the opportunity to define themselves by their occupation and what they do, not just by the label of a particular disability. Public health can be a key player in addressing inequities of people with disabilities by recognizing the need in all aspects of programming, with a particular emphasis on efforts that are directed at workforce.

Resources

Assistive Technology State Program Directory: https://www.at3center.net/stateprogram

Centers for Independent Living: https://www.ilru.org/projects/cil-net/cil-center-and-association-directory

One Stop Career Centers: https://www.careeronestop.org/LocalHelp/local-help.aspx

RETAIN: https://www.dol.gov/odep/topics/SAW-RTW/how-to-apply.htm

Vocational Rehabilitation: https://www2.ed.gov/programs/rsabvrs/index.html

Universal Design: https://universaldesign.org

References

Accenture. (2018). *Getting to equal: The disability inclusion advantage.* Author. Retrieved from https://www.accenture.com/_acnmedia/pdf-89/accenture-disability-inclusion-research-report.pdf

ADA National Network. (n.d.). *Reasonable accommodations in the workplace.* Retrieved from https://adata.org/factsheet/reasonable-accommodations-workplace

Administration for Community Living. (2019). *Partnerships for employment.* Retrieved from http://partnershipsinemployment.com/

American Public Health Association. (2019). *Community health workers.* Retrieved from https://www.apha.org/apha-communities/member-sections/community-health-workers

Antosh, A., Blair, M., Edwards, K., Goode, T., Hewitt, A., Izzo, M., & Wehmeyer, M. (2013). *A collaborative interagency, interdisciplinary approach to transition from adolescence to adulthood.* Silver Spring, MD: Association of University Centers on Disabilities.

APSE. (2019). *Mission, vision & values.* Retrieved from https://apse.org/about/mission-vision/

APSE. (n.d.). *Statement on employment first.* Retrieved from https://apse.org/employment-first/employment-first-statement/

Association of University Centers on Disabilities. (2019). *Including people with disabilities—Public health workforce competencies.* Retrieved from https://www.aucd.org/template/page.cfm?id=830

Ben-Shalom, B. (2016). *Steps states can take to help workers keep their jobs after injury, illness or disability.* Final report submitted to the U.S. Department of Labor, Office of Disability Employment Policy. Washington, DC: Mathematica Policy Research.

Bureau of Labor Statistics. (2019). *Number of jobs, labor market experience and earnings growth.* Retrieved from https://www.bls.gov/news.release/pdf/nlsoy.pdf

Burgstahler, S. (2009). Universal design of instruction (UDI): Definition, principles, guidelines, and examples. Retrieved from http://www.washington.edu/doit/Brochures/Academics/instruction.html

Carter, E., Austin, D., & Trainor, A. (2012). Predictors of postschool employment outcomes for young adults with severe disabilities. *Journal of Disability Policy Studies, 23,* 50–63.

CDC. (n.d.). *Cost as a barrier to care for people with disabilities: A tip sheet for public health professionals.* Retrieved from https://www.cdc.gov/ncbddd/disabilityandhealth/documents/cost_barrier-tip-sheet%2D%2D_phpa_1.pdf

Centers for Disease Control and Prevention. (n.d.-a). *Health equity.* Retrieved from https://www.cdc.gov/chronicdisease/healthequity/index.htm

Centers for Disease Control and Prevention. (n.d.-b). *Workplace health promotion.* Retrieved from https://www.cdc.gov/chronicdisease/resources/publications/factsheets/workplace-health. htm?CDC_AA_refVal=https%3A%2F%2Fwww.cdc.gov%2Fchronicdisease%2Fresources%2 Fpublications%2Faag%2Fworkplace-health.htm

Doren, B., Gau, J., & Lindstrom, L. (2013). The relationship between parent expectations and postschool outcomes of adolescents with disabilities. *Exceptional Children, 79*(1), 7–24.

Holub, T., Lamb, P., & Bang, M. Y. (1998). Empowering all students through self-determination. In C. Jorgensen (Ed.), *Restructuring high schools for all students: Taking inclusion to the next level* (pp. 183–208). Baltimore, MD: Paul Brookes.

Houtenville, A., & Boege, S. (2019). *Annual report on people with disabilities in America: 2018.* Durham, NH: University of New Hampshire, Institute on Disability.

KentuckyWorks. (n.d.). *Evidence based strategies for successful transition. Partnerships in employment proposal.* Lexington: Human Development Institute, University of Kentucky.

Leslie, M. J., Sheppard-Jones, K., & Bishop, M. (under review). *Implications of the opioid crisis for the American disability community.* Rehabilitation Research, Policy and Evaluation.

Linn, M. W., Sandifer, R., & Stein, S. (1985). Effects of unemployment on mental and physical health. *American Journal of Public Health, 75*(5), 502–506.

Lobianco, T., & Kleinert, H. (2013). *HDI Winter 2013 Research Brief: Factors and strategies in successful post-school transitions.* Lexington: Human Development Institute, University of Kentucky.

Lollar, D. (2008). Rehabilitation psychology and public health: Commonalities, barriers and bridges. *Rehabilitation Psychology, 53*(2), 122–127.

National Academies of Sciences, Engineering, and Medicine. (2018). *People living with disabilities: Health equity, health disparities, and health literacy: Proceedings of a workshop.* Washington, DC: The National Academies Press. https://doi.org/10.17226/24741

National Governors Association. (2012). *A better bottom line: Employing people with disabilities.* Washington, DC: Author.

Neuhauser, F. (2016). The myth of workplace injuries: Why we should eliminate workers' compensation for 90% of workers and employers. *Perspectives, 1*, 21–33.

Nye-Lengerman, K., & Nord, D. (2016). Changing the message: Employment as a means out of poverty. *Journal of Vocational Rehabilitation, 44*, 243–247.

National Institute on Drug Abuse. (2018). Opioid overdose crisis. National Institute on Drug Abuse: Advancing Addiction Science. Retrieved from https://www.drugabuse.gov/drugs-abuse/ opioids/opioid-overdose-crisis.

Osburn, J. (2007). An overview of SRV theory. *The SRV Journal, 1*(1), 4–13.

Otto, N. (2017). *Avoidable turnover costs employers big.* Retrieved from https://www.benefit-news.com/news/avoidable-turnover-costing-employers-big?brief=00000152-14a7-d1cc-a5fa-7cffccf00000&utm_content=socialflow&utm_campaign=ebnmagazine&utm_source=twitter&utm_medium=social

Patterson, L. (2018). The disability rights movement in the United States. In M. R. Rembis, C. K. Kudlick, & K. E. Nielsen (Eds.), *The Oxford handbook of disability history* (pp. 439–457). New York, NY: Oxford University Press.

Rubin, S., Roessler, R., & Rumrill, P. (2016). *Foundations of the vocational rehabilitation process* (7th ed.). Austin, TX: Pro-Ed.

Rueda, S., Raboud, J., Mustard, C., Bayoumi, A., Lavis, J. N., & Rourke, S. B. (2011). Employment status is associated with both physical and mental health quality of life in people living with HIV. *AIDS Care, 23*(4), 435–443.

Sanford, J. A. (2016). Universal design as a human factors approach to return to work interventions for people with a variety of diagnoses. In I. Z. Schultz & R. J. Gatchel (Eds.), *Handbook of return to work* (pp. 403–422). New York, NY: Springer.

Saunders, S. L., & Nedelec, B. (2014). What work means to people with work disability: A scoping review. *Journal of Occupational Rehabilitation, 24*(1), 100–110.

Schultz, I. Z., Chlebak, C. M., & Stewart, A. M. (2016). Impairment, disability and return to work. In I. Z. Schultz & R. J. Gatchel (Eds.), *Handbook of return to work* (pp. 3–27). New York, NY: Springer.

Shogren, K., Wehmeyer, M., Palmer, S., Rifenbark, G., & Little, T. (2015). Relationships between self-determination and postschool outcomes for youth with disabilities. *Journal of Special Education, 48,* 256–267.

Smart, J. (2016). *Disability, society, and the individual* (3rd ed.). Austin, TX: Pro-Ed.

Story, M. F., Mueller, J. L., & Mace, R. L. (1998). *The universal design file: Designing for people of all ages and abilities.* Raleigh, NC: Center for Universal Design, NC State University.

Strauser, D. R. (2014). *Career development, employment and disability in rehabilitation: From theory to practice.* New York, NY: Springer.

Switzer, J. V. (2003). *Disabled rights: American disability policy and the fight for equality.* Washington, DC: Georgetown University Press.

Test, D. (2012). *Evidence-based instructional strategies for transition.* Baltimore, MD: Paul Brookes.

Towles-Reeves, E., Kearns, J., Flowers, C., Hart, L., Kerbel, A., Kleinert, H., … Thurlow, M. (2012). *Learner characteristics inventory project report (A product of the NCSC validity evaluation).* Minneapolis, MN: University of Minnesota, National Center and State Collaborative.

U.S. Department of Health and Human Services. (2018). *Employment. In healthy people 2020.* Retrieved from https://www.healthypeople.gov/2020/topics-objectives/topic/social-determinants-health/interventions-resources/employment

Wagner, M., Newman, L., Cameto, R., Levine, P., & Garza, N. (2006). *An overview of findings from wave 2 of the National Longitudinal Transition Study-2 (NLTS2).* Menlo Park, CA: SRI.

Wehmeyer, M., & Palmer, S. (2003). Adult outcomes for students with cognitive disabilities three-years after high school: The impact of self-determination. *Education and Training in Developmental Disabilities, 38*(2), 131–144.

Wehmeyer, M. L., Palmer, S. B., Shogren, K., Williams-Diehm, K., & Soukup, J. (2013). Establishing a causal relationship between intervention to promote self-determination and enhanced student self-determination. *The Journal of Special Education, 146*(4), 195–210.

Whitehouse, E., Ingram, K., & Silverstein, B. (2016). *Work matters: A framework for states on workforce development for people with disabilities.* Washington, DC: Office of Disability Employment Policy State Exchange on Employment and Disability.

Winsor, J., Butterworth, J., & Boone, J. (2011). Jobs by 21 partnership project: Impact of cross-system collaboration on employment outcomes of young adults with developmental disabilities. *Intellectual and Developmental Disabilities, 49,* 274–284.

World Health Organization. (2011). *World report on disability.* Retrieved from www.who.int/disabilities/world_report

World Health Organization. (2018). *Disability and health.* Retrieved from https://www.who.int/en/news-room/fact-sheets/detail/disability-and-health

Chapter 16
Preparing a Disability-Competent Workforce

Adriane Griffen and Susan Havercamp

16.1 Workforce Capacity Opportunity

Public health is inclusive and collaborative, involving a diverse workforce of practitioners ranging from professionals with expertise in health promotion to healthcare providers. Many programs and efforts are intended to reach and serve everyone living in the community, yet people with disabilities are often overlooked in public health planning and programs. A fully prepared workforce would be comprised of this wide range of professionals who have the capacity to include people with disabilities in public health efforts. Workforce capacity may be built through promoting readiness for the change of inclusion of people with disabilities, practical collaboration experiences with partners, and learning from the act of working with people with disabilities in public health efforts. These workforce capacity building efforts may be embedded into existing professional training in order to reach a diverse group of public health professionals. Public health professionals may include any provider who supports health promotion through accessing quality health care. The current public health workforce has an opportunity to more fully embrace the meaning of public health by including people with disabilities in efforts that serve the whole community.

A. Griffen (✉)
Association of University Centers on Disabilities, Silver Spring, MD, USA
e-mail: agriffen@aucd.org

S. Havercamp
Nisonger Center, The Ohio State University, Columbus, OH, USA
e-mail: susan.havercamp@osumc.edu

© Springer Science+Business Media, LLC, part of Springer Nature 2021
D. J. Lollar et al. (eds.), *Public Health Perspectives on Disability*,
https://doi.org/10.1007/978-1-0716-0888-3_16

16.2   Public Health Overview and Relation to Disability

Public health may be understood as a spectrum—from health promotion to health care. One may view public health as the science and art of preventing disease, prolonging life, and promoting health and efficiency through an organized community effort (Winslow, 1920); however, this presents a potential conflict with respect to people with disabilities. Historically, the public health system was conceptualized as a tool to prevent disabilities, rather than a tool to promote the health of people with disabilities (Lollar & Crews, 2003). People with disabilities were not considered a demographic group to be included in public health programs (US Department of Health and Human Services, 2000, 2005); rather disability was viewed only as a negative health outcome to be prevented (Lollar & Crews, 2003; US Department of Health and Human Services, 2008). The Surgeon General's Call to Action to Improve the Health of Persons with Disabilities (2005) and the Healthy People 2010 (US Department of Health and Human Services, 2000) introduced new ideas about disability. These documents made it clear that public health strategies should be tailored to the needs of people with disabilities. Disability may be considered just one of many demographic characteristics attributed to a person, similar to gender, race, or ethnicity (Krahn, Walker, & Correa-De-Araujo, 2015).

16.3   People with Disabilities: A Growing Demographic in the US

Approximately 61 million, or one in four, Americans have some type of disability such as mobility, sensory, or intellectual or developmental limitation (Okoro, Hollis, Cyrus, & Griffin-Blake, 2018). People with disabilities comprise a significant portion of any community that public health professionals might serve. People with disabilities may live full lives in the community as our coworkers, neighbors, family, and friends. More people in the Southern region of the USA are living with a disability compared to the Northern region (Okoro et al., 2018).

16.4   Health Disparities for People with Disabilities

People with disabilities report poorer health than people without disabilities and face structural, programmatic, and attitudinal barriers to health promotion (Wingo & Rimmer, 2018). People with disabilities have higher rates of health risks compared to people without disabilities including poor access to health care, unhealthy diets, lack of physical activity, increased obesity and cardiovascular disease, and poor emotional and social support (Havercamp & Scott, 2015). These disparities are partially attributed to social determinants of health such as lower levels of education, high unemployment, and low household income (Krahn et al., 2015).

People with disabilities are overrepresented in the healthcare system due, in part, to high rates of chronic health conditions (Emerson, et al., 2016; Havercamp, Scandlin, & Roth, 2004; Havercamp & Scott, 2015). Despite having a greater need for healthcare services, people with disabilities have poorer access to health care compared to people without disabilities (Armour, Swanson, Waldman, & Perlman, 2008; Havercamp, Scandlin, & Roth, 2004; Havercamp & Scott, 2015; Reichard, Stolzle, & Fox, 2011). Compared to people without disabilities, people with disabilities report barriers to accessing quality health care, dissatisfaction with the care they receive (Armour et al., 2008; Havercamp, Scandlin, & Roth, 2004; Reichard, Stolzle, & Fox, 2011), and high rates of unmet healthcare needs (Havercamp & Scott, 2015). These disparities are largely attributed to negative attitudes and assumptions about people with disabilities that are widely held in society.

Negative attitudes toward and assumptions about disabilities have an adverse effect on the health and quality of health care for people with disabilities. The perception of disability often elicits pity, compassion, and the desire to be helpful, but it also often elicits distinctly negative reactions such as disgust or anxiety. These negative perceptions can be understood as unconscious but strongly held biases against people with disabilities. Negative perceptions are widely held in Western society across genders, ethnicities, age groups, and political orientations and even among participants who themselves have disabilities (Nosek et al., 2007; Wilson & Scior, 2014). Although largely unconscious, negative attitudes are associated with the tendency to blame individuals for their disabling conditions and to avoid contact with people who have disabilities (Park, Faulkner, & Schaller, 2003).

Healthcare providers are not protected from prevalent social attitudes and biases. In fact, students are drawn to the health profession and trained to restore their patients to full health. Unfortunately, this purpose proves challenging when confronted with a person who has a permanent disability. Healthcare providers may feel frustrated or defeated at the outset because public health has already failed to prevent or heal the disability (Lollar & Crews, 2003). Negative attitudes have been reported by medical students (Mitchell, Hayes, Gordon, & Wallis, 1984; Tervo, Azuma, Palmer, & Redinius, 2002), nursing students, other health professional students (Tervo, Palmer, & Redinius, 2004), physicians (Bond, Kerr, Dunstan, & Thapar, 1997), and nurses (Matziou et al., 2009). The negative attitudes interfere with the ability of health professionals to establish effective communication and provide quality health care to diverse populations.

One fundamental barrier is the perception that the person with a disability differs in significant and meaningful ways from other patients or the health professional. These assumptions, though unconscious, are prevalent when serving people from different ethnic or racial backgrounds and when serving people with disabilities (Chadd & Pangilinan, 2011). Healthcare professionals often feel that it is more difficult and less appealing to care for people with disabilities.

The "inability assumption" about people with disabilities limits the quality of health care they receive. People without disabilities often tend to underestimate the abilities of people with disabilities, assuming lower levels of cognitive ability, independence, and interest in improving and maintaining current function. Adults with disabilities are often perceived as childlike (Robey, Beckley, & Kirschner, 2006) and asexual (Milligan & Neufeldt, 2001; Shakespeare, 2000). These assumptions may contribute to the finding that women with disabilities are screened for colon cancer at similar rates as their nondisabled peers but are less likely to be screened for breast cancer and cervical cancer (Andresen et al., 2013; Pharr & Bungum, 2012). The sexual health of women with intellectual disability is particularly neglected (Greenwood & Wilkinson, 2013) in terms of screening for breast and cervical cancer (Havercamp & Scott, 2015). Assuming that the patient is extremely limited, an inaccurate assumption often made by health professionals is that people with disabilities are incapable of contributing to their own health or healthcare plan and decisions. The health professional acts with benevolence on behalf of people with disabilities but is less likely to ask for or listen to the individual's point of view. While a person's best interests may be in mind, inaccurate assumptions and biases limit the quality of health care provided to people with disabilities.

A third assumption that reflects a negative bias and that directly affects health care is the belief that quality of life is severely compromised by disability (Albrecht & Devlieger, 1999). When asked to imagine their life after acquiring a paralyzing injury, healthcare providers estimated their life would be barely worth living. Only 18% of emergency care providers including emergency nurses, technicians, residents, and attending physicians, imagined they would be glad to be alive after sustaining a spinal cord injury. This is in stark contrast to the 92% of spinal cord injury survivors who reported having a good quality of life (Gerhart, Koziol-McLain, Lowenstein, & Whiteneck, 1994). This misconception directly affects patient care by limiting the type, scope, and aggressiveness of treatment options considered. One study found that 71% of pediatric residents questioned the aggressive treatment of children with severe disabilities (Edwards, Davidson, Houtrow, & Graham, 2010), and only 22% of emergency care providers reported they would want to be treated with "everything possible to ensure survival" after a severe spinal cord injury (Gerhart et al., 1994). Drainoni et al. (2006) reported a case of a woman with intellectual disability and advanced breast cancer. Her physician determined that surgical intervention was not warranted due to her already low quality of life (owing to her disability). She died within a year.

16.4.1 Communication

Negative attitudes and assumptions interfere with effective communication between health professionals and people with disabilities. People with disabilities complain that healthcare encounters feel rushed and that physicians do not spend enough time to communicate effectively (Harrington, Hirsch, Hammond, Norton, & Bockenek, 2009; Kroll, Beatty, & Bingham, 2003; McKee, Barnett, Block, & Pearson, 2011; Morrison, George, & Mosqueda, 2008). Deaf patients complain about difficulty understanding their healthcare provider. They report that health professionals speak too quickly and use unfamiliar vocabulary. Although the use of an ASL interpreter increases use of preventive care including colonoscopy, flu shot, and cholesterol screening among deaf people, interpreter services are not always provided even when requested by the individual (Harrington et al., 2009). People with disabilities described negative experiences in the healthcare system, creating a loss of trust in healthcare providers and even fear of certain health providers and settings (Neri & Kroll, 2003). As noted in the World Report on Disability (World Health Organization, 2011), negative experiences with the healthcare system, such as experiencing disrespect, insensitivity, and devaluation, may lead people with disabilities to avoid seeking care and rely upon self-diagnosis and treatment.

It is interesting to note how people with disabilities may define wellness. A recent social media Twitter chat hosted by the Association of University Centers on Disabilities (AUCD) engaged the overall disability community in a conversation on the meaning of wellness. People with disabilities who participated shared values of wellness, connecting with resources, and access to health care and health promotion services. Other themes shared by people with disabilities included the importance of having a sense of belonging, caring for body and mind, disability being part of being well, and the acknowledgment of visible and invisible disabilities (AUCD webinar, #IDefineMyWellness, October 29, 2019).

16.5   Need for Disability Training

Disability should be included in public health training because 25% of the population experiences disability and would benefit from skilled health and public health professionals. Despite this growing population of people who live with a disability, most public health professionals receive little to no disability training. A recent survey of Council on Education for Public Health (CEPH) accredited schools and programs showed that about half include disability content in at least one class, with most disability content being offered in graduate-level curricula (Sinclair, Tanenhaus, Courtney-Long, & Eaton, 2015). Content on disability often appeared in elective, rather than required courses, and therefore, many public health students learn nothing about people with disabilities in their professional training.

16.6   New Curricula Frameworks

The US healthcare system is insufficiently prepared to recognize and address the needs of people with disabilities (Ankam et al., 2019). Because people with disabilities live in every community and have a full range of health needs, every public health practitioner and clinician needs to demonstrate comfort and competence in treating this population (Ankam et al., 2019). Disability training is needed to improve the health and health care of people with disabilities. Health professionals must recognize and mitigate the barriers facing people with disabilities in health promotion program participation and accessing quality health care (Ankam et al., 2019; Wingo & Rimmer, 2018).

Competency-based education maps the specific health needs of the population (e.g., people with disabilities) to a set of competencies, or skills, for the workforce in training. These expectations are then used to develop learning objectives and corresponding curricular elements designed to produce the requisite knowledge, values, and skills in the learners to achieve these competencies (Gruppen, Mangrulkar, & Kolars, 2012). Disability competencies may then guide the development and evaluation of disability training programs.

Two sets of disability competencies have been developed to guide disability training: *Including People with disabilities: Public Health Workforce Competencies* and *Core Competencies on Disability for Health Care Education*. The *Including People with disabilities: Public Health Workforce Competencies* support inclusive health promotion and awareness of access to health care developed for the current public health workforce, while the *Core Competencies on Disability for Health Care Education* were developed to train future healthcare providers to provide quality care to patients with disabilities. Both the *Public Health Workforce Competencies* and the *Health Care Education Competencies* emphasize opportunities to include a disability perspective that aligns with current professional practice and training standards, with a fundamental focus on disability inclusion. Both frameworks address disability as a demographic characteristic that contributes to diversity and intersects with all ages, races, ethnicities, genders, sexual identities, and languages. Another shared principle is that disability does not necessarily limit health or quality of life and that people with disabilities benefit from health promotion activities. Both sets of *Competencies* emphasize that, with appropriate supports and services, people with disabilities can live long healthy and happy lives (Table 16.1).

16.7   Development and Alignment with Training Standards

The *Public Health Workforce Competencies* were developed by a national committee comprised of disability and public health experts, including the Association of University Centers on Disabilities (AUCD), CDC's National Center on Birth Defects and Developmental Disabilities (NCBDDD), and CDC's Office for State, Tribal, Local, and Territorial Support. Professional partners, including the American Public Health Association Disability Section and the Alliance for Disability in Health Care Education, provided guidance and feedback and helped with dissemination.

Including People with disabilities: Public Health Workforce Competencies outlines knowledge and practice skills that public health professionals need to include people with disabilities in the core public health functions. Strategies and real examples of how people with disabilities can be successfully included in public health activities are also provided. The *Public Health Workforce Competencies* provide foundational knowledge about the relationship between public health programs and health outcomes among people with disabilities and are relevant to professionals already working in the public health field and to public health training programs. The *Public Health Workforce Competencies* aim to expand workforce skills and

Table 16.1 Public Health Workforce Competencies and Core Competencies—disability inclusion areas of emphasis by spectrum of public health

	Spectrum of public health	
	Health promotion	Health care
Disability inclusion areas of emphasis	*Including People with disabilities: Public Health Workforce Competencies*	*Core Competencies on Disability for Health Care Education*
	Web: disabilityinpublichealth.org	Web: https://nisonger.osu.edu/education-training/ohio-disability-health-program/corecompetenciesondisability/
Disability may be experienced across the lifespan. People with disabilities may live healthy lives, just like anyone else.	**Competency 1: Discuss disability models across the lifespan** Learning objectives: 1.1. Compare and contrast different models of disability 1.2. Define model(s) of disability for a particular scope of work or population served 1.3. Describe the social determinants of health and how they affect health disparities for people with disabilities	**Competency 1: Contextual and conceptual frameworks on disability** Acquire a conceptual framework of disability in the context of human diversity, the lifespan, wellness, injury, and social and cultural environments
People with disabilities are an important demographic in society.	**Competency 2: Discuss methods used to assess health issues for people with disabilities** Learning objectives: 2.1. Identify surveillance systems used to capture data that includes people with disabilities 2.2. Recognize that disability can be used as a demographic variable	**Competency 1: Contextual and conceptual frameworks on disability** Acquire a conceptual framework of disability in the context of human diversity, the lifespan, wellness, injury, and social and cultural environments **Competency 2: Professionalism and patient-centered care** Demonstrate mastery of general principles of professionalism, communication, respect for patients, and recognizes optimal health and quality of life from the patient's perspective

(continued)

Table 16.1 (continued)

	Spectrum of public health	
	Health promotion	Health care
A combination of health promotion, laws, communities, organizations, and accessibility standards impact health outcomes for people with disabilities.	**Competency 3: Identify how public health programs impact health outcomes for people with disabilities** Learning objectives: 3.1. Recognize health issues of people with disabilities and health promotion strategies that can be used to address them 3.2. Use laws as a tool to support people with disabilities 3.3. Recognize accessibility standards, universal design, and principles of built environment that affect the health and quality of life for people with disabilities 3.4. Explain how public health services, governmental programs, and nongovernmental/community-based organizations interact with disability 3.5. Describe how communities (places where people live, work, and recreate) can adapt to be fully inclusive of disability populations	**Competency 2: Professionalism and patient-centered care** Demonstrate mastery of general principles of professionalism, communication, respect for patients, and recognizes optimal health and quality of life from the patient's perspective **Competency 3: Legal obligations and responsibilities for caring for patients with disabilities** Understand and identify legal requirements for providing health care in a manner that is, at minimum, consistent with federal laws such as the Americans with Disabilities Act (ADA), Rehabilitation Act, and Social Security Act to meet the individual needs of people with disabilities

(continued)

Table 16.1 (continued)

	Spectrum of public health	
	Health promotion	Health care
People with disabilities need access to high-quality health care, just like anyone else.	**Competency 4: Implement and evaluate strategies to include people with disabilities in public health programs that promote health, prevent disease, and manage chronic and other health conditions** Learning objectives: 4.1. Describe factors that affect healthcare access for people with disabilities 4.2. Use strategies to integrate people with disabilities into health promotion programs 4.3. Identify emerging issues that impact people with disabilities 4.4. Define how environment can impact health outcomes for people with disabilities 4.5. Apply evaluation strategies (needs assessment, process evaluation, and program evaluation) that can be used to demonstrate impact for people with disabilities	**Competency 4: Teams and systems-based practice** Engage and collaborate with team members within and outside their own discipline to provide high-quality, interprofessional team-based health care to people with disabilities **Competency 5: Clinical assessment** Collect and interpret relevant information about the health and function of patients with disabilities to engage patients in creating a plan of care that includes essential and optimal services and supports **Competency 6: Clinical care over the lifespan and during transitions** Knowledgeable about effective strategies to engage patients with disabilities in creating a coordinated plan of care with needed services and supports

practices to enable public health professionals to successfully develop programs and activities that include people with disabilities. Practitioners may use this resource to enhance disability inclusion skills among staff engaged in practice-based public health efforts. The *Public Health Workforce Competencies* can also be embedded into existing public health curricula and training programs and fit seamlessly within the larger domains of the core public health functions.

To increase the capacity of public health providers to include people with disabilities in their public health plans and efforts, *Including People with disabilities: Public Health Workforce Competencies* offers the following core areas:

Competency 1: Discuss disability models across the lifespan.

Competency 2: Discuss methods used to assess health issues for people with disabilities.

Competency 3: Identify how public health programs impact health outcomes for people with disabilities.

Competency 4: Implement and evaluate strategies to include people with disabilities in public health programs that promote health, prevent disease, and manage chronic and other health conditions.

The *Including People with disabilities: Public Health Workforce Competencies* are available at https://disabilityinpublichealth.org.

These *Public Health Workforce Competencies* align with and compliment broad public health competencies such as the Association of Schools and Programs of Public Health, Association of Schools and Programs of Public Health (ASPPH) Areas of Study, Public Health Accreditation Board, Public Health Foundation Core Competencies, the Council on Education for Public Health (CEPH), and the ten Essential Public Health Services. In addition, they foster workforce capacity-building priorities, such as those described in Healthy People (see Table 16.2). The Core Competencies for Public Health Professionals (Public Health Competencies) (Web: accessed September 23, 2019: http://www.phf.org/resourcestools/Documents/Core_Competencies_for_Public_Health_Professionals_2014June.pdf) represent a consensus set of skills needed for the broad practice of public health as defined by the Council on Linkages Between Academia and Public Health Practice (Council on Linkages). These public health competencies highlight disability awareness as a skill needed across all levels of professional practice: from Tier 1, Front Line Staff/Entry Level to Tier 2, Program Management/Supervisory Level, to Tier 3, Senior Management/Executive Level.

16.8 Core Competencies on Disability for Health Care Education

The *Core Competencies on Disability for Health Care Education* establish the baseline expertise required to provide quality health care to patients with disabilities. The intent of these *Health Care Education Competencies* is to provide broad disability standards to guide healthcare education. The Alliance for Disability in Health Care Education, a nonprofit group comprised of interprofessional health educators, developed these competencies to increase healthcare providers understanding in order to provide quality health care to patients with disabilities. These *Health Care Education Competencies* were designed to apply to people with all types of disabilities (e.g., mobility disabilities, developmental disabilities, mental health disabilities) and to future healthcare providers across disciplines (e.g., medicine, nursing, social work, nutrition, speech, and hearing). The Alliance partnered with Ohio Disability and Health Program at the Ohio State University Nisonger Center to solicit feedback and refine the *Health Care Education Competencies* with input from a broad group of disability stakeholders. A consensus on the core Health Care Education Competencies was achieved through an iterative structured feedback process that included people with disabilities, family members, disability and health experts, health educators, and health care providers. An overwhelming majority (91%) shared that the *Health Care Education Competencies* were relevant to education across health disciplines (91%). The *Disability Competencies for Health Care Education* are available at https://go.osu.edu/corecompetenciesdisability-learnmore.

Table 16.2 Including People with disabilities: Public Health Workforce Competencies Alignment with Public Health Training Standards

Including People with disabilities: Public Health Workforce Competencies	Core Competencies (PHF Council on Linkages) ASPPH areas of study/CEPH learning domains Essential Public Health Services (PHAB)
Competency 1: Discuss disability models across the lifespan Learning objectives: 1.1. Compare and contrast different models of disability 1.2. Define model(s) of disability for a particular scope of work or population served 1.3. Describe the social determinants of health and how they affect health disparities for people with disabilities	Policy Development/Program Planning Skills (PHF) Communication Skills (PHF) Cultural Competency Skills (PHF) Community Dimensions of Practice Skills (PHF) Leadership and Systems Thinking Skills (PHF) Health administration (ASPPH) Develop policies and plans that support individual and community health efforts (PHAB) Enforce laws and regulations that protect health and ensure safety (PHAB) Link people to needed personal health services and assure the provision of health care when otherwise unavailable (PHAB) Multicultural studies and minority health and health disparities (ASPPH) Public health leadership (ASPPH) Mobilize community partnerships to identify and solve health problems (PHAB) Assure a competent public and personal healthcare workforce (PHAB) Social determinants of health (ASPPH) Public health practice (ASPPH)
Competency 2: Discuss methods used to assess health issues for people with disabilities Learning objectives: 2.1. Identify surveillance systems used to capture data that includes people with disabilities 2.2. Recognize that disability can be used as a demographic variable	Analytical/Assessment Skills (PHF) Public Health Sciences Skills (PHF) Biostatistics (ASPPH/CEPH) Monitor health status to identify and solve community health problems (PHAB) Epidemiology (ASPPH/CEPH) Diagnose and investigate health problems and health hazards in the community (PHAB)

(continued)

Table 16.2 (continued)

Including People with disabilities: Public Health Workforce Competencies	*Core Competencies* (PHF Council on Linkages) ASPPH areas of study/CEPH learning domains *Essential Public Health Services (PHAB)*
Competency 3: Identify how public health programs impact health outcomes for people with disabilities Learning objectives: 3.1. Recognize health issues of people with disabilities and health promotion strategies that can be used to address them 3.2. Use laws as a tool to support people with disabilities 3.3. Recognize accessibility standards, universal design, and principles of built environment that affect the health and quality of life for people with disabilities 3.4. Explain how public health services, governmental programs, and nongovernmental/community-based organizations interact with disability 3.5. Describe how communities (places where people live, work and recreate) can adapt to be fully inclusive of disability populations	*Analytical/assessment skills (PHF)* *Community Dimensions of Practice Skills (PHF)* *Public Health Sciences Skills (PHF)* Health education/behavioral sciences (ASPPH/CEPH) *Research for new insights and innovative solutions to health problems (PHAB)* Communication sciences and disorders and informatics (ASPPH) *Inform, educate, and empower people about health issues (PHAB)*
Competency 4: Implement and evaluate strategies to include people with disabilities in public health programs that promote health, prevent disease, and manage chronic and other health conditions Learning objectives: 4.1. Describe factors that affect healthcare access for people with disabilities 4.2. Use strategies to integrate people with disabilities into health promotion programs 4.3. Identify emerging issues that impact people with disabilities 4.4. Define how environment can impact health outcomes for people with disabilities 4.5. Apply evaluation strategies (needs assessment, process evaluation, and program evaluation) that can be used to demonstrate impact for people with disabilities	*Community Dimensions of Practice Skills (PHF)* *Public Health Sciences Skills (PHF)* *Financial Planning and Management Skills (PHF)* *Leadership and Systems Thinking Skills (PHF)* Health services administration (CEPH)public health leadership (ASPPH) Public health practice (ASPPH) *Evaluate effectiveness, accessibility, and quality of personal and population-based health services (PHAB)*

16.8.1 Development and Alignment with Training Standards

The *Core Competencies for Disability in Health Care Education* were developed to guide future health professionals to provide effective, interprofessional team-based health care to patients with disabilities across the lifespan. Interprofessional education occurs when students from two or more professions learn about, from, and with each other to enable effective collaboration and improve health outcomes. The Interprofessional Education Collaborative (IPEC) works across public health and healthcare professions with the opportunity for professional enrichment on better integrating and coordinating the education of members of the healthcare team to provide more collaborative and patient-centered care (Accessed October 11, 2019: https://www.ipecollaborative.org/about-ipec.html). Founding members include the American Association of Colleges of Nursing, the American Association of Colleges of Osteopathic Medicine, the American Association of Colleges of Pharmacy, the American Dental Education Association, the Association of American Medical Colleges, and the Association of Schools of Public Health. IPEC works to ensure that new and current health professionals are proficient in the competencies essential for patient-centered, community- and population-oriented, interprofessional, collaborative practice. As shown in Table 16.3, the *Health Care Education Competencies* align closely with the Core Competencies for Interprofessional Collaborative Practice (IPEC).

16.9 Progress Toward Disability Inclusion in Public Health

Efforts from professional organizations may serve as drivers to support disability inclusion in public health. Two such efforts come from the Public Health Accreditation Board and the American Medical Association. The Public Health Accreditation Board (PHAB) is planning to add disability inclusive health in Version 2.0 of the PHAB standards for accreditation, estimated release of 2021 (October 24, 2018 Inclusive Health Expert Panel Meeting, Alexandria, VA: https://phaboard.org/wp-content/uploads/2.0_InclusiveHealthSummary.pdf; personal correspondence September 23, 2019). The disability inclusive health goal will promote the inclusion of people with disabilities in the planning and execution of public health efforts. These inclusive health standards will be woven across several PHAB domains, including (1) conduct and disseminate assessments focused on population health status and public health issues facing the community; (2) investigate health problems and environmental public health hazards to protect the community; (3) inform and educate about public health issues and functions; (4) engage with the community to identify and address health problems; (5) develop public health policies and plans; and (6) promote strategies to improve access to healthcare services.

Another example of a training driver from a professional entity is the American Medical Association (AMA) resolution on including developmental disabilities in

Table 16.3 *Health Care Education Competencies* alignment with core competencies for Interprofessional Collaborative Practice (IPEC)

IPEC Competencies	Alignment between the *Disability in Health Care Education Competencies* and IPEC Competencies	Elements unique to the *Disability in Health Care Education Competencies*
Values/Ethics for Interprofessional Practice (IPEC Competency 1)	Place patient at the center of all care decisions and delivery (IPEC VE1) (Disability 4.2) Consider the cultural beliefs and values of the individual in all forms of patient care (IPEC VE3, VE4) (Disability 2.7, 6.4) Establish a trusting professional relationship with client (IPEC VE6) (Disability 2.4, 2.5)	Include social and physical environment as factors in determining patient and population health status (Disability 5.10, 5.11) Understand established frameworks and models of disability and regard disability as a diversity/cultural identity (Disability 1.1, 1.6) Consider social determinants of health in clinical decisions and provision of care (Disability 1.5, 2.8)
Roles/Responsibilities (IPEC Competency 2)	Engage an interprofessional team of providers when developing strategies to meet health needs of specific patients and populations (IPEC RR3, RR7) (Disability 4.1, 6.5) Participate in professional development and to enhance team performance and collaboration (IPEC RR8) (Disability 3.6) Utilize individual abilities of team members to provide best possible care to the patient (IPEC RR9) (Disability 4.2, 6.1)	Recognize systems of community-based services and supports outside of the healthcare system as patient care resources (Disability 4.5) Health promotion strategies and preventative screenings should be recommended to patients with disabilities at the same timing and frequency as they would other patients (Disability 6.2, 6.8) Provide accessible office environment and diagnostic/screening equipment for all patients (Disability 3.1, 3.3)
Interprofessional Communication (IPEC Competency 3)	Encourage ideas and feedback from each team member in order to provide the best possible patient-centered care (IPEC CC4, CC5) (Disability 2.6, 4.4) Use respectful language appropriate for a given situation (IPEC CC6) (Disability 2.2) Choose terminology and communication methods that are understandable to patient and caregivers (IPEC CC1, CC2) (Disability 3.2)	Regard the patient with disabilities as the central member of the healthcare team (Disability 5.1) Avoid making assumptions about a patient based on implicit bias or perceived ability level (Disability 2.1) Anticipate needs of patients who use alternative formats and methods to access health information and services (Disability 3.2, 3.4)

(continued)

Table 16.3 (continued)

IPEC Competencies	Alignment between the *Disability in Health Care Education Competencies* and IPEC Competencies	Elements unique to the *Disability in Health Care Education Competencies*
Teams and Teamwork (IPEC Competency 4)	Demonstrate skills in building effective teams of health and other professionals (IPEC TT1) (Disability 6.5) Engage a diverse group of health and other professionals to inform and collaborate on patient-centered care plans and outcomes (IPEC TT3, TT10) (Disability 4.5, 6.7) Consider both evidence-based best practices and client preferences when making decisions about plan of care for patient (IPEC TT4) (Disability 6.4)	Understand barriers/challenges to creating a person-centered healthcare system (Disability 4.3) Ensure that all members of a healthcare team and support staff are able to provide disability competent care (Disability 3.5) Identify situations where a caregiver can provide information necessary to complete a full health assessment or intervention (Disability 5.2)

curriculum in undergraduate, graduate, and continuing medical education of physicians (AMA HOD Official A-17 Proceedings Report, 2017: https://www.ama-assn.org/sites/ama-assn.org/files/corp/media-browser/public/hod/a17-resolutions.pdf). This AMA resolution encourages the Liaison Committee on Medical Education, Commission on Osteopathic College Accreditation, and allopathic and osteopathic medical schools to develop and implement curriculum on the care and treatment of people with developmental disabilities. Further, the Accreditation Council for Continuing Medical Education, specialty boards, and other continuing medical education providers are also encouraged to develop and implement continuing education programs that focus on the care and treatment of people with developmental disabilities (DD). This is especially significant as people with DD are living well into adult life, with the great majority receiving their health care in integrated community and primary care settings rather than specialized centers (Patja, Iivanainen, Vesala, Oksanen, & Ruoppila, 2000).

16.9.1   Competency Alignment to Prepare a Broad Workforce

Aligning disability competencies with those of PHAB, AMA, Council on Linkages, and IPEC presents an opportunity to expand training opportunities to keep the health workforce on the cutting edge of our country's population needs. With one in four Americans having a disability, all health practitioners need to have familiarity with disability in order to improve population health. Given the broad application of health competencies from health promotion to health care, an equally broad workforce is needed with sophisticated knowledge of the entire community—including people with disabilities—as well as specific strategies to include people with disabilities in efforts for the general community.

16.10 Strategies for Integrating Disability into Professional Education and Training

A common myth held among health educators is that adding disability content requires removal of some other content. Given that people with disabilities are part of every community everywhere, connections may be made in integrating disability into professional evaluation and training on any aspect of service for the whole community. A few critical strategies have been used by professional educators to successfully include disability content into training of public health professionals. Whichever strategy is utilized, ongoing learning opportunities are essential for training disability competent health professionals.

16.10.1 Strategy 1: Weave Disability Perspective Throughout Training

There are many opportunities to embed a disability perspective into public health and healthcare education. Rather than viewing disability as a separate topic to be addressed in a special class or activity, one may weave a disability perspective throughout the curriculum. Any health topic is relevant to people with disabilities. Disability awareness may be integrated into any public health course or training that reviews planning, health equity, social determinants of health, ethics, maternal and child health, aging, or epidemiology. Teaching public health students and training staff about disabilities is critical to having a prepared workforce that can serve the whole community.

Three key public health topics or hooks for connecting this disability perspective with general public health educational efforts have been articulated by a national learning group facilitated by the Association of University Centers on Disabilities (AUCD).

1. *Epidemiology and surveillance*: Any time the surveillance needs of the community are addressed, it is an opportunity to integrate a disability perspective. Health data needs to reflect all demographics in the community, including people with disabilities.
2. *Health equity*: People with disabilities experience health inequities and may be addressed alongside any other marginalized populations. People with disabilities

are the largest minority group, comprising 25% of the US population, and a group that anyone can join at any time.

3. *Social determinants of health*: The lived experience of disability may be viewed as an important part of the social determinants of health framework as sectors like housing, transportation, education, and employment have an opportunity to embed a disability perspective in their efforts in order to better serve the whole community. Often, people with disabilities are not included within this framework yet are often negatively impacted by these different social determinants. When a system is designed with people with disabilities in mind, it is better for everyone.

Strategy highlight: The Capacity-Building Toolkit for Including Aging and Disability Networks in Emergency Planning Federal law (Section 2814 and 2802 of the Public Health Service Act (2013)) describes requirements to address the needs of at-risk individuals, including older adults and people with disabilities, in the event of a disaster or public health emergency. *Capacity-Building Toolkit for Including Aging and Disability Networks in Emergency Planning* (*https://www.naccho.org/uploads/downloadable-resources/Capacity-Building-Toolkit-for-Aging-and-Disability-Networks-2-5-19.pdf,* accessed October 14, 2019), developed by the National Association of County and City Health Officials (NACCHO), serves as a resource to guide the aging and disability networks in increasing their ability to plan for and respond to public health emergencies and disasters. This toolkit guides programs that serve people with access and functional needs, including older adults and people with disabilities, through the emergency planning process of preparedness, response, recovery, and mitigation activities.

16.10.2   Strategy 2: Add Disability Content to Public Health and Healthcare Education Standards

Embedding dedicated disability content into public health and healthcare education is another strategy to educate students on disability awareness, while fulfilling competencies for general training.

Strategy highlight: The University of Connecticut offers an online, graduate-level Certificate of Interdisciplinary Disability Studies in Public Health. In addition to public health students, the Certificate serves individuals in the professional and paraprofessional workforce in medicine, dentistry, nursing, social work, law, education, psychology, political science, physical therapy, occupational therapy, and speech/language/hearing sciences. The ten Essential Public Health Services are the framework for the Certificate program. The Certificate is comprised of four courses: (1) Foundations of Public Health and Disability; (2) Epidemiology of Disability, (3) Disability Law, Policy, Ethics, and Advocacy; and (4) Public Health Interventions in Disability. Students may take the Foundations of Public Health and Disability course in fulfillment of a requirement for their respective field or take the entire series of four courses and receive the Certificate. This may serve as a model for implementing disability content in existing public health and allied health curricula. See Sect. 16.13 for other disability inclusion training offerings for the public health workforce.

16.10.3   Strategy 3: Add Disability Competencies into Education Standards

Currently, disability competencies are not included in the education standards for accreditation or licensure for schools and programs of public health or healthcare education for any discipline. If disability learning objectives were required, every professional student would graduate with basic disability competence. Efforts to align disability competencies with existing educational standards and to secure endorsements from disability and professional associations (see https://go.osu.edu/corecompetenciesdisability-learnmore) bring us closer to this goal. An approach to including intellectual and developmental disability content in medical education is being explored with pilot efforts across the country guided by the American Academy of Developmental Medicine and Dentistry (AADMD) and through pilot efforts in regions of the country with a higher disability prevalence guided by AUCD.

16.11   Workforce Supports for Including People with Disabilities: How to Take Action

Emerging research shows five conditions to support inclusion of people with disabilities and sustain public health leaders in this change of perspective and how to take action. These five conditions or supports include (1) facilitative leadership, (2) taking advantage of timing, (3) sufficient support, (4) systematic reflection, and (5) alignment with personal commitment and interest (Griffen, Risley, Petros, & Welter, 2018).

Facilitative leadership is exemplified by leaders guiding conversations with intention. Leaders should be familiar with facilitation tools and use them appropriately. How leaders lead and facilitate is unique to each individual. Leaders may be successful in including people with disabilities when they are able to take what they have heard through genuine, present listening and take action. The expectation is that people with disabilities are included at every level, from planning to running an effort.

Taking advantage of timing is a critical condition to support inclusion of people with disabilities. Through knowing target partner groups, active networking, and building one's network, public health practitioners may be able to gauge when the time is best to start a new program or piggyback on an existing effort to include people with disabilities. Reaching out to potential partners is a great way to get started on the journey to take advantage of upcoming opportunities.

Thinking of support more globally than just in terms of finances helps public health leaders be aware of all the resources available. Connecting and collaborating with colleagues in a shared area of interest not only help practitioners gain perspective from others and share experiences but also may reinforce efforts to include people with disabilities. This broader perspective enables practitioners to access expertise on disability inclusion through growing their networks.

Another way to engage networks and groups is through systematic reflection. Systematic reflection encourages individual as well as collective thinking to take place within a limited amount of time. The Action Learning process has been shown to be an effective public health leadership tool to guide systematic reflection (Center for Health Leadership and Practice, Public Health Institute: Web: http://www.phi. org/focus-areas/?program=center-for-health-leadership-and-practice, Accessed October 7, 2019), as it includes a continuous cycle of taking action, dedicated reflection, documenting learnings, and planning to link learning and future action (Marquardt, 2011).

Taking actions toward including people with disabilities in public health efforts also attracts practitioners who are invested in implementing positive changes. Alignment with personal commitment and interest has been shown to be an effective support for public health practitioners to strive to include people with disabilities in their efforts. This alignment with personal commitment and interest drives real-world experiences of trial and error of including people with disabilities in efforts, as well as the ability to learn from these experiences to make improvements.

Overall, these five areas contribute to successful outcomes in serving the whole community—including people with disabilities—and may even be helpful in other areas, such as reaching underserved or unserved populations. Inclusion of people with disabilities is a system-wide quality improvement the public health field is poised to make with passionate and well-trained professionals.

16.11.1 Factors of Readiness, Capacity Building, and Capacity

Critical readiness, capacity building, and capacity factors may serve as a framework on how public health practitioners may move forward with efforts to include people with disabilities. Essential factors of readiness for change include recognition of the need to coordinate with other partners, contact and interactions with organizations, and positive perception as well as quality interactions with partners. Steps toward capacity building and implementation of actually including people with disabilities in public health efforts may be supported by engagement in a network, practical collaboration experience, continuing education, and critical reflection. Knowledge of people with disabilities as a priority population, along with dedicated staff and funds, supports the capacity to include people with disabilities in public health efforts (Griffen et al., 2018).

Awareness of the need for these factors of readiness, capacity building, and capacity and five supports for inclusion of people with disabilities further supports public health practitioners to have an openness to learning and seek educational opportunities.

16.12 Future Workforce

The public health workforce needs to reflect the whole community. Addressing attitudinal barriers that do not support inclusion of people with disabilities is an essential training goal. Students with disabilities should be able to access education and training, just as anyone else. If the future workforce reflected population demographics, there would be practitioners with disabilities across the broad spectrum of public health to include health promotion and allied health practitioners. It is important to remove barriers to enrollment so that the future public health workforce will have lived disability experience. A saying within the disability community is "Nothing about us without us," and this applies to the composition of the public health workforce as well to extend lived experience to public health research, policy, and practice.

16.12.1 A Note on Resilience

Inclusion of people with disabilities in public health efforts is still an emerging area of focus for the field. Professionals will have to maintain a sense of resilience as they strive to implement efforts that improve service to the whole community, including people with disabilities. One tool that may help in this pursuit is Action Learning (Marquardt, 2011), a process that includes a continuous cycle of (1) taking action, (2) dedicated reflection, (3) documenting learnings, and (4) planning to link learning and future action. Action Learning may be used to solve real-world problems in an iterative process, with a focus on learning and sharing learnings as a benefit that may help enhance efforts on the adaptive change of including people with disabilities in public health efforts. There is no one correct way to include people with disabilities in these efforts. Rather, each professional must strive to acknowledge the critical need to include everyone in the community and remain resilient in this pursuit, while incorporating lessons learned and continuing to take action. Public health is for everyone.

16.13 Learn More

Here are a few ways to learn more about disability inclusion in public health:

1. Visit with People Living with Disabilities

    There is no substitute for learning about lived experience through the perspective of someone who has a disability. It is important for students to meet actual people with disabilities to gain comfort and challenge limiting assumptions. Set up an appointment with a partner group to meet people with disabilities. Ask about what a typical day is like, and look for the combination of health promotion, laws, communities, organizations, and accessibility standards that impact health outcomes for people with disabilities.

2. Leadership Reflection

Inclusion of people with disabilities is a system-wide quality improvement the public health field is poised to make with passionate and well-trained professionals. In what leaders or organizations do you see evidence of Adaptive Leadership Supports for Disability Inclusion? These include (1) facilitative leadership, (2) systematic reflection, (3) support, (4) personal interest and commitment, and (5) taking advantage of timing.

3. Seek Partners and Support

Many partners in the disability and public health field use evidenced-based strategies to develop and increase the ability of public health professionals to include people who have disabilities (see Table 16.4). Public health professionals would be wise to consider engaging these partner organizations in state, regional, and local efforts in order to get connected with people with disabilities in the region, as well as to become aware of current efforts. These partners may be able to collaborate and serve as trusted advisors to keep public health workforce on the cutting edge of our country's population needs, as well as involve people with disabilities in planning and execution of efforts in an effort to embody the disability community saying, "Nothing about us without us."

4. Keep Learning

Stay on the cutting edge of public health needs, and continue to learn about including people with disabilities in public health efforts. There are several freely available, continuing education disability inclusion training options offered by partner organizations online. See Table 16.5 for a list of several disability inclusion options to explore.

Table 16.4 Disability in Public Health Partners

Organization	Website
American Academy of Developmental Medicine and Dentistry (AADMD)	aadmd.org
American Association on Health and Disability (AAHD)	aahd.us
American Public Health Association (APHA) Disability Section	www.apha.org/apha-communities/member-sections/disability-section
Association of University Centers on Disabilities (AUCD)	aucd.org
National Association of Councils on Developmental Disabilities (NACDD)	nacdd.org/councils
National Center on Health, Physical Activity and Disability (NCHPAD)	nchpad.org
National Council on Independent Living (NCIL)	ncil.org
Special Olympics, Center for Inclusive Health	inclusivehealth.specialolympics.org

Table 16.5 Free disability inclusion training options online

Organization	Training description	Web link
National Association of County and City Health Officials	*Health and Disability 101 Training for Health Department Employees* provides foundational knowledge about people with disabilities, the health disparities that they experience, and how local health department staff can include people with disabilities in their public health programs and services	http://bit.ly/HealthDisability101
Ohio Disability and Health Program, Nisonger Center, University Center for Excellence in Developmental Disabilities (UCEDD) at The Ohio State University. Approved for continuing education by the Centers for Disease Control and Prevention	*Part I: Persons with Physical and Sensory Disabilities (WB2695) and Part II: People with Developmental Disabilities (WD4234)* are designed to increase the capacity of healthcare providers to provide quality health care for persons with disabilities	https://nisonger.osu.edu/education-training/ohio-disability-health-program/disability-healthcare-training/

Organization	Training description	Web link
Resources for Integrated Care, a collaboration between the Medicare-Medicaid Coordination Office (MMCO) in the Centers for Medicare & Medicaid Services (CMS), The Lewin Group, and the Institute for Healthcare Improvement	*Disability-Competent Care*, a participant-centered model that focuses on the eventual goal of supporting individuals to achieve maximum function. The model is delivered by an interdisciplinary team whom recognizes and treats each individual as a unique person, not their diagnosis or condition	https://www.resourcesforintegratedcare.com/concepts/disability-competent-care
TRAIN Learning Network from the Public Health Foundation	*Disability Training for First Responders: Serving People with disabilities* provides information and best practices to ensure the safety of people with disabilities and EMS, Firefighters, Law Enforcement, and other Allied Health Professionals	https://www.train.org/odh/course/1072437/compilation
TRAIN Learning Network from the Public Health Foundation	*Disability Training for Emergency Planners: Serving People with disabilities* provides information and best practices to ensure the safety of people with disabilities and Emergency Planners	https://www.train.org/odh/course/1058486/

References

Albrecht, G. L., & Devlieger, P. J. (1999). The disability paradox: High quality of life against all odds. *Social Science & Medicine, 48*(8), 977–988.

Andresen, E. M., Peterson-Besse, J. J., Krahn, G. L., Walsh, E. S., Horner-Johnson, W., & Iezzoni, L. I. (2013). Pap, mammography, and clinical breast examination screening among women with disabilities: A systematic review. *Womens Health Issues, 23*(4), e205–e214.

Ankam, N. S., Bosques, G., Sauter, C., Stiens, S., Therattil, M., Williams, F. H., … Mayer, R. S. (2019). Competency-based curriculum development to meet the needs of people with disabilities: A call to action. *Academic Medicine, 94*(6), 781–788.

Armour, B. S., Swanson, M., Waldman, H. B., & Perlman, S. P. (2008). A profile of state-level differences in the oral health of people with and without disabilities, in the US, in 2004. *Public health reports, 123*(1), 67–75.

Bond, L., Kerr, M., Dunstan, F., & Thapar, A. (1997). Attitudes of general practitioners towards health care for people with intellectual disability and the factors underlying these attitudes. *Journal of Intellectual Disability Research, 41*(Pt 5), 391–400. http://www.ncbi.nlm.nih.gov/pubmed/9373819

Chadd EH, Pangilinan PH. (2011). Disability attitudes in health care: a new scale instrument. *Am J Phys Med Rehabil, 90*(1):47–54. https://doi.org/10.1097/PHM.0b013e3182017269

Drainoni, M.-L., Lee-Hood, E., Tobias, C., Bachman, S. S., Andrew, J., & Maisels, L. (2006). Cross-disability experiences of barriers to health-care access: Consumer perspectives. *Journal of Disability Policy Studies, 17*(2), 101–115.

Edwards, J. D., Davidson, E. J., Houtrow, A. J., & Graham, R. J. (2010). Pediatric resident attitudes toward caring for children with severe disabilities. *American Journal of Physical Medicine & Rehabilitation, 89*(9), 765–771. https://doi.org/10.1097/PHM.0b013e3181ec9936

Emerson, E., Hatton, C., Baines, S., & Robertson, J. (2016). The physical health of British adults with intellectual disability: cross sectional study. *International journal for equity in health, 15*(1), 11.

Gerhart, K. A., Koziol-McLain, J., Lowenstein, S. R., & Whiteneck, G. G. (1994). Quality of life following spinal cord injury: Knowledge and attitudes of emergency care providers. *Annals of Emergency Medicine, 23*(4), 807–812.

Greenwood, N. W., & Wilkinson, J. (2013). Sexual and reproductive health care for women with intellectual disabilities: A primary care perspective. *International Journal of Family Medicine, 2013*, 1–8.

Griffen, A., Risley, K., Petros, M., & Welter, C. (2018). Inclusion wheel: Tool for building capacity and public health leaders to serve people with disabilities. *Health Promotion Practice, 21*, 209. https://doi.org/10.1177/1524839918788578

Gruppen, L. D., Mangrulkar, R. S., & Kolars, J. C. (2012). The promise of competency-based education in the health professions for improving global health. *Human Resources for Health, 10*, 43.

Harrington, A. L., Hirsch, M. A., Hammond, F. M., Norton, H. J., & Bockenek, W. L. (2009). Assessment of primary care services and perceived barriers to care in persons with disabilities. *American Journal of Physical Medicine & Rehabilitation, 88*(10), 852–863. https://doi.org/10.1097/PHM.0b013e3181b30745

Havercamp, S. M., Scandlin, D., & Roth, M. (2004). Health disparities among adults with developmental disabilities, adults with other disabilities, and adults not reporting disability in North Carolina. *Public health reports, 119*(4), 418–426.

Havercamp, S. M., & Scott, H. M. (2015). *National health surveillance of adults with disabilities, adults with intellectual and developmental disabilities, and adults with no disabilities.* Disability and Health Journal, 8(2), 165–172.

Krahn, G. L., Walker, D. K., & Correa-De-Araujo, R. (2015). Persons with disabilities as an unrecognized health disparity population. *American Journal of Public Health, 105*, S198–S206. https://doi.org/10.2105/AJPH.2014.302182

Kroll, T., Beatty, P. W., & Bingham, S. (2003). Primary care satisfaction among adults with physical disabilities: The role of patient-provider communication. *Managed Care Quarterly, 11*(1), 11–19.

Lollar, D. J., & Crews, J. E. (2003). Redefining the role of public health in disability. *Annual Review of Public Health, 24,* 195–208. https://doi.org/10.1146/annurev.publhealth.24.100901.140844

Marquardt, M. (2011). *Optimizing the power of action learning* (2nd ed.). Boston, MA: Nicholas Brealey Publishing.

Matziou, V., Galanis, P., Tsoumakas, C., Gymnopoulou, E., Perdikaris, P., & Brokalaki, H. (2009). Attitudes of nurse professionals and nursing students towards children with disabilities. Do nurses really overcome children's physical and mental handicaps? *International Nursing Review, 56*(4), 456–460. https://doi.org/10.1111/j.1466-7657.2009.00735.x

McKee, M. M., Barnett, S. L., Block, R. C., & Pearson, T. A. (2011). Impact of communication on preventive services among deaf American Sign Language users. *American Journal of Preventive Medicine, 41*(1), 75–79. https://doi.org/10.1016/j.amepre.2011.03.004

Milligan, M. S., & Neufeldt, A. H. (2001). The myth of asexuality: A survey of social and empirical evidence. *Sexuality and Disability, 19*(2), 91–109. https://doi.org/10.1023/A:1010621705591

Mitchell, K. R., Hayes, M., Gordon, J., & Wallis, B. (1984). An investigation of the attitudes of medical students to physically disabled people. *Medical Education, 18*(1), 21–23.

Morrison, E. H., George, V., & Mosqueda, L. (2008). Primary care for adults with physical disabilities: Perceptions from consumer and provider focus groups. *Family Medicine, 40*(9), 645–651.

Neri MT, Kroll T. (2003) Understanding the consequences of access barriers to health care: experiences of adults with disabilities. *Disability and rehabilitation, 25*(2):85–96.

Nosek, B. A., Smyth, F. L., Hansen, J. J., Devos, T., Lindner, N. M., Ranganath, K. A., et al. (2007). Pervasiveness and correlates of implicit attitudes and stereotypes. *European Review of Social Psychology, 18,* 1–53. https://doi.org/10.1080/10463280701489053

Okoro, C. A., Hollis, N. D., Cyrus, A. C., & Griffin-Blake, S. (2018). Prevalence of disabilities and health care access by disability status and type among adults—United States, 2016. *MMWR Morbidity and Mortality Weekly Report, 67,* 882–887. https://doi.org/10.15585/mmwr.mm6732a3

Patja, K., Iivanainen, M., Vesala, H., Oksanen, H., & Ruoppila, I. (2000). Life expectancy of people with intellectual disability: A 35-year follow-up study. *Journal of Intellectual Disability Research, 44*(5), 591–599.

Pharr, J. R., & Bungum, T. (2012). Health disparities experienced by people with disabilities in the United States: A behavioral risk factor surveillance system study. *Global Journal of Health Science, 4*(6), 99–108. https://doi.org/10.5539/gjhs.v4n6p99

Park JH, Faulkner J, Schaller M. Evolved disease-avoidance processes and contemporary antisocial behavior: Prejudicial attitudes and avoidance of people with physical disabilities. *J Nonverbal Behav. 2003;27*(2):65–87. doi:10.1023/A:1023910408854.

Reichard A, Stolzle H, Fox MH. Health disparities among adults with physical disabilities or cognitive limitations compared to individuals with no disabilities in the United States. *Disability and health journal. 2011 Apr 1;4*(2):59–67.

Robey, K. L., Beckley, L., & Kirschner, M. (2006). Implicit infantilizing attitudes about disability. *Journal of Developmental and Physical Disabilities, 18*(4), 441–453. https://doi.org/10.1007/s10882-006-9027-3

Shakespeare, T. (2000). Disabled sexuality: Toward rights and recognition. *Sexuality and Disability, 18*(3), 159–166. https://doi.org/10.1023/A:1026409613684

Sinclair, L. B., Tanenhaus, R. H., Courtney-Long, E., & Eaton, D. K. (2015). Disability within US Public Health School and Program Curricula. *Journal of Public Health Management and Practice, 21*(4), 400–405. https://doi.org/10.1097/PHH.0000000000000114

Tervo RC, Palmer G, Redinius P. (2004) Health professional student attitudes towards people with disability. *Clin Rehabil, 18*(8):908–915.

U.S. Department of Health and Human Services. (2000). *Healthy people 2010. With understanding and improving health and objectives for improving health* (2nd ed.. 2 vols). Washington, DC: U.S. Government Printing Office.

U.S. Department of Health and Human Services. (2005). *The Surgeon General's call to action to improve the health and wellness of persons with disabilities*. Washington, DC: Office of the Surgeon General, US Department of Health and Human Services.

U.S. Department of Health and Human Services: The Secretary's Advisory Committee on National Health Promotion and Disease Prevention Objectives for 2020. (2008). *Phase I report: Recommendations for the framework and format of Healthy People 2020. Section IV. Advisory Committee findings and recommendations*. Washington, DC: U.S. Department of Health and Human Services.

Wilson, M. C., & Scior, K. (2014). Attitudes towards individuals with disabilities as measured by the implicit association test: A literature review. *Research in Developmental Disabilities, 35*(2), 294–321. https://doi.org/10.1016/j.ridd.2013.11.003

Wingo, B., & Rimmer, J. (2018). Emerging trends in health promotion for people with disabilities. *International Journal of Environmental Research and Public Health, 15*(4), 742. https://doi.org/10.3390/ijerph15040742

Winslow, C. E. A. (1920). The untilled field of public health. *Modern Medicine, 2*, 183–191.

World Health Organization. (2011). *World report on disability*. Geneva: World Health Organization.

Index

Printed in the United States
by Baker & Taylor Publisher Services